Psychoactive Drugs
Harm Reduction:
From Faith to Science

Psychoactive Drugs and Harm Reduction: From Faith to Science

Edited by

NICK HEATHER, ALEX WODAK,
ETHAN A. NADELMANN and PAT O'HARE

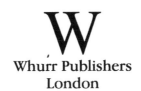

Whurr Publishers
London

Preface

This book is based loosely on the Third International Conference on the Reduction of Drug-related Harm held in Melbourne, Australia at the end of March, 1992. It is the second book to arise from this series of conferences, the previous volume having been based on the first conference in Liverpool in 1990 (O'Hare et al., 1992).

All keynote speakers at the Melbourne conference contributed chapters to this book. In addition, several other conference speakers, whose presentations coincided with the plans of the editors, were asked to contribute chapters. However, pains have been taken to avoid producing yet another regurgitation of conference proceedings. In the first place, the contents have been organised coherently into sections rather than being presented in an arbitrary order; second, the structure of the book follows themes identified by the conference organisers as being of particular relevance to the field of harm reduction at its present stage of development; last, the book has been closely edited and final versions of several chapters differ substantially from the material presented at the conference.

The theme that gives the book its subtitle was taken from an address given by John Strang at the First International Conference on the Reduction of Drug-related Harm in Liverpool. This is the idea that, despite the growing popularity of the harm-reduction approach to drug-related problems, there has been a disappointing lack of rigour in the definition of key terms and concepts, and not enough careful evaluation of harm-reduction policies and programmes. If the principles and objectives of harm reduction are to exert their rightful influence on prevention and treatment in the drugs field, and be taken seriously by policy makers and treatment providers, enthusiastic advocacy must now be supplemented by conceptual clarity combined with sound empirical evidence of effectiveness. In short, faith in harm reduction must be augmented by the traditional virtues of scientific method.

This point has been made previously in writings on harm reduction and, indeed, found expression in the previous volume coming from the international harm reduction conference series (see O'Hare et al., 1992). However, the organisers of the Melbourne meeting chose to make this the major theme of the conference and, to this end, invited Strang to deliver an Opening Address on this general topic. A revised version of this address is reproduced here as the opening chapter in Part I.

Not all chapters in the book confine themselves to this central issue of increased scientific rigour in the harm-reduction movement but many incorporate this theme within the focus of their concerns or contain material highly relevant to it. Moreover, several contributors, including Strang in Chapter 1, call for more extensive evaluation of harm-reduction approaches. Indeed, until the necessary evidence is available, the benefits of harm reduction will have to be taken on trust. As conceptual clarity is a prerequisite for evaluation, researchers and policy makers need to be able to distinguish reliably between harm-reduction and alternative approaches to drug use and drug problems. What is distinctive about the harm-reduction approach to drug problems?

In our view, the essential feature of harm reduction is that it involves an attempt to ameliorate the adverse health, social or economic consequences of mood-altering substances without necessarily requiring a reduction in the consumption of these substances. Thus, harm reduction is distinguished from other and more conventional approaches to psychoactive drugs simply by its emphasis on decreasing problems resulting from consumption rather than on decreasing consumption itself.

The remaining two chapters in Part I on *Concepts and Definitions* both provide their respective authors' characterizations of harm reduction and their attempts to clarify various strands of thought that may have become confused. Thus in Chapter 2, Stephen Mugford asks whether those who support what he calls the typical position on harm reduction are fully aware of the implications of their view. In this challenging chapter, Mugford argues that there are serious problems with the way in which harm reduction is currently conceived and with the policies that flow logically from it. In Chapter 3, Ethan Nadelmann confronts the vexed question of the relationship between 'harm reduction' and the legalisation of presently illicit drugs; in so doing, he identifies a range of commonalities and differences between various positions in drug policy field, particularly with respect to the situation in the USA.

Part II of the book presents four different perspectives on harm reduction from various professional and academic viewpoints. Chapter 4, by the Hon. Peter Staples MP, gives a view of harm reduction from the Minister for Aged, Family and Health Services in the Commonwealth government of Australia – in other words, from the

Minister responsible for overseeing the National Campaign Against Drug Abuse. Staples' chapter stresses the fact that 'harm minimisation' is the official aim of the Australian national campaign. This is followed in Chapter 5 by an historical perspective from Virginia Berridge who traces the origins of harm minimization to developments long before the advent of the AIDS epidemic. In Chapter 6, Julian Cohen provides an educationist's perspective on harm reduction, together with a very practical account of Harm Reduction Drugs Education in the Tameside region of the UK. Finally in this section, Jean-Paul Grund and colleagues in Chapter 7 describe a methodological approach to the understanding of drug use from the perspective of 'Experimental Comparative Ethnography', using the key concept of 'rituals of regulation'.

Part III is devoted to the topic of *Harm-reduction Policies*. First, in Chapter 8, David Hawks explores the impediments that might exist to the global adoption of harm-reduction policies. In Chapter 9, based on their current research, Robert MacCoun and his colleagues from the RAND Drug Policy Research Center discuss both the promise and the drawbacks of using cross-national comparisons to examine the effects of drug policies. Then, in an international collaboration in Chapter 10, two policemen, Tjibbe Reitsma from Rotterdam and Derek O'Connell from Merseyside, describe how law enforcement serves in their respective areas as a harm-reduction strategy. Duncan Chappell and Heather Strang from the Australian Institute of Criminology in Canberra provide an introduction and commentary to this discussion. In Chapter 11, Erik Fromberg argues that prohibition is a necessary stage in the acculturation of 'foreign' drugs in any society and uses the example of the history of cannabis in the Netherlands as an illustration of his thesis. The section concludes with an account by Gabrielle Bammer and her co-workers in Chapter 12 of their research into the feasibility of conducting a trial of prescribed heroin in the Australian Capital Territory.

Another major theme of the Melbourne conference was that the relevance of harm-reduction principles and methods to the licit drugs, particularly alcohol and nicotine, had been neglected. There has been an unfortunate tendency to think of harm reduction, if not as solely confined to the prevention of spread of HIV infection among injecting drug users, then certainly as applying almost entirely to illicit substances such as heroin, cocaine and cannabis. This ignores the fact that in most countries of the world legal drugs are responsible for far greater adverse health, social and economic consequences than illegal drugs. As a result, Part IV of the book on *Applications to Specific Substances* includes chapters by Michael Russell (Chapter 13) on the potential of forms of nicotine replacement as a mean of reducing smoking-related harm and by Nick Heather (Chapter 14) on the application of harm-reduction principles to the treatment of alcohol problems. The remaining chapters in the section cover psychostimulants (Patricia Erickson: Chapter 15), cannabis (John Morgan and colleagues: Chapter 16) and MDMA (Ecstasy) (Peter McDermott and colleagues: Chapter 17).

A further important theme of the conference was that previous discussions of harm reduction had tended to ignore its relevance to the situation of developing countries of the world. Consequently, Part V is given over to a consideration of the relevance of harm-reduction principles, practices and related issues to the developing parts of the globe. Any conference or publication that deserves to be considered 'international' must surely be conscious of the fact that 80% of the world's population lives in developing countries. Alcohol- and drug-related problems are increasing more rapidly in many developing countries where there are far fewer resources to respond to these problems than in the industrialised world. Moreover, as Anthony Henman (Chapter 18) points out, developed countries may have as much to learn about harm reduction from developing countries as the reverse. Henman's chapter is mainly concerned with the inimical effects of drug policies originating from the developed world on the welfare of developing countries. This is followed in Chapter 19 by a discussion of harm-reduction policies and programmes in developing countries by Naotaka Shinfuku, the Regional Adviser in Mental Health and Drug Dependence for the WHO Western Pacific Region. This region of the world is the focus for Chapter 20 by Sally Casswell on efforts to ameliorate harm due to legal drug use in the developing countries of the Pacific. The section is brought to a conclusion with an account by Alex Wodak and colleagues in Chapter 21 of 'the gathering storm' associated with HIV infection in developing countries.

The topic of HIV infection in developing countries is also included by Don Des Jarlais and Sam Friedman in their international perspective on HIV AIDS and drug use (Chapter 22). However, the main reason for devoting Part VI to *Harm Reduction and HIV/AIDS* is a recognition of the simple fact that, although its application should be interpreted in the broadest possible terms, interest in harm reduction was greatly accelerated by the advent of the HIV epidemic and this remains the most important single category of drug-related harm to which harm-reduction policies are currently directed. Furthermore, Des Jarlais and Friedman argue that the perceived success of harm-reduction practices in this area will have powerful consequences for the acceptance of the entire approach. This final section of the book is concluded by a review of research by Matt Gaughwin and David Vlahov in Chapter 23 on the crucial topic of HIV transmission in correctional centres and by a personal account by David Herkt in Chapter 24 of the role of peer-based user groups in the fight against AIDS in Australia.

Participants at the Melbourne conference, as at previous conferences in this series, represented a wide range of professional and personal interests, attitudes to drug use, and basic perspectives on harm reduction and its implications for controversial issues, such as the advantages of drug policy reform. Nevertheless, despite these differences – which are inevitable in any conglomeration of relatively new ideas – we do think it appropriate and helpful to speak of a harm-reduction movement.

This movement is perhaps unified in a negative sense by its opposition to ineffective, wildly irrational and often harm-augmenting 'drug war' policies and 'zero-tolerance' attitudes, and by a general consensus that saner solutions to the problems posed by psychoactive drugs must be available and must soon be found. But there is also wide agreement among those who would consider themselves adherents of harm reduction that societies must come to terms with the fact that human beings always have, and probably always will, use psychoactive substances and that this is not necessarily a bad thing. Whether one wishes to call this a 'paradigm shift', as Erickson does (see Chapter 15), or uses some other term, there is little doubt that it marks an important turning-point in the history of formal theories and responses to drugs and drug-related harm. While Virginia Berridge (Chapter 5) is correct to point out that harm reduction has a long pedigree in the drugs field, the contrast between 'use reduction' and 'harm reduction' approaches to the amelioration of the adverse consequences of psychoactive drug use has never been sharper. We will be satisfied if the present volume contributes in some measure to the orderly development of this harm-reduction movement.

Since this book would not have been possible without the Third International Conference on the Reduction of Drug-related Harm, the editors wish to thank all those who contributed in many different ways to its success. We would especially like to thank Bill Stronach and Caroline Thompson for shouldering the main burden of organisation, and Nick Crofts for his contributions to the Programme Committee which are reflected in this book. The Convening Organizations for the conference were the Alcohol and Drug Foundation, Victoria and the Mersey Drug Training and Information Centre.

Reference

O'Hare, P.A., Newcombe, R., Matthews, A., Buning, E.C. and Drucker, E. (1992). *The Reduction of Drug-related Harm*. London: Routledge.

Nick Heather
Alex Wodak
Ethan Nadelmann
Pat O'Hare

Dedication

The Third International Conference on the Reduction of Drug-related Harm, held in Melbourne in 1992, provided the occasion for the first presentation of the *Rolleston Awards for Achievement in Harm Reduction*. There were two recipients: Les Drew received the National Section award in recognition of the critical part he played, during his 14-year tenure as Senior Advisor on Alcohol and Drugs to the Commonwealth Minister for Health, in establishing harm reduction as a central element of Australian drug control policy; David Purchase received the International Section award in recognition of his role in creating one of the first needle and syringe exchanges in the USA in Tacoma, Washington, and on behalf of all US pioneers of needle and syringe exchanges.

The Rolleston Awards are named after Sir Humphrey Rolleston, a former President of the Royal College of Physicians in Britain, who chaired the Ministry of Health's Departmental Committe on Morphine and Heroin Addiction from 1924 to 1926. The Rolleston Committee, as it is popularly known, was highly influential in shaping the course of drug policy in the UK during this century. Its recommendations established the principle of harm reduction in drug control policy long before the term itself was coined.

This book is dedicated to Les Drew and David Purchase, first winners of the Rolleston Awards for Harm Reduction.

Contents

Contributors

Gabriele Bammer, Research Fellow, National Centre for Epidemiology and Population Health, Australian National University, Canberra, Australia

Andrew Bennett, Deputy Director, Mersey Drug Training and Information Centre, Liverpool, UK

Virginia Berridge, Senior Lecturer in History and Co-director, AIDS Social History Programme, Department of Public Health and Policy, London School of Hygiene and Tropical Medicine, University of London, London, UK

Sally Casswell, Director, Alcohol and Public Health Research Unit, Department of Community Health, University of Auckland, Auckland, New Zealand

Duncan Chappell, Director, Australian Institute of Criminology, Canberra, Australia and Professor of Criminology, Simon Fraser University, Burnaby, British Columbia, Canada

Gregory B. Chesher, Honorary Research Fellow, National Drug and Alcohol Research Centre, University of New South Wales, Sydney, Australia

Julian Cohen, Freelance Consultant and Trainer and Drugs Education Co-ordinator, Tameside Education Authority, Tameside, UK

Nick Crofts, Head, Epidemiology and International Health, Macfarlane Burnet Centre for Medical Research, Melbourne, Australia

Don C. Des Jarlais, Director of Research, Chemical Dependency Institute, Beth Israel Medical Center, and Professor of Community Medicine, Mt Sinai School of Medicine, New York, USA

Martin de Vries, Professor of Social Psychiatry and Director, International Institute for Psycho-social and Socio-ecological Research, State University of Limburg, Maastricht, The Netherlands

Bob Douglas, Professor and Director, National Centre for Epidemiology and Population Health, Australian National University, Canberra, Australia

Patricia G. Erickson, Senior Scientist, Addiction Research Foundation, Toronto, and Adjunct Professor, Department of Sociology, University of Toronto, Ontario, Canada

Robert Fisher, Associate Professor of Psychiatry, School of Medicine, Vanderbilt University, Nashville, Tennessee, USA

Samuel R. Friedman, Senior Principal Investigator, National Development and Research Institutes, New York, USA

Erik Fromberg, Project Manager, Nederlands Instituut voor Alcohol en Drugs, Utrecht, The Netherlands

Matt Gaughwin, Visiting Fellow, National Centre for Epidemiology and Population Health, Australian National University, Canberra, Australia

Jean-Paul C. Grund, Director, DV8 Research Training and Development, and Researcher, Addiction Research Institute, Medical and Health Sciences Faculty, Erasmus University, Rotterdam, The Netherlands

David Hawks, Professor of Addiction Studies and Director, National Centre for Research into the Prevention of Drug Abuse, Curtin University, Perth, Australia

Nick Heather, Professor of Drug and Alcohol Studies and Director, National Drug and Alcohol Research Centre, University of New South Wales, Sydney, Australia

Anthony Henman, Director, Drug Reform, Monmouth, UK

David Herkt, Project Worker, Australian IV League, Canberra, Australia

James P. Kahan, Senior Scientist, Drug Policy Research Center, The RAND Corporation, Santa Monica, California, USA

Charles D. Kaplan, Co-ordinator, Drug Use and Abuse Research, International Institute for Psycho-social and Socio-ecological Research, State University of Limburg, Maastricht, The Netherlands

Robert J. MacCoun, Behavioral Scientist, Drug Policy Research Center, The RAND Corporation, Santa Monica, California, USA

Peter McDermott, Editor, *International Journal of Drug Policy*, Liverpool, UK

Alan Matthews, Freelance Researcher, Liverpool, UK

Michael Moore, Member, Legislative Assembly for the Australian Capital Territory, Canberra, Australia

John P. Morgan, Professor of Pharmacology, City University of New York Medical School, New York, USA

Stephen Mugford, Senior Lecturer, Department of Sociology, Australian National University, Canberra, Australia

Ethan A. Nadelmann, Assistant Professor of Politics and Public Affairs, Woodrow Wilson School of Public and International Affairs, Princeton University, New Jersey, USA

Derek O'Connell, Superintendent of Police, Mersey CID Drug Squad, Merseyside, UK

Pat O'Hare, Director, Mersey Drug Training and Information Centre, Liverpool, UK

Tjibbe Reitsma, Superintendent of Police, City of Rotterdam Police, Rotterdam, The Netherlands

Peter Reuter, Co-director, Drug Policy Research Center, The RAND Corporation, Santa Monica, California, USA

Diane Riley, Senior Analyst, Canadian Centre on Substance Abuse and University of Toronto, Toronto, Ontario, Canada

Michael A.H. Russell, Professor of Addiction and Honorary Director, ICRF Health Behaviour Unit, The Maudsley Institute of Psychiatry, London, UK

Aaron J. Saiger, Resident Consultant, Drug Policy Research Center, The RAND Corporation, Santa Monica, California, USA

Naotaka Shinfuku, Regional Adviser, Mental Health and Drug Dependence, World Health Organization, Western Pacific Region, Manila, Philippines

The Honourable Peter Staples, Minister for Aged, Family and Health Services, Commonwealth Department of Community Services and Health, Canberra, Australia

Heather Strang, Executive Research Officer, Australian Institute of Criminology, Canberra, Australia

John Strang, Getty Senior Lecturer in the Addictions, National Addiction Centre, The Maudsley Institute of Psychiatry, London, UK

David Vlahov, Associate Professor of Epidemiology, School of Hygiene and Public Health, The Johns Hopkins University, Baltimore, Maryland, USA

Alex Wodak, Director, Alcohol and Drug Services, St Vincent's Hospital, Sydney, Australia

Acknowledgements

Chapter 5

I am grateful to the Nuffield Provincial Hospitals Trust for supporting the AIDS Social History Programme and to Ingrid James for secretarial assistance.

Chapter 7

We would like to thank the drug users who participated in this study. This research was supported by a grant from NWO (grant no. 900-556-039). Opinions expressed in the chapter do not necessarily reflect the policy of the supporting organisation.

Chapter 8

I am grateful to my colleagues Wendy Loxley, Claudia Ovenden, Alison Marsh and David Moore for their comments on a draft version of this paper. This is not to say however that they necessarily agree with the views expressed!

Chapter 9

This research was supported by a grant from the Alfred P. Sloan Foundation. We thank Ethan Nadelmann and Thomas Schelling for providing useful comments.

Chapter 13

I am grateful to the Medical Research Council and the Imperial Cancer Research Fund for generous financial support, Wilhelmina Maisey for secretarial assistance and Martin Jarvis for helpful comments on the manuscript.

Chapter 15

The author appreciates the comments of Yuet Cheung, Bruce Alexander and the Editors. The computer graphics were ably prepared by Joan Moreau.

The longitudinal research on Canadian cocaine users was supported by the National Health Research and Development Program, Health and Welfare Canada (Project Number 6606-3929-DA).

The views expressed in this chapter are those of the author and do not necessarily reflect those of the Addiction Research Foundation.

Chapter 17

The authors would like to apologise unreservedly to S-Express, Bob Dylan, E-Zee Posse, Diana Ross and the Supremes, and the Jimmy Castor Bunch for the cavalier misappropriation of their lyrics, and to Michele Durkin and Jenny O'Connor for their invaluable help in planning and executing the *Chill Out* information campaign, and for their staunch support during the media's ferocious attack upon the agency and its director.

Part I
Concepts and Definitions

Chapter 1
Drug Use and Harm Reduction: Responding to the Challenge

JOHN STRANG

Faith must be replaced by science: so it was argued in the opening address at the *First International Conference on the Reduction of Drug-Related Harm* in 1990: 'The time has come for the debate around harm reduction to move from something akin to religious dogma to a sounder scientific basis. The religious passion may have been important at one stage but a move to objective and scientific study of the policy and practice dimensions of harm reduction is now required.'

Much has happened in the intervening two years, and the attempts at clarification in this chapter owe much to various explorations of theory and practice from around the world.

The reader of this book may be part of a broader treatment, policy or research community which has become interested in harm reduction from varied backgrounds. Each individual may carry the baggage of different perspectives on the use of drugs and associated problems. Some carry the baggage of their views of treatment, or perhaps on the shortcomings of treatment availability; others carry the baggage of their views on the morality of drug taking and associated behaviours; or perhaps their views on free will and the rights of the individual; or perhaps on the legalisation of drugs. What is the characteristic that binds together the harm-reduction movement? And what are the areas of disagreement or lack of resolution which require further exploration or research? The true champion of harm reduction is not necessarily anti-drugs; nor necessarily pro-drugs. He or she expresses support, opposition or indifference to a proposed public or personal health approach or a proposed legal or social response solely on the basis of the extent to which it increases or decreases the amount of harm consequent upon the drug use in question. A pre-determined position on drug use as intrinsically 'bad' or 'good' has no meaning in this context, where the response is determined solely by the extent of observed or anticipated harm which results from the drug use. Thus the champion of harm reduction is neither for nor against increased civil rights for drug users; neither for nor against the increased availability of drug substitu-

3

tion programmes or drug-free programmes; neither for nor against the legalisation or decriminalisation of drug use; neither for nor against diversions from the criminal justice system – except insofar as one or other of these choices influences the nature and extent of harms consequent upon the drug use.

An approach of harm minimisation is applicable to all psychoactive drugs. Indeed, not only is it applicable to all drugs, but it could be strongly argued that it is one of the foundation stones for all personal and public policy and treatment responses. Harm reduction in the drugs field has a history which goes back well before the last few years (see Berridge, Chapter 5, this volume). In the late 1960s and early 1970s, several drug clinics and day centres in London taught injecting technique and included fixing rooms in which the addicts could inject. When and why these fixing rooms were abandoned is not well documented. Underground drug literature gave clear harm-reduction advice (e.g. the 'Speed kills' campaign in the late 1960s). In the UK, the Institute for the Study of Drug Dependence (ISDD) looked at harm reduction as it might be applied within a school setting for reducing the extent and severity of harm from sniffing volatile solvents (ISDD, 1976, 1980). Harm reduction was behind the removal of controls on the public sale of needles and syringes from supermarkets in Italy after the hepatitis B epidemic of the 1970s (Tempesta and Di Gianntonio, 1990). It was at the forefront of the review of drug strategy in The Netherlands in the early 1980s and was formally adopted, becoming the rationale behind not only the low-threshold methadone programmes but also the initial needle and syringe exchange programmes established by the 'Junkiebonden' and subsequently by the statutory services (see Buning, 1990; Engelsman, 1991).

There are many within the drugs field who would argue that the effort to clarify the concepts, define the terms, and introduce measures of harm reduction is but a distraction from the important task of implementing harm-reduction practices. They may argue that these approaches are self-evidently worthwhile. In the present climate in some countries, this argument may be sufficient – at least for the time being. However, in the harsher climate of other countries or other times, the rhetoric of the zealot will be insufficient. The lack of a clear set of concepts and definitions of harm reduction is likely to stand as a distinct problem in the development of this area of policy and practice. Newcombe (1992) has argued that 'developing precise concepts (of the reduction of drug-related harm) is important because it allows us to measure the effectiveness of harm-reduction interventions, and measurement is the basis of evaluation', and that 'the main function of the harms/benefits model is to help policy makers and service providers decide which harms they are attempting to reduce, so that scientific evaluation is possible'. Despite determined and sometimes articulate defence of this different perspective on drug taking, the absence of a legitimising ideology will interfere with the development of harm reduction and its incorporation into practice, research and training, affecting both personal and public health policy.

Harm or Risk?

What is harm, and how does it relate to risk? Risk reduction and harm reduction are terms which are often used as if they were synonymous. Harm must surely be our target. Support for competing proposals should be determined by the extent to which they reduce or increase the amount of harm accrued by the individual, the community or society.

Risk relates to the possibility that an event might occur; harm might be seen as the event itself or as relating to the event. There may be times when we choose to look at ways of reducing risk, but this would only be because we felt that this was a more useful 'handle' on the possible harm which may be incurred. Risk would, to some extent, be seen as a surrogate for the harm incurred (or likely to be incurred), again at the level of the individual, community or society.

One of the troubles with the measurement of harm is that it may not be directly or easily measurable. For example, there may be a convoluted relationship between the original behaviour and the manifest harm, which may appear at a distance in time (e.g. several years later), may be deliberately concealed (e.g. as a result of the stigma associated with sexually transmitted diseases), or may be most evident in hidden populations (e.g. among prostitutes or among groups who do not have orthodox access to health care).

What is the relationship between drug use and harm?

Risk behaviour does not necessarily result in harm. For example, there are many 80 year olds who still smoke 20 cigarettes per day and are still offensively fit and healthy. Similarly, there are still individuals who ride their motor bikes or mountain bikes without a crash helmet or drive their cars without seat belts, and many of these individuals will succeed in evading the associated harm. Nevertheless, the observed individual variability does not alter the robustness of the relationship that exists between the behaviour and the likelihood of harm being accrued.

What types of relationship can be identified between the drug-taking behaviour and the harm? Some relate to the substance itself (i.e. the drug being used), such as some types of liver damage and brain damage associated with use of alcohol or barbiturates. Others are associated with the technique of drug use (e.g. the paraphernalia used), such as hepatitis B or HIV infection from sharing injection equipment, or the asphyxiation of the aerosol sniffer from laryngospasm resulting from

the cold jet on the back of the throat. There would seem to be at least
one further type of relationship which can be identified, in which the
harm is associated with the context in which the drug is used – for
example, drink–driving accidents.

Risk: a discrete or cumulative event?

How does risk mount up over time? If the risk of contracting hepatitis
B or HIV from a single episode of sharing a needle or a syringe can be
calculated, then what are the laws which govern how to calculate the
cumulative risk as this behaviour continues? Drug workers, policy makers and researchers in the drugs field have not yet begun serious consideration of cumulative risk. Drug users themselves, on the other
hand, are already making up their own minds: if Charlie has been having unprotected sex with his girlfriend Jenny and has been sharing needle and syringe with his regular buddy Henry, then he may decide that
it is OK to carry on with the behaviour – in effect, he may be forming
the view that the continuation of the behaviour does not represent any
increase in the cumulative total of the risk to which he has already
exposed himself.
   It is probable that risk per event of drug use is not constant. First,
engagement in a novel form of drug use is probably associated with
higher levels of risk for some sorts of harm – for example, the harm of
accidental overdose or the harm of hepatitis B or HIV infection.
Subsequent repeat of the risk behaviour may result in some accumula-
tion of the total risk to which the individual has been exposed, but the
additional risk per additional event may be less than on the initial occasion for a number of reasons. If exposure to the virus has not occurred
with a sexual or injecting contact, then it may be that it has been established as a non-infectious contact; or an alternative explanation for this
reduced additional risk may relate to the acquisition of a degree of
expertise in the use of the drug (for example, learning syringe-cleaning
strategies or learning how to titrate dose against effect with intravenous
injection of a new drug). Thus paradoxically, as the cumulative total of
risk increases with repeated episodes, it may be the case that the risk
per episode may decrease as the user moves from novice to more regular user. Finally, it may be that risk per event then increases again for
some individuals, as their concern, cognitive vigilance and/or caution
become reduced – for example, due to sustained intoxication or in
association with compromise in atypical circumstances, such as during
withdrawals in police custody or prison.

Harm: a discrete or cumulative event?

Some harm can indeed be regarded as a single event of harm – for example, the risk of a road traffic accident for the drink driver, or the risk of hepatitis B or HIV infection for the injecting drug user. In other instances, the harm itself is clearly cumulative – for example, the liver damage seen with alcoholic cirrhosis. Although we have just identified infection with hepatitis B or HIV as a single event, we may reach a different conclusion when we turn to a consideration of disease progression, when we find that the cumulative effect of specific co-infections, or of general immunological insult, may increase the likelihood of HIV-related chronic hepatitis or of progression of asymptomatic HIV-seropositivity to AIDS.

Harm Reduction and Harm Minimisation

These two terms are frequently used as if they were synonymous. However, it may be more valuable to use them to refer to different sorts of consideration. Harm reduction might perhaps be regarded as something that is essentially operational (for example, harm-reduction policies, harm-reduction programmes etc.), whereas harm minimisation might be the overall goal or end point to be aimed for. Harm-reduction strategies are then seen as the means by which the goal of harm minimisation might be achieved. Thus a harm-minimisation policy or approach might reasonably comprise various harm-reduction elements.

Consideration of an overall approach of harm minimisation leads one to take a 'balance sheet' perspective in which there may be advantages and disadvantages, or harms and benefits, associated with a particular harm-reduction element. These can then be considered first at the individual level of harm minimisation, and second at the public level of harm minimisation (the balance of benefits and harms for the population as a whole, acknowledging the possibility of cases of individual overall harm provided it leads to overall public benefit).

The same consideration that has been given above to the concepts of harm reduction and harm minimisation can presumably be applied to harm augmentation and harm maximization. Whilst it is unlikely that such policies or practices would be embraced deliberately, perhaps the main importance of these concepts is to draw the attention of policy makers and practitioners to the impact of their decisions on the resulting harm to individuals and society as a whole.

Personal versus public health perspectives

It has been a fortunate and convenient coincidence that many of the proposed responses to the problem of HIV infection among injecting drug users have simultaneously satisfied personal health and public health considerations.

Consider, for example, the intravenous barbiturate problem in the UK and Australia during the 1970s and early 1980s. Indeed, a more contemporary example of the barbiturate dilemma is currently available in the UK. Since the mid 1980s there has been extensive intravenous use of benzodiazepines (Strang, Sievewright and Farrell, 1992). Temazepam capsules were available in the form of liquid-filled capsules (known as 'soft eggs') which were then injected through a wide-bore needle. As a result of concerns about this developing epidemic and reports of associated physical complications, the manufacturers reformulated the preparation so that it was no longer so easy to inject by replacing the liquid-filled capsule with a Gelthix formulation in which the contents of the capsule now resembled candle wax. Since this reformulation two years ago, the injecting of temazepam capsules has continued, with injecting drug users variously reporting softening of the capsules in a microwave or physical manipulation of the Gelthix contents so that they can inject the temazepam through a wide-bore needle. Not surprisingly, the early reports are of increased morbidity associated with such injecting, but data are not available on the extent to which the injecting of temazepam may have become less common. In some cities in the UK, there are preliminary reports that temazepam injecting continues at a similar level, whereas elsewhere there has been a substantial reduction in the number of new drug users reporting recent injecting of temazepam. It may well be that the reformulation has resulted in increased harm to those individuals who continue with the behaviour, but decreased harm for the majority of drug users who have been deflected on to more established drugs of intravenous use. Time will tell whether this control-orientated intervention has increased or decreased harm for specific individuals, and has increased or decreased overall harm.

What are the dimensions of harm?

What different axes or dimensions may be considered to help in accurate description (and hopefully quantification) of harm?

At its simplest level, if harm can be incurred as a one-off event or, in other circumstances, is cumulative, then this provides us with a single crude dimension of severity of harm, with some harms being spread along a continuum (for example, degree of liver damage, degree of family breakdown, degree of social dislocation, degree of criminalisation of the local community, degree of economic impact at the national level). Describing harm along such a continuum does not necessarily mean that the affected population is evenly distributed along this continuum; it may well be that there is a clustering of individuals or populations at one or other point on the continuum (perhaps, most probably, at the extremes). If *infection* with HIV or hepatitis B virus is considered, then this would be an example of a harm where the population under study existed at one or other end of the continuum. (Indeed, the concept of continuum becomes meaningless when there are only the two possible positions or categories). However, when the consideration shifts to HIV *disease* or hepatitis B *disease*, then it may become more meaningful to return to a continuum, with a substantial proportion of the population at one end of the continuum as asymptomatic seropositives, and the remaining positive population spread along the continuum according to the extent of progression of disease.

But this approach requires a vision of harm as unidimensional. Whilst it may be convenient in general conversation to consider the quantification of harm in this simple way, it soon becomes apparent that this is an insufficient approach for more detailed study. For a nociometer or a harm-gauge to be useful, it will need to be an instrument that is more adaptable than a simple Geiger counter which bleeps away in the presence of harm. Like the Geiger counter itself, it may be possible to examine the phenomenon on different scales, and for there to be a degree of quantification to this examination. Descriptions of the 'problem drinker' and 'problem drug taker' have involved some attempt to identify the nature of the harm, an attempt to identify the particular drug-taking behaviour with which the harm appears to be associated. More recently Dorn (1992) has suggested that the various dimensions of harm which may be considered cover personal harm, social harm, legal harm and financial harm.

Newcombe (1992) has recently described two axes – the type of harm (health, social or economic) and the level at which the harm is experienced (individual, community or societal). Even by use of this simple three-by-three matrix, the discussion becomes more meaningfully descriptive when considering the nature of an existing harm, or the extent to which it may be possible for this to be influenced. Moving on from this two dimensional model to include axes for the timing of onset of the harm (short-term through to long-term onset), the duration of the harm (temporary through to permanent harm), and a measure of intensity of this harm, then significant progress has been made in quantifying the harm being considered.

As harm reduction comes of age, it will need to be accompanied by the routine and widespread incorporation of measures of the harms which are occurring and which we wish to influence. Some of these harms will be easy to measure in visible populations, but problems will be encountered in estimating the extent of harm in hidden populations. (For a recent discussion of drug use and HIV risk in hidden populations, see Lambert (1990).) Problems will also be encountered with the identification and quantification of harms where there is a time lag between the critical event and the visible expression of the harm (for example, the late onset of lung cancer and coronary heart disease among cigarette smokers, and the time lag between HIV infection and hepatitis B infection and the development of AIDS and chronic hepatitis respectively). Other harms may prove difficult to measure because they are experienced by individuals, groups or organisations who are not the identified drug users (for example, social and family distress and influences on household burglaries or the national economy).

Possible Influences on Harm

The influence of availability

With illicit drugs, availability is all too often seen as having a fairly direct, inverse relationship with interdiction efforts. In fact, real availability is influenced by many other factors, including the geographical distribution of the product, the cost per unit dose, the regularity of supply etc. For example, there is presumably no question as to whether gold and silver are available within our societies, but the everyday obstacles involved in accessing these products, the limited outlets and the cost deterrents all contribute to an eventual set of circumstances which is little different to non-availability.

To what extent does the availability of one product (and the way in which this availability is achieved) have an impact on the availability of another product? For example, the argument (perhaps most famously from Amsterdam) that it is possible to achieve a separation of the cannabis market from the market in other illicit drugs would be an illustration of the case where manipulating the form of one availability may have an influence on the actual availability of other drugs. This leads on to consideration of the different ways in which availability can be managed, ranging from the extremes of total prohibition to unrestricted open access (see next section).

With respect to the issue of needle and syringe availability in the UK, most attention has been paid to the new needle and exchange schemes (see Stimson et al.,1988, 1990), although it is important to consider also the extensive over-the-counter purchase of needles and syringes from community pharmacists (see Glanz, Byrne and Jackson, 1989). Availability of needles and syringes is presumably only one part (and possibly often a small part) of the role of the needle and syringe exchange scheme. If the simple provision of needles and syringes is seen as the main or only function of the exchange scheme, then one can readily envisage a time when the human component may be replaced by machine – for example, the various dispensing machines which are being developed to provide clean needles and syringes on the basis of direct provision, sale or exchange. If there is more to the operation of a needle and exchange scheme than the simple provision or exchange of equipment (as would presumably be held to be the case by most practitioners who have had links with exchange schemes), then it becomes necessary to identify these other components; and, hopefully through this clarification, it may be possible to enhance the efficacy of these additional components and avoid a preoccupation with the simple provision or collection of equipment.

Methods of controlling availability

At the 1989 Melbourne conference on *Options for Drug Control*, Rolfe (unpublished background papers) outlined the following options for control and controlled availability: (1) harsher penalties (use?; possession?; supply?); (2) prescription of the drug (which drugs?; in which forms?; with what dosage restrictions?; to which individuals or categories of individual?); (3) licensing of the drug (as for 2); (4) regulation of supply of the drug (commercial sale?; government monopoly?); (5) decriminalisation (discretionary non-enforcement?; partial prohibition?). Rolfe's proposals seem to have been influenced considerably by the policy options for cannabis described by the South Australian Royal Commission (1979), but with the additional consideration of options for prescribed availability. The particular advantage of this approach is that it avoids a damaging polarisation of the debate and the risk that only two extremes are considered.

Within this framework, controlled availability may need particular attention, as it is clearly an area in which planners and practitioners are likely to be actively involved. Controlled availability might be defined as 'the prescription by a medical practitioner of a specified drug of addiction to a person known to be an addict with the objective of reducing the adverse health, social and economic consequences of illicit drug use' (A. Wodak, personal communication, 1992). Contained within this proposed definition are an identification of the drug to be made available (and presumably the form in which it would be made available), the means by which it would be made available (prescription by a medical practitioner), the identification of 'caseness' of the individual to whom the drug would be available (an addict), and the objective underlying this controlled availability (reducing the adverse consequences).

The influence of price

Despite the repeated contention, from drug workers as well as drug users, that drug takers will only change their use of drug when they are 'ready to do so' or when they 'really wish to do it for themselves', economists (e.g. Wagstaff and Maynard, 1988, 1989) have repeatedly drawn attention to the importance of cost as a proportion of available surplus income and its influence on per capita consumption when measured at the population level. Thus the starting point for a discussion on the influence of price should perhaps be that increased price is likely to lead to decreased use. However, what is the nature of the relationship between cost and use of the drug? Is use evenly distributed across the population, and are economically driven changes in drug use seen evenly across this population? Might there be evidence of substantial benefit to one part of the population, with a neutral or even deleterious effect on other parts of the population? It is also important to examine the links within the relationship between price and use of the drug. For some harms, the concern may be entirely to do with the amounts of the substance which are used (the relationship between cost and levels of cirrhosis may be an example of this more straightforward relationship). But for other harms (such as infection with hepatitis B or HIV), the harm may be mediated through changes in the route of drug use, and hence an economic change which results in change of pattern of drug use or change of route of drug use may be a change of particular importance; for example, if there is a sharp increase in price or decrease in purity such that the heroin-smoking addict may move to more efficient technology of administration such as injecting, then, despite a possible reduction in the amount of drug being used, the harm accrued may be greatly increased.

The influences of different products in the marketplace

Different forms of drug may be associated with different harms, purely by virtue of their possible means of administration. The availability of smoking-only heroin in the market-place would not be associated with risks of hepatitis B or HIV infection in the same way as the availability of injection-only heroin or of versatile forms of black market heroin which can be taken by either route. At present, control strategies of the Customs and police pay little attention to the route of administration of the drug seized; a seizure of 10 kg of heroin is not accompanied by a consideration of the routes by which this heroin might have been used, nor a consideration of the influence on the dynamics of the black market in the days or weeks that follow the seizure. It is possible to envisage a scenario where the well-intentioned seizure of quantities of smoking heroin may leave the heroin-smoking addict compromised and may inadvertently lead to first injection; and conversely it could be argued that the effective interdiction of injection-only heroin and its consequent removal from the marketplace, combined with sufficient supplies of smoking-only heroin, might even encourage healthy changes from injecting to smoking as a pattern of use. This whole area appears to have received little attention and might be worthy of more specific consideration, with input from studies of markets of legal drugs and other consumer products. The case for discussion is not that economic factors do not decrease or increase the extent of consumption, but that the relationship between this changed level of consumption and the harms accrued has not been sufficiently investigated; if less alcohol, nicotine, temazepam or heroin are used by the population, then what impact will this have on different forms of harm which may occur?

Do changes or transitions occur in risk behaviour and harm accrued; and, if so, what may influence these transitions?

Attention has recently been drawn to significant changes which may occur in the nature of ongoing drug use, and one particular form of change which is an area of new, invigorated study is the transition in route of drug use (see Des Jarlais et al., 1992; Griffiths et al., 1992; Strang et al., 1992a – for discussion of the significance of the transitions and presentation of preliminary data from the USA and UK). For example, route of first heroin use in London is no longer by intravenous injection; whereas 90% of those initiated into heroin prior to 1980 had first injected the drug, the intravenous route is extremely rare for heroin users who have been initiated in recent years, with more than 90% of new users during the last few years taking their first heroin by 'chasing the dragon' (Strang et al., 1992b). Although 'chasing the dragon' has been found to be a robust pattern of heroin use even after dependence and high-dose intake have been established (Gossop et al., 1988), data are now emerging to indicate the considerable extent to which heroin users in the community may undergo a transition from one route to another (and perhaps back again at a later date), just as has previously been reported for treatment populations (Griffiths et al., 1992; Strang, Heathcote and Watson, 1987). Non-treatment populations of heroin users are now being studied (Des Jarlais et al., 1992; and London Heroin Transitions Study – ongoing). Of particular relevance to the feasibility of harm-reduction strategies is the finding that 'reverse transitions' had occurred (a 'reverse transition' being a move from a more harm-laden form of drug use such as injecting back to a non-injecting route, thus apparently moving back up 'the slippery slope'). Transitions were reported by 89 of the 200 heroin users interviewed in London, and a third of the reported transitions were 'reverse transitions'. What are the factors that may reduce the likelihood of a harm-augmenting transition; or, conversely, what influences can be brought to bear to increase the likelihood of a 'reverse transition'? In future study of transitions and the factors that influence them, it might also be meaningful to regard the move from intravenous heroin use to oral methadone as a transition.

The influence of dependence on transitions

This discussion of harms associated with drug use has largely been conducted without considering the influence of dependence. Quite apart from arguments about dependence as a psychological and physical harm in its own right, it may well be that the extent to which dependence pre-exists may have a significant modulating effect on the influence of other factors, such as changes in availability or price. If the heroin smoker runs out of smokable heroin and is offered only intravenous heroin, or if the heroin injector who has always been scrupulously hygienic is imprisoned and can only administer heroin from borrowed needle and syringe, then might the degree of dependence and/or the extent of withdrawal phenomena influence the likelihood of this harm-augmenting transition? This area should surely warrant more specific study, as it may draw our attention to areas of particular influence – for example, the provision of substitute opiates at times of drug droughts on the street, or the prevention of emergence of withdrawal symptoms which would develop following incarceration.

The Harm-reduction Movement and other Lobbying Groups

Consideration should also be given to the extent to which there is a necessary relationship between harm reduction and various other perspectives (such as civil rights, treatment availability, legal sanctions etc.).

The legalisation debate

There is often confusion between calls for harm minimisation (with specific harm-reduction elements in policy and practice) and calls for the legalisation or decriminalisation of some or all aspects of use, possession, supply etc. of drugs that are currently illegal. This confusion is dangerous, not only because it derives from sloppy thinking, but also because it may generate an opposition to harm-reduction proposals which actually emanates from a position contrary to legalisation. What drugs are being considered, and what forms of the drug (e.g. oral, intravenous, smokable etc.)? Is the call for open availability or less restrictions on availability (for example, access according to age, established addict status, established injector status etc.), and is the call for more fundamental changes in the present legal structure (e.g. legalisation) or modification of the present legal position, possibly accompanied by changes in the application of the law (for example, decriminalisation, perhaps accompanied by diversions out of the criminal justice system)? Although the law may be an ass, there are times when it may be a surprisingly subtle ass (Hawks, 1976).

Harm reduction and the prescribing debate

The issues here are similar to those in the preceding section. There may be areas of overlap between the two debates but they are not the same debate. For some advocates, the provision or non-provision of substitute drugs seems to encompass almost all harm reduction. In fact, the greatest harm reductions have probably been achieved in areas where prescribing is a marginal consideration – for example, the public education about the risks of cigarette smoking, the risks of sharing needles and syringes, and the subsequent substantial changes in the smoking and injecting practices of the populations involved in these behaviours, either ceasing the practices or moving to adaptations of the practice so as to avoid or reduce the likelihood of accruing harm. In the drug users' comic 'Smack in the Eye', Grandpa Smackhead Jones warns younger and less experienced drug injectors of the particular dangers of injecting tablets of dextromoramide (Palfium) with its allegedly greater risk of inadvertent overdose, but he does not need to recommend prescribing of substitute drugs in order to give this harm-reduction advice (Gillman, 1992). From the professional end, Fraser and George (1992) describe the incorporation of harm-reduction elements in the role of the police force, and Stover and Schuller (1992) describe how abstinence-orientated services have taken on board AIDS prevention and associated harm-reduction goals so as to enable the drug user to survive the phase of drug dependence without irreversible damage to health.

Harm reduction and the debate about pleasure-promotion

Advocacy for harm-reduction measures is not synonymous with condoning or promoting pleasure-seeking, nor opposing it. Confusion most commonly arises when it is contended that attempts to obstruct or prohibit pleasure-seeking may result in harm-augmentation or harm-maximisation. The point to be made from the standpoint of harm reduction is that this adverse effect must be corrected, and this point can perhaps be made most cogently by separating it from an argument either for or against pleasure-promotion. Both the hedonist and the puritan can apply harm reduction.

Harm reduction and the rights of individuals to self-determination

Here again, the same point must be made. These confusions only weaken the harm-minimisation position. There are those who would support impassioned calls for the rights of individual drug users to be recognised, alongside a call for them to be integrated and assimilated into broader society without discrimination or ostracisation. But regardless of whether this position should be supported or not, it is a debate that should be clearly placed outside the debate about the worth or otherwise of harm-reduction strategies. From the pure harm-reduction perspective, the support of the personal freedoms of one or other group of drug users should be determined solely by the extent to which one or other course of action can be shown to result in an over-all reduction of harm accrued.

Harm reduction and the focus on abstinence: are they opposites or not?

Abstinence is an excellent means of achieving harm reduction and harm minimisation insofar as the abstinence can be securely achieved and robustly held. The problem arises with the higher number of instances of failures to attain abstinence or the breakdown of the absti-nence. Indeed, it may even be the case that the pursuit of abstinence results in a more catastrophic return to drug use when it occurs (the 'abstinence violation effect' described by Marlatt and Gordon (1985)). From the harm-reduction perspective, the same position should be taken in this debate as in the other areas of overlap, in that the approach for the individual or the population should be supported solely according to the extent to which there are changes in the harms under consideration.

Indeed, there are dangers in identifying harm-reduction practices as being opposites to abstinence-orientated approaches, for there may be firmly abstinent programmes which can nevertheless incorporate important harm-reduction measures. For example, the first week or two after incarceration in prison may be a time of atypical risk behav-iour in addicted heroin users, who may be so compromised by their withdrawal symptoms that they inject or share needles and syringes for the first time. Thus the policy document in England (instructing med-ical practitioners working in prisons that they should provide appropri-ate methadone detoxification) may represent a small but highly significant introduction of a new service (Prision Medical Service, 1991).

There is a real risk that the pure consideration of harm reduction will be confused or diluted by the introduction of other concepts or debates, and it may prove vital to the healthy survival of the harm-reduction debate for it to be conducted at a distance from the other debates, which may perhaps be related but not the same. Consider, for example, the extensive opposition to harm-minimisation policy proposals in the US. It seems clear that much of the opposition to harm minimisation is in fact an opposition to actual or perceived calls for drug legalisation; there is confusion of the debates to the detriment of the development of harm-minimisation policies and practices. It is for these reasons (among oth-ers) that some articulate advocates of harm minimisation have concluded that 'there is a need to distinguish and distance harm-minimisation pro-posals from proposals for legalisation' (Dorn, 1992).

Are There Possible Easy Gains?

Some of the responses that could be considered stand as opportunities for reducing harm at no cost. (In this context, cost is not seen as a financial cost but as a cost in terms of other harms accrued). Attention could profitably turn to examples of uncontroversial harm-reduction measures, which are perhaps overlooked precisely because they are not controversial.

For example, what about the designated driver programme promoted by the Alcohol and Drug Foundation in Australia? With a mixture of carrot and stick, bars and hotels are invited to participate in a 'voluntary' scheme in which the bouncer approaches a group of drinkers who arrive together and suggests that they should decide at this early stage in the evening which of them will be driving for the rest of the evening, and then the management of the establishment provides free non-alcoholic drinks to this designated driver. Or what about the addition of vitamin supplements, such as thiamine, to alcoholic beverages, as has been proposed now for some years, but for which there has never quite been a sufficient push for the idea to be translated into practice? Or what about the provision of hepatitis B immunisation to injecting drug users who are so far uninfected? From the point of view of harm reduction, the case for such interventions seems incontestable; they stand as examples of all benefit and minimal cost. These would surely be excellent vanguard projects for a harm-reduction movement.

Some thought should also be given to more controversial options – for example, the possible distribution of supplies of naloxone (the opiate antagonist) to opiate users who may at some later date be able to give a life-saving injection of the drug to a fellow drug user who inadvertently overdoses, as has recently been put forward (Strang and Farrell, 1992).

Perhaps consideration should even be given by interdiction forces (e.g. Customs and police) to the selective application of their efforts, so as, for example, to target intravenous types of opiate (black market heroins for injecting and diverted pharmaceutical drugs) rather than smokable, oral or sniffable forms. This might prevent sudden imbalances in the market such that the dependent heroin smoker can only obtain drugs for injecting, and may even nudge or provoke the injector to move across to non-injecting routes such as smokable heroin, oral methadone or codeine.

Why is more attention not paid to these areas? They may be less glamorous, but they offer the prospect of very real benefits for large numbers of drug users at low cost. Whether in a clinical, policy or political setting, the advocate of harm-reduction practices would be more assured of winning the case when arguing for such straightforward initiatives (and such initial successes may then set the tone for subsequent, more difficult considerations). Thus it is disappointing to see the limited extent to which these more clear-cut benefits of harm reduction have not been achieved, and it is particularly disappointing to see the low level of advocacy for such incontestable developments. What irony that the advocate of harm reduction often overlooks these obvious proposals and chooses instead to invite opposition to proposals which are seen as more controversial!

Conclusions

There are perhaps three points which need particular emphasis.

First, the lack of a clear set of concepts and definitions of harm reduction is likely to stand as a distinct problem in the development of this area of policy and practice. Notwithstanding the existence of impassioned and sometimes articulate advocates of this different perspective on drug taking, the lack of a legitimising ideology will stand as an obstacle to the longer-term development of harm reduction as a credible and perhaps dominant perspective on drug use. Hence it will stand in the way of its incorporation into strategies of practice, research and training at the levels of both personal and public health policy. In particular, if there are serious proposals to promote policy and practice which lead to reductions in harm, then they will need to be accompanied by a clear understanding about which harms need to be considered and what framework is required to explore the various dimensions of harm. For example, should there not be development of measures along these dimensions that could be easily and routinely applied in clinical and policy practices?

Second, the central identity of the harm-reduction movement requires clarification. What links should be established with other lobbying or advocacy groups in the drugs field? The harm-reduction movement may choose to form alliances with groups working to other agendas, but this can only be on a conditional basis, subject to evidence that is at least indicative that the proposed alliance does indeed reduce harm (and probably still reduces harm even when considered across populations and over time). Thus either legalisation or prohibition (or any proposal in between) may be incorporated with a preferred strategy for harm reduction, once it has been established that the proposed approach does indeed reduce harm. Indeed, if the policy and practice of harm reduction is to be taken seriously, then there is no choice but to be driven by the evidence which will become available in the future on the efficacy of these different approaches as harm-reduction strategies.

Third, and finally, should there not be action on some of the less controversial proposals that are more easy to implement for harm reduction? For example, why is it that there is still not widespread hepatitis B testing and vaccination for injecting drug users, or the addition of thiamine supplements to beers? The reductions in harm would be great and at minimal cost, and these options may represent excellent vanguard projects for the harm-reduction movement.

The harm-reduction field has gathered an expanded and powerful following over the last few years and has the opportunity to become a dominant influence on practice, research and training in the drugs field, but only if it can establish a sound scientific basis for the policy and practice measures that are proposed.

References

Buning, E. (1990). The role of harm reduction programmes in curbing the spread of HIV by drug injectors. In J. Strang and G.V. Stimson (Eds), *AIDS and Drug Misuse: The Challenge for Policy and Practice in the 1990s*. London: Routledge.

Des Jarlais, D.C., Casriel, C., Friedman, S. and Rosenblum, A. (1992). AIDS and the transition to illicit drug injection: Results of a randomised trial prevention program. *British Journal of Addiction*, 87, 493–498.

Dorn, N. (1992). Clarifying policy options on drug trafficking: Harm minimization is distinct from legalisation. In P. O'Hare, R. Newcombe, A. Matthews, E.C. Buning and E. Drucker (Eds), *The Reduction of Drug-related Harm*. London: Routledge.

Engelsman, E. (1991). Drug use and the Dutch: A matter of social well being and not primarily a problem for the police and the court. *British Medical Journal*, 302, 484–485.

Fraser, A. and George, M. (1992). The role of the police in harm reduction. In P. O'Hare, R. Newcombe, A. Matthews, E.C. Buning and E. Drucker (Eds), *The Reduction of Drug-related Harm*. London: Routledge.

Gillman, M. (1992). Smack in the eye! In P. O'Hare, R. Newcombe, A. Matthews, E.C. Buning and E. Drucker (Eds), *The Reduction of Drug-related Harm*. London: Routledge.

Glanz, A., Byrne, C. and Jackson, P. (1989). Role of community pharmacies in prevention of AIDS among injecting drug misusers: Findings of a survey in England and Wales. *British Medical Journal*, 209, 1076–1079.

Gossop, M., Griffiths, P. and Strang, T. (1988). Chasing the dragon: characteristics of heroin chasers. *British Journal of Psychiatry*, 83, 1159–1162.

Griffiths, P., Gossop, M., Powis, B. and Strang, J. (1992). Extent and nature of transitions of route among heroin addicts in treatment: Preliminary data from the Drug Transitions Study. *British Journal of Addiction*, 87, 485–492.

Hawks, D. (1976). The law relating to cannabis 1964–1973: How subtle an ass? In J.P.D. Graham (Ed.), *Cannabis and health*. London: Academic Press.

Institute for the Study of Drug Dependence (1976). Not to be sniffed at? *Druglink*, 6, 1–2.

Institute for the Study of Drug Dependence (1980). *Teaching About a Volatile Situation: Suggested Health Education Strategies for Minimizing Casualties Associated with Solvent Sniffing*. London: ISDD.

Lambert, E. (Ed.). (1990). *The Collection and Interpretation of Data from Hidden Populations*. NIDA Research Monograph Series 98. Washington DC: US Government Printing Office.

Marlatt, G.A. and Gordon, J.R. (Eds). (1985). *Relapse Prevention: Maintenance Strategies in the Treatment of Addictive Behaviours*. New York: Guilford.

Newcombe, R. (1992). The reduction of drug-related harm: A conceptual framework for theory, practice and research. In P. O'Hare, R. Newcombe, A. Mathews, E. Buning and E. Drucker (Eds), *The Reduction of Drug-related Harm*. London: Routledge.

Prison Medical Service (Home Office) (1991). *Management and Throughcare of Durg Users*. London: Home Office.

South Australian Royal Commission into Non-Medical Use of Drugs (1979). *Final Report* (Professor Sackville, Chairman). Adelaide: The Commission.

Stimson, G., Alldritt, L., Dolan, K. and Donoghoe, M. (1988). Syringe exchange schemes for drug users in England and Wales. *British Medical Journal*, 296, 1717–1719.

Stimson, G., Donoghoe, M., Lart, R. and Dolan, K. (1990). Distributing sterile needles and syringes to people who inject drugs: The syringe-exchange experiment. In J. Strang and G. Stimson (Eds), *AIDS and Drug Misuse. The Challenge for Policy and Practice in the 1990s*. London: Routledge.

Stover, H. and Schuller, K. (1992). AIDS prevention with injecting drug users in West Germany: A user-friendly approach on a municipal level. In P. O'Hare, R. Newcombe, A. Matthews, E. Buning and E. Drucker (Eds), *The Reduction of Drug-related Harm*. London: Routledge.

Strang, J., Des Jarlais, D., Griffiths, P. and Gossop, M. (1992a). The study of transitions in the route of drug use: The route from one route to another. *British Journal of Addiction*, 87, 473–486.

Strang, J. and Farrell, M. (1992). Harm minimisation for drug users: When second best may be best first. *British Medical Journal*, 304, 1127–1128.

Strang, J., Gossop, M., Griffiths, P. and Powis, B. (1992b). First use of heroin: Changes in route of administration over time. *British Medical Journal*, 304, 1222–1223.

Strang, J., Heathcote, S., and Watson, P. (1987). Habit-moderation in injecting drug addicts. *Health Trends*, 19, 16–18.

Strang, J., Sievewright, N. and Farrell, M. (1992). Intravenous and other novel abuses of benzodiazepines: The opening of Pandora's box? *British Journal of Addiction*, 87, 1373–1376.

Strang, J., Stimson, G.V. and Des Jarlais, D.C. (1992). What is AIDS doing to the drug research agenda? *British Journal of Addiction*, 87, 343–346.

Tempesta, E. and Giannantonio, M. (1990). The Italian epidemic: a case study. In J. Strang and G. V. Stimson (Eds), *AIDS and Drug Misuse: The Challenge for Policy and Practice in the 1990s*, pp. 108–117. London: Routledge.

Wagstaff, A. and Maynard, A. (1988). *Economic Aspects of the Illicit Drug Market and Drug Enforcement Policies in the United Kingdom*. Home Office Research Study No. 95. London: Her Majesty's Stationery Office.

Wagstaff, A. and Maynard, A. (1989). Economic aspects of illicit drug problems: summary of report. *British Journal of Addiction*, 84, 461–466.

Chapter 2
Harm Reduction: Does It Lead where Its Proponents Imagine?

STEPHEN MUGFORD

This chapter is a friendly polemic on 'harm reduction'. It is polemical because I suggest that there are serious problems with the way that harm reduction is conceived and with the policies which flow from it if coherently applied. It is 'friendly' because it is directed chiefly at friends and allies as well as at my own earlier writings on the topic which share the weaknesses I document. Along the way, however, I direct barbs at my 'enemies'. I begin by characterising a position that I think typical of many harm reductionists and then critique it.

I suggest that harm reduction has four elements: a moral stance, a description of a problem, a suggested solution and a pay-off.

Moral stance

Drug use is viewed as neither right nor wrong in itself. Rather, drug use is evaluated in terms of harm to others and, to some extent, harm suffered by users. The latter is regrettable, but acceptable if it arises from 'informed choice'. Laws are appropriate to prevent harm to third parties and to reduce the exploitation of users by producers/sellers but not as primary barriers to informed use.

Description of a problem

The current drug laws which prohibit the use of drugs like heroin, cocaine and cannabis are mistaken. They do not achieve what their protagonists claim are their goals (drug free societies and the like); rather they create a vast black market with profits for suppliers, hazards for users and corruption of the control systems. Internationally, drug trafficking distorts producer economies and increases exploitation. In user countries, the (selective) prosecution of laws produces injustice and misery and (especially in the USA) is connected to racial inequality and repression. Nonetheless, since powerful drugs can cause serious harm and, given that the bulk of harm arises from 'legal' drugs, simple 'legalisationist' models are not generally viewed as the answer to drug problems.

21

Solution

This lies in calculating the harm that arises from drug use and pursues the reduction – ideally the minimisation – of such harm. Harm, like drug use itself, is not seen as eliminable but an optimum state of minimum harm may, by careful monitoring, be approached. Many protagonists believe that this morally neutral stance also confers a long range political benefit. By eschewing a 'pro-drugs' position one may seize the 'middle ground' and cash in on the growing sense that 'prohibition has failed and that we have to try something new'.

Pay-off

Since drug prohibition is frequently used as a tool for racist exploitation and for the maintenance of political power by right wing forces who (cynically) take the moral high ground on drugs as a cover for other purposes, promoting harm reduction (and hence undermining that right wing position) puts one 'on the side of the angels' – in favour of individual liberty, against exploitation and against the unreasonable extension of police powers etc.

The core arguments of my chapter can be summarised in relation to this sketch. First, I accept the description of the problem. Although there are many details to clarify, this is a useful overview. By the same token, I find the moral stance broadly defensible. Thus I have nothing further to say about them here.

I used to accept, also, the proposed solution and imagined pay-off, but I am now deeply suspicious of them. Harm reduction, I shall argue, must be viewed more critically, lest it lead in quite unanticipated – and unwelcome – directions. My critique falls into two parts. In the first, I try to think through exactly what harm reduction would look like in practice. In the second, I develop some philosophical and theoretical arguments.

Harm Reduction in Practice

To begin with, if harm reduction is to have any utility it must aggregate different kinds of harm. Policies that reduce one kind of harm at the expense of greater increases in other kinds must be suspect. Would we accept that it was worthwhile to save 20 lives which might have been lost by the use of impure drugs if the alternative cost was 100 lives lost through 'drugged driver accidents'? Of course not, but here like (lives) is compared with like. What if there are 20 lives saved but the alternative cost is 2000 people addicted to a drug, or 200 lost person years of productivity?

Two alternatives to this conundrum present themselves. *Either* we cannot measure different harms on one central scale, in which case harm reduction is a hollow claim, *or* we must find a universal and trans-contextual 'scale' to assess harm. In modern society, there is only one such universal scale – monetary values. Money, that neutral, rational, grey and amoral commodity, is the measure of all things (Marx, 1976; Simmel, 1978; see also Turner, 1986.) Harm reduction, then, must offer cost-benefit analyses of drug policies, otherwise harm is left unmeasured and one cannot make harm-*reduction* choices.

If we accept the task of a cost-benefit analysis, further questions arise. Central to these are the overall distribution of costs under different regimes of regulation and the question of how one might need to shift individual drug use patterns in order to move in harm-reduction directions. Let me take these in turn.

What is the overall distribution of costs under different regimes of regulation?

I have suggested two axes of differentiation of drug-related harm (Mugford, 1991a, b). The first axis concerns whether harm is suffered by the user (*direct harm*) or another person/group (*indirect harm*). The second axis concerns those harms that are *intrinsic* to use and those that are *extrinsic*. (An example of the latter would be HIV transmission through shared needles because needle exchanges have been banned.) Cross-connection of these two axes yields four types of harm which are differently distributed (Mugford, 1991b), for there are two very general relations between harm and regulation*. First, intrinsic-direct harm rises with use and in turn use tends to rise with availability. That is, there is a straight line function for the harm/regulation relation. In Figure 2.1 this is the line a–b. Second, other forms of harm tend to be distributed according to a U curve (c–d in Figure 2.1). It follows that the best *general* model for the harm/regulation relation is the sum of these two – namely the J curve from c to e.

This is the *general* argument. For any given drug the exact functions will vary. In addition, since we know that people switch their drug use from one drug to another depending on price and availability, the varied J curves for drugs would need to be summed to an overall (and currently undescribed) aggregate J. In the absence of extensive studies to document variation and substitution, however, we may reasonably assume that the net effect will be roughly as shown in Figure 2.1.

The main policy implication of Figure 2.1 is obvious. Harm reduction involves searching for the point at the bottom of the curve. That is, moving away from both prohibition *and* legal sale. If, however, these

---

*I sketch this very briefly here, for reasons of brevity. The argument is developed more fully in Mugford (1991b, 1992).

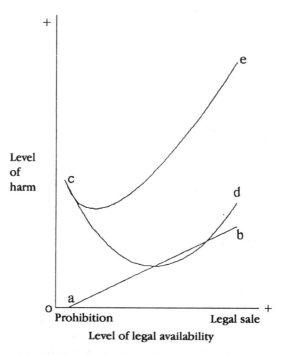

Figure 2.1 Legal availability and level of harm

are the only options available (for either ideological or other reasons), the overall harm point of prohibition (c) is lower than that which characterises complete legalisation (e). It follows that, compared to open sale, prohibition can be presented as a harm-reduction measure – and such presentation is neither incoherent nor deceitful. This is not to say prohibitionists are not incoherent and deceitful; at times they are both (see O'Malley and Mugford, 1991b). Nonetheless, a rational, hard-nosed prohibitionist could profitably employ the harm-reduction platform, as I suspect many are beginning to realise.

This is not the only interesting implication of Figure 2.1, however. The J curve reminds us of the distribution of current drug harm where most arises from legally available alcohol and tobacco (point e), not illicit drugs. Serious harm reductionism, therefore, should concentrate on legal drugs, since that is where the greatest savings lie. In the USA, for example, one should direct efforts not to stopping the 'War on Drugs' – destructive and hypocritical though it may be – but to strangling the tobacco and alcohol industries. And so on.

Thus, harm reduction might lead to much less effort being directed at reducing prohibitions and much more at increasing drug controls on the licit drugs. Serious harm reductionists could find their efforts directed not at reforming the laws on marijuana, cocaine and heroin, nor in civil libertarian campaigns against the 'War on Drugs' but in designing better anti-drug messages, stronger tobacco smoking bans and so forth.

How should one shift drug use patterns of individuals in order to move in harm-reduction directions?

Within a given regime of regulation and for any given drug, how are use patterns distributed? I suggest that the 'Ledermann curve' is the best start point here. Writing about alcohol, Ledermann (1956) argued that use followed a mathematical function (log normal) and that the key parameter of the mean level of alcohol consumption determined the length of the 'tail' of the curve and hence the proportion of problem users found under the extreme of that curve. The policy conclusion, if the model holds, is that to reduce problem levels of drinking we must shift mean consumption downwards and increase the proportion of alcohol abstinent people.

This model may be overly determinist and efforts have been made to modify it or improve upon it (see e.g. Tan, Lemmens and Koning, 1990). However, there is no reason to reject the broad thrust of the argument. Indeed, Tan and co-workers (1990) in reviewing the more sociological alternative of O. J. Skog (e.g. Skog, 1980) – who centres upon drinking norms and behaviour – conclude that empirical research seems to establish two major findings for alcohol:

> (1) The consumption level of all types of drinkers … seems to increase with an increasing mean level of consumption. This may be regarded as an expression of the collective nature of drinking behaviour.
> (2) In a population with a changing mean consumption, the relatively low and medium drinkers seem to show a proportionally larger change in consumption than heavier drinkers.
>
> *(Tan et al., 1990, p.746)*

While the differences between Ledermann and Skog are profound in theoretical terms and lead to different statistical projections, the overall model does not differ greatly when used as a crude policy guide. A generalised model, derived in part from Ledermann, Skog and other writers on alcohol consumption, is offered in Figure 2.2, but with an additional twist.

Figure 2.2 suggests that for any social activity there will be a roughly normal distribution of individuals around the average. Why then is the curve 'truncated' where alcohol (or other drug use) is concerned? This is because *behaviourally* one cannot go 'further' than not drinking. Nonetheless, the teetotal segment of the population (the cross-hatched segment) can be extrapolated leftward at the *belief* level, from a larger number who 'don't drink', to a smaller number who 'don't-drink-and-think-no-one-else-really-should', to the small minority who would

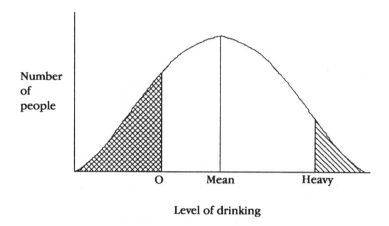

Figure 2.2 Drinking patterns as a normal curve

actively ban all drinking. At the other extreme, we find heavy and problem drinkers (the shaded segment).

In the absence of alternative models supported by research data, we
should apply the underlying logic of Figure 2.2 to all drugs*. Of course,
abstinence levels will be located in very different places, and the proportions distributed between 'don't use', 'don't-use-and-think-no-one-
else-really-should' and those who would actively ban all use will vary
enormously depending on the drug. But, for all that, we can still use
the model productively. Applying the logic of Figure 2.2, we can recre-
ate a series of Ledermann style curves (see Figure 2.3).

If the curve shown in Figure 2.3 as a solid line is broadly descriptive
of drug use in general we can identify two ways to move towards harm
reduction. We may pay attention to those heavy users who are in the
problem zone. Alternatively, we may think about the gain to be made
by lowering use levels generally, thus making small gains at the individual level but large gains in aggregate.

Let us start with heavy/problem users whose individual use levels
are high and who are thus likely to suffer serious harm. Although few
in number, these users nonetheless represent a disproportionate share

*Astute critics might now say that I have twice followed the same path – that of setting up a
hypothetical model, applying it in the absence of anything better and then acting as if the
conclusions that followed from it were justified because the model is presumed to hold. To
this my retort is simple – show me better assumptions, clearer logic, usable data and I will
happily modify or even abandon my position. Meanwhile, this is the best I can find and certainly a great deal better than copious rhetoric unaccompanied by any clear thinking through
to possible conclusions. See Weatherburn (1992) and Mugford (1992) for a debate that raises
some of these issues.

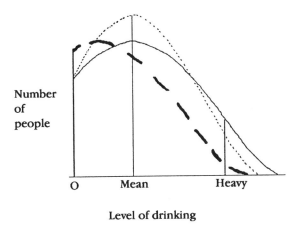

Figure 2.3 Some applications of a Ledermann style curve

of problems. It follows that reducing their use would be a positive harm-reduction step; but how can we do this? One option is to imagine shifting the main curve (the solid line) towards the second curve in Figure 2.3 (the dotted line). This shift leaves the proportion of non-users unaffected, does not alter the use level of modal users, but shifts heavy users back towards safer use. This sounds good, but while it may be possible, I have seen no persuasive evidence that demonstrates a shift from dangerous use while leaving relatively safe use untouched.

More plausible as a strategy is to attempt to shift the entire curve to the left – the dashed line in Figure 2.3. By moving the curve this way we achieve three things: we increase abstinence, we lower modal levels of use and we reduce the number of problem uses(rs). Such curve shifting has been discussed recently by Hackler (1991), who bases his work on earlier Canadian writings concerning drug use.

As Hackler argues, such curve shifting makes large aggregate gains by shifting all individuals. With drug use, although heavy users represent disproportionate levels of harm per capita, in aggregate terms moderate users represent the bulk of harm, simply because there are so many more of them. *Thus, shifting the whole curve to the left is the better harm-reduction option.* With alcohol, for example, we cease to concentrate upon the heavy drinker, instead focusing on the 'civilised drinker' (Kreitman, 1986).

This strategy is counter-intuitive to the way we think in individualist cultures, for it involves putting the aggregate good ahead of the freedom of a drug user to choose to use a drug safely. Moreover, such logic easily leads us to the view expressed recently by several prominent anti-drug American officials who have said that recreational users bear more responsibility for drug problems than do 'junkies'. This view – which raises the hackles of the harm reductionists I know – can be generated quite sensibly by applying the logic contained in Figure 2.3.

In short, whether we concentrate upon the overall model in Figure 2.1 or the distribution model in Figure 2.3, rational reasoning takes us down paths that most harm reductionists have not trodden and are opposed to treading. How can this happen?

Simply put, I have so far equated harm reduction with cost-benefit analysis, but I have examined only *costs*. Nowhere does 'benefit' come into the equation. Where illicit drug use is concerned, there is only one kind of benefit that currently could be counted – pleasure. Whereas with alcohol and tobacco one could make a series of plausible arguments about gross domestic product (GDP), about 'the industry', about employment and taxation revenues, with illegal drugs these benefits are not counted. We are left with pleasure – which is difficult to defend in the sober, rational discourse that harm reduction would like to be. But there are many reasons to suppose that drug use is better comprehended by a theoretical position that understands drug use in terms of commodified excitement typical of a modern culture (O'Malley and Mugford 1991a; forthcoming), something which I have documented empirically for at least one substantial group of users (Dance and Mugford, 1992).

However, excitement and pleasure are not benefits that harm reductionists want to champion. Yet unless one can defend pleasure and with it moments of non-rational hedonist risk-taking (and possibilities of irresponsibility), any cost-benefit analysis of drug use will inevitably drift towards the evaluation of costs alone. In the case of illicit drugs, such a position necessarily drifts towards anti-drug, even prohibitionist sentiments. Thus an attempt to develop harm reduction as a coherent policy position leads to some difficulties for those whose views I outlined earlier*. In following such a logic, moreover, one departs from the logic traditionally at the core of utilitarianism which sought to balance private pleasures against public harm†.

These 'internal' problems I have outlined in this section do not exhaust the difficulties of harm reduction. I now turn to some 'external' difficulties.

---

*In very recent times, a new breed of harm reductionist is jumping on the band wagon. So far as I can see, this breed consists largely of young, humourless, bureaucratic employees whose slogan might be *In Nike veritas*, whose view of all drugs is neo-Puritanical and who see harm reduction as a way to rid the world of a variety of evil practices. When, a decade or more ago, it was popular to pursue a relaxation of severe anti-marijuana legislation by comparing the drug with alcohol and tobacco, few of us imagined that our logic would be captured by those crying, 'You are right, they are very similar. Ergo, we must ban alcohol and tobacco too!!'.

†I am grateful to Jack Barbalet for making this point to me very lucidly.

Theoretical and Philosophical Problems.

There are numerous philosophical and theoretical problems that harm reduction confronts and I cannot possibly *argue* them in the space remaining to me. I therefore simply *list* three key points.

The political problems of harm reduction

Harm-reduction logic must use money as a measure of harm (cost) and develop utilitarian calculations to guide policy. In this case, the utilitarian catch-cry of 'the greatest happiness of the greatest number' is replaced by the version 'the least harm of the least number'. Such a version, however, neither escapes the problems of utilitarianism nor avoids producing new ones. I have shown that it falls into one major trap by not valuing pleasure, but even if this were rectified, utilitarianism has never solved the problem of aggregating different types of pleasure and happiness (MacIntyre, 1981) and could not solve the problems of aggregating the different types of cost/harm. For example, what if one's analysis showed that the death of a few, young, uneducated and unemployable black men in a run-down area of an American city involved less aggregate cost than legalising drug X and suffering a nationwide loss of productivity of two days per person per annum? Obviously, the former outcome is 'harm reducing' and should be preferred on aggregate harm-reduction grounds.

This unpalatable conclusion is a *necessary* outcome of a utilitarianism that eschews any moral choice about which activities are morally acceptable and imagines that it 'merely offers a neutral cost-benefit analysis' of the phenomena at hand. In short, one cannot avoid making and defending choices about what is good, what is acceptable, what is 'permissible-albeit-risky' and what is unacceptable. A common modern fantasy is that we can avoid such choices by hiding behind moral neutrality. The pay-off in the case of harm reduction might seem to be that we can capture the middle ground and avoid alienating people who would reject anything that seemed to champion drug use. But the 'middle ground' option does not work in this case. It is not simply that we risk inconsistency – I think it was Winston Churchill who said pithily that he would rather be right than consistent – but because when we do not specify that pleasure is a 'benefit' in our cost-benefit analyses and when we do not issue moral challenges to other viewpoints on drugs, we simply allow those alternatives to counter-colonise what we invent. All they need do is take harm reduction seriously and follow it to the logical anti-drug conclusion.

The naivety of 'liberation'

Harm reductionists are often naive about their political claims. They champion, for example, the reduction of prohibition and the replacement of criminal statutes on drug use with either legal or 'de-criminalised' controls. They imagine that these changes must represent less control by the State over the individual and hence be liberating. In doing so, they speak and write as if the last two decades of debate about 'social control' and 'governmentality' had not taken place. To mention two of a myriad of possible examples, Stan Cohen (1985) claims that new forms of control are not an exercise in reducing the powers of the State but might better be viewed as an exercise in 'widening the net' of social control and at the same time making the 'mesh' of the net finer. And Rose, following the seminal work of Michel Foucault, outlines the issue of governmentality thus:

> For all systems of rule in the West since about the eighteenth century, the population has appeared as the terrain of government *par excellence*. Not the exercise of sovereignty ...[nor] the management of the life of the nation as if it were a family...but the regulation of the processes proper to the population, the laws that modulate its wealth, health, longevity ...its capacity ... to engage in labour and so forth.

> Two features of government are of particular significance ... On the one hand, to govern a population one needs to isolate it as a sector of reality, to identify certain characteristics and processes proper to it... to make its features notable, speakable, writable, ...

> On the other hand, governing a population requires knowledge of a different sort. To make calculations about a population necessitates the highlighting of certain features of that population as the raw material of calculation... Knowledge here takes a very physical form; it requires the transcription of such phenomena as a birth, a death, a marriage, an illness ... Calculation, that is to say, depends upon processes of 'inscription' which translate the world into material traces: written reports, drawings, maps, charts, and, pre-eminently, numbers.

> *(Rose, 1988, pp.5–6)*

At least some forms of drug control proposed by harm reductionists (e.g. licences to purchase powerful drugs, computer records of transactions to monitor use levels and/or detect diversion to those not entitled to use) could easily be seen both as increased control in the sense referred to by Cohen and as contributing to inscription. Indeed, if one takes seriously the argument that prohibition is deficient precisely because it cedes controls that governments normally have over consumption and allows drug users to disappear from sight – arguments that I have often heard and repeated – one is *ipso facto* supporting the extension of State power and the ability to govern.

The point here is not to promote mindless anarchism, nor to advance a paranoid conviction that 'all government is bad government'.

It is simply to point to a vital area of debate which harm reductionists should engage with. In the absence of such debate, we risk falling into the view that all politics are party politics, to imagine for example that a shift from nasty, right wing, Republican (Tory etc.) administrations to caring, liberal-left Democrat (Labour etc.) administrations exhausts the relevant range of options, without wondering if all forms of administration may share some characteristics with which we have difficulty.

The limits of 'reason'

It is clear that harm reduction is lodged firmly in the post-Enlightenment discourses that see policy as a matter for rational discourse between reasonable men. (The gender attribution is not a careless slip.) There is a strong sense in harm reduction debates that they remain untouched by the ferment in modern philosophy and social theory that centres upon post-modernism and feminism in particular. Harm reductionists often write and think within the discourse of what Toulmin (1990) calls 'high modernity', a position that is characterised by an obsession with certainty, systematicity and the idea of a 'clean slate'. To this systematising tendency, Toulmin opposes the need for our practical philosophy to return to concerns with reasonableness, by attending to such things as the local, the timely, the particular and the oral.

In the area of concern to which this paper is addressed, this would mean a concern with involving oneself in a wide variety of actions to scrutinise, challenge, modify and improve drug policies, rather than a concern with developing an over-arching critique or defence of any one type of policy. It might, for example, abandon as sterile the idea of debating the value of prohibition-in-general, taking the view that no intelligible answer could ever be produced to this problem, preferring instead the evaluation of specific prohibitions. Or it might accept that rather than designing the 'right' system, it is best in practice to muddle along using existing systems – to think, for instance, that any official distribution of drugs to 'registered users' cannot avoid leaking at the edges, but that far from being a problem such a leak might be the least harmful way to meet the inevitable demand that the system neglects. After all, the drugs that leak are pure, the market does not generate large profits, organised crime sees little advantage in participating and so forth*. This is messy, untidy and anti-systematic, and might be useful for just such reasons.

A greater sensitivity to post-modern and feminist concerns, a willingness to abandon the Enlightenment project, would also give a solid

---

*This example was suggested to me in conversation with Peter Cohen, who characterised the Dutch model as incorporating such deliberate and constructive sloppiness.

intellectual base to the democratic intent of many harm reductionists who want to empower otherwise exploited drug users and allow their voices to be heard, but who often cannot find out how to do this in practice. Harm reduction is all too often a white, middle-class, male enterprise.

Such a tolerance for diversity of voices is also essential if we are to have any chance of allowing a wide ranging debate on what 'harm' really is. What I think we have done is to try to 'close out' some of the more absurd claims of the right wing prohibitionists, with their rhetoric about 'nations' and 'families', and in so doing closed out a large number of other views as well.

Conclusion

I have tried to show that for those who would question existing drug laws and who wish to improve drug policy by making it more humane, more respectful of civil liberties and more democratic, the harm-reduction banner is a dubious flag to fly. It looked like a good emblem, and it may still be a useful rallying point, but the very notion of harm reduction necessarily brings with it an intellectual baggage train which contains many things which aid the enemy, not our cause.

If we want to say that drug laws are not good laws, that drug use is acceptable (even if we do not advocate it), that civil liberties are more important than drug busts, that current drug enforcement in the USA is about white, middle-class fears and exploitations, not justice – and so forth – then let us say exactly those sorts of things. The idea that we should say these things as footnotes to a middle ground thrust for 'harm reduction' is a seductive trap. Marsha Rosenbaum has said that the lovely thing about 'harm reduction' as a phrase is that it is such a great 'sound bite'. Everyone thinks they know what it means and it seems reasonable to everyone, and this is a view I long shared. But now I think the sound bite is haunting us, much as simple political slogans (such as 'Read my lips') come to haunt the politicians who uttered them. It is time to think the problem of drug policy beyond 'harm reduction' – before we are caught regretting we ever said it.

References

Cohen, S. (1985). *Visions of Social Control: Crime, Punishment and Class-ification*. Cambridge: Polity Press.

Dance, P. and Mugford, S.K.(1992). The St Oswald's Day celebrations: 'Carnival' versus 'sobriety' in an Australian drug enthusiast group. *Journal of Drug Issues*, 22, 591–606.

Hackler, J. (1991). The reduction of violent crime through economic equality for women. *Journal of Family Violence*, 6, 199–216.

Kreitman, N. (1986). The preventive paradox. *British Journal of Addiction*, **81**, 353–363.

Ledermann, S. (1956). *Alcool, Alcoolisme, Alcolisation*, vol. 1. Paris: Presses Universitaires de France.

MacIntyre, A. (1981). *After Virtue: A Study in Moral Theory*. Notre Dame, IN: University of Notre Dame Press.

Marx, K. (1976) *Capital: A Critique of Political Economy*, vol. 1. (Introduced by Ernest Mandel, translated by Ben Fowkes.) London: Penguin Books in association with New Left Books.

Mugford, S.K. (1991a). Drug policy and harm reduction:Towards a unified policy for legal and illegal drugs. In T. Carne, L. Drew, J. Mathews, S.K. Mugford and A. Wodak (Eds), *An Unwinnable War: The Politics of Drug Decriminalisation*, pp. 33–50. Sydney: Pluto Press.

Mugford, S.K. (1991b). Drug legalization and the 'Goldilocks' problem: Thinking about the costs and control of drugs. In M.B. Krause and E.P.Lazear (Eds), *Searching for Alternatives: Drug Control Policy in the United States*, pp. 33–50. Stanford: Hoover Institution Press.

Mugford, S.K. (1992). Crime and the partial legalisation of heroin: Comments and caveats. *Australian and New Zealand Journal of Criminology*, **25**, 27–40.

O'Malley, P.T. and Mugford, S.K. (1991a). The demand for intoxicating commodities: Implications for the 'War on Drugs'. *Social Justice: A Journal of Crime, Conflict and World Order*, **18**, 49–75.

O'Malley, P.T. and Mugford, S.K. (1991b). Moral technology: The political agenda of random drug testing. *Social Justice: A Journal of Crime, Conflict and World Order*, **18**, 122–146.

O'Malley, P.T. and Mugford, S.K. (1993). Crime, excitement and modernity. In G Barak (Ed.), *Varieties of Criminology*, in press. New York: Praeger.

Rose, N. (1988). *Governing the Soul: The Shaping of the Private Self*. London: Routledge.

Simmel, G. (1978). *The Philosophy of Money*. (Translated by Tom Bottomore and David Frisby.) London: Routledge and Kegan Paul.

Skog, O. (1980). Social interaction and the distribution of alcohol consumption. *Journal of Drug Issues*, **10**, 71–92.

Tan, E.S., Lemmens, P.H.H.M. and Koning, A.J. (1990). Regularity in alcohol distributions: Implications for the collective nature of drinking behaviour. *British Journal of Addiction*, **85**, 745–750.

Toulmin, S. (1990). *Cosmopolis: The Hidden Agenda of Modernity*. New York: Free Press/Macmillan.

Turner, B.S. (1986). Simmel, rationalisation and the sociology of money. *Sociological Review*, **38**, 93–114.

Weatherburn, D. (1992). Crime and the partial legalisation of heroin. *Australian and New Zealand Journal of Criminology*, **25**, 11–26.

Chapter 3
Progressive Legalizers, Progressive Prohibitionists and the Reduction of Drug-related Harm*

ETHAN A. NADELMANN

To legalize or not to legalize? That, as two pairs of drug policy sceptics have recently written, is not really the right question (Zimring and Hawkins, 1992; Kleiman and Saiger, 1990). The appropriate question is much broader, and it is one that incorporates the 'legalize or not' question with respect to particular psychoactive drug products: what, simply stated, are the best means to regulate the production, distribution and consumption of the great variety of psychoactive substances available today and in the foreseeable future? For a variety of reasons, the efforts of myself and others to answer that highly complex question have been captured by the label of 'legalization'. The term itself proved immensely successful in drawing the attention of tens of millions in the United States and elsewhere to what was at once a radical sounding but quite sensible critique of drug prohibition policies. However, it exacted a stiff price with its implication that the only alternative to current policies was something resembling contemporary alcohol and tobacco control policies. Few of those publicly associated with 'legalization' in fact advocated such an alternative, but this wrong impression has stuck in the public mind.

The fact of the matter is that 'legalization' has always meant different things to different people (Wisotsky, 1986; Hamowy, 1987; Trebach, 1987; Nadelmann, 1988a,b, 1989; Boaz, 1990; Ostrowski, 1990; Trebach and Zeese, 1990a,b, 1991; Miller, 1991; Krauss and Lazear, 1991). From my perspective, it has been first and foremost a critique of drug prohibitionist policies that stresses the extent to which most of what people commonly identify as part and parcel of 'the drug problem' are in fact the results of those policies. The widespread failure to perceive the extent and content of this causal relationship, and to distinguish between the problems that stem from the misuse of drugs *per se* and those that stem from drug prohibitionist policies, remains the single greatest obstacle to any significant change in drug prohibition

*Portions of this chapter appear in slightly revised form in Nadelmann (1992).

policies around the world. The recognition of this causal relationship does not, it should be stressed, lead automatically to a public policy recommendation that all of drug prohibition should be abandoned. But it does suggest that alternative policies less dependent upon prohibitionist methods are likely to prove more effective.

'Legalization' also implies a set of policy objectives at odds with governments' frequently proclaimed objectives of fighting a 'war against drugs' and creating a 'drug-free society'. Any drug control strategy, I and others have argued, should seek to minimize both the negative consequences of drug use and the negative consequences of the policies themselves. This is as true of public policies with respect to alcohol, tobacco and caffeine as it is of policies directed at limiting the misuse of cannabis, cocaine, amphetamine, opiates, hallucinogens and all other drugs. It is imperative, for instance, that any drug control policy distinguishs between casual drug use that results in little or no harm to anyone, drug misuse that causes harm primarily to the consumer, and drug misuse that results in palpable harm to others – and then focuses primarily on the last of these, secondarily on preventing the misuse of drugs, and little if at all on casual drug use. It is also imperative that any drug control policy be assessed not only in terms of its success in reducing drug abuse but also in terms of its direct and indirect costs.

Implicit in the 'legalization' critique of US and foreign drug control policies are in fact two different types of arguments. At one level, it points out the ways in which drug prohibition *per se* is responsible for many drug-related problems. By criminalizing the production, distribution and use of particular drugs, drug prohibition fundamentally transforms the nature of the drug markets, the ways in which people consume drugs, the lenses through which much of society views 'the drug problem', and the range of policies deemed appropriate for dealing with drug abuse. On another level, however, the critique advances a far more modest claim, which is that there are better and worse types of drug prohibition, with the Dutch 'harm reduction' approach epitomizing the former and the American 'war on drugs' the latter. Indeed, for many of those characterized as advocates of drug legalization, the Dutch model offers an alternative that is preferable not only to current US policies but also to the extreme libertarian model. The ideal set of drug control policies, from this perspective, can be found somewhere between the Dutch example and the libertarian model.

Harm Reduction and Legalization

The 'harm reduction' (or 'harm minimization') approach emerged in the Netherlands and the UK during the 1970s and early 1980s, although previous manifestations date back decades (Velleman and Rigby, 1990;

Berridge, Chapter 5, this volume). It has since become increasingly influential both in those countries, and in other parts of Europe and Australia, as public health and other officials have recognized the need for more innovative and less punitive policies to stem the transmission of the HIV virus by, and among, illicit drug users (Strang and Stimson, 1990; O'Hare et al., 1992). 'Harm reduction' policies seek to reduce the harms that result from illicit drug use. Rather than attempt to wean all illicit drug addicts off drugs by punitive means, 'harm reduction' policies begin with the acknowledgement that some users cannot be persuaded to quit and then seek to reduce the likelihood that they will contract or spread diseases such as hepatitis and AIDS, 'overdose' on drugs of unknown purity and potency, or otherwise harm themselves or others. Proponents of 'harm reduction' policies typically favor an assortment of drug treatment programs including methadone and other maintenance programs. They insist on the need for needle exchange programs; they recommend public health and community outreach efforts to maintain contact between health service providers and illicit drug users; and they demand that drug policies acknowledge, both in law and policy, the human rights of drug users. Also implicit in most 'harm reduction' approaches is the notion of 'normalization', which posits that the harms associated with illicit drug use are best minimized by integrating drug users into normal society rather than isolating them in separate clinics, programs, markets and neighborhoods (Van de Wijngaart, 1988).

The relationship between the 'harm reduction' approach and the notion of drug legalization remains ambiguous. Some proponents of 'harm reduction' vigorously oppose any broader trend toward disassembling the drug prohibition system (Dorn, 1992; Pearson, 1992; Strang, Chapter 1, this volume). They are quick to point out that much of the opposition they have encountered stems from fears and perceptions that the 'harm reduction' approach represents no more than a stepping stone to legalization. Others insist that this approach taken to its logical and sensible conclusion would more closely resemble a legal regulatory regime than the current prohibition system. Any harm reduction strategy, they argue, must seek to reduce not just the harms to users but also the many other negative consequences of drug prohibition: the violence that attends illicit drug markets; the corruption of public officials; the *de facto* subsidy of organized crime; the incarceration of hundreds of thousands of people; the deprivation of individual liberties; and so on. All agree, however, that modest efforts to reduce the negative consequences of *status quo* policies are better than no efforts whatsoever.

Given the substantial intellectual, ideological and institutional overlap between 'legalization' and 'harm reduction', little can be gained by attempting to tease out their differences. Indeed, such is the diversity of opinion among self-described 'legalizers', and among self-described advocates of 'harm reduction', that any distinctions based upon these two terms would amount to little more than crude caricatures. The more useful distinction, I suggest below, is between pro-legalization advocates of harm reduction and anti-legalization advocates of harm reduction – or what I refer to respectively as progressive legalizers and progressive prohibitionists.

Before developing this distinction, however, it is important to acknowledge the political, strategic and semantic components of the tensions and alliances between 'legalization' and 'harm reduction'. The advantage of 'harm reduction' or 'harm minimization' as a slogan or policy label is obvious. Who, in their right mind, could oppose the notion of reducing harm? It is easily embraced by government officials and others who favor less emphasis on criminal justice policies and more emphasis on public health approaches, and not readily disavowed even by those who prefer more punitive drug control methods. It is sufficiently vague that people with very different ideas about drug policy feel comfortable embracing it as their label. And it conveys a sense of British or Dutch 'sensibility' that can prove irresistible to those who view the ideological excesses of drug war rhetoric with a sceptical eye. Given its rhetorical advantages, the principal challenge confronted by opponents of punitive policies lies in promoting their definitions of 'harm reduction' in the public, political and policy arenas.

The ascendancy of the language of 'harm reduction' within Europe and Australia contrasts markedly with the failure of the same language to take hold in the United States of America. The closest analogy in the USA is the language of public health, with its emphasis on drug treatment. However, whereas most interpretations of 'harm reduction' begin with the acknowledgement that some people cannot be persuaded to abstain from drugs, most public health formulations emphasize notions of disease, contagion and curative abstinence. Absent as well from the American context is the association of human rights and illicit drug use. The discourse of rights in the United States is almost entirely bound up with the Constitution, which has provided the central reference point for all assertions and rejections of individual rights since the nation's origins. Most Americans instantly associate 'human rights' with foreign policy, and violations of human rights with the abuses of foreign governments against their citizens. Organizations that promote the civil rights of homosexuals have made some progress in recent years with their claims that discrimination against them is not just a constitutional issue but also a matter of human right, but illicit drug users can claim no progress in this regard. In Europe, by contrast, references to the 'human rights of drug users' can be heard with increasing frequency.

What distinguishes the American debate over drug policy from debates elsewhere is the dominating influence of 'legalization' as both a buzz word and a radical alternative to current drug control policies. The reasons for this are many. In an arena of public policy powerfully shaped by media sensationalism and political rhetoric, both the idea and the language of 'legalization' have proved to be immensely appealing to media interests. 'Should Drugs Be Made Legal?' surely provided a much more enticing, and profitable, cover story for *Time* magazine in mid-1988 than would have 'Reducing Drug-Related Harm' (*Time*, May 30, 1988). Legalization as a principle also appeals to both the powerful libertarian strain in right-wing American politics and the more general national confidence in free market forces. William Buckley, Milton Friedman and George Shultz – to name the most prominent Republicans who have publicly declared themselves favorably disposed to drug legalization – are listened to and respected by millions of Americans on the right of the political spectrum. For many Americans tired of complex problems and yearning for simple solutions, the prospect of 'legalization' appears to offer a quick and simple solution. Unlike most Europeans, Americans share a collective national consciousness of a prior drug prohibition (from 1920 to 1933) as well as its conspicuous failure and repeal. And whereas most Europeans do not identify drug-related violence as a central dimension of the drug problem, most Americans (and, for that matter, Colombians) are accustomed to drawing a very strong connection between illicit drugs and violence. This is a problem for which legalization, but not 'harm reduction' as it is conventionally defined, offers a clear solution.

The advantages of 'drug legalization' over 'harm reduction' as a critique of the 'war on drugs' are thus twofold. From a rhetorical perspective, it provides the sort of sensational and radical language required to attract the attention of the American media. And from an analytical perspective, it focuses attentions not just on the excesses of the 'war on drugs' but also on the ways in which drug prohibition *per se* is responsible for drug-related crime and many other drug-related problems. Its disadvantages, however, are substantial. Both rhetorically and politically, it suggests an all-or-nothing choice between the 'war on drugs' and a policy of making everything from marijuana to crack cocaine available like beer and cigarettes. Critics of the 'war on drugs' in search of arguments and proposals for more humane, sensible and politically feasible approaches to the drug problem find the implications of the legalization critique of the drug war too tough to digest either politically or pragmatically. And proponents of the 'war on drugs' see legalization as a useful tag with which to label and hence dismiss even modest 'harm reduction' initiatives such as needle exchange programs.

Opponents of the 'war on drugs' in the USA now face the challenge of injecting the language of 'harm reduction' into popular American discourse on drug policy. The principal obstacle, apart from the rhetorical weakness of the phrase in the American context, is the intense moralism that characterizes both debates and policies regarding illicit drugs in the USA. 'Harm reduction' offers a language that is wonderfully neutral, but also vulnerable to debasement by those who continue to favor repressive measures for dealing with drug abuse. The even greater challenge thus involves promoting the ideas and ideals that underlie 'harm reduction' – in particular those that emphasize the inevitability and ineradicability of drug use, the recognition that abstinence is not the only solution to drug abuse, and the notion that 'drug users are people too'.

Legalizers, Prohibitionists and the Common Ground

Notwithstanding the diversity of opinions associated with the notion of 'harm reduction', one can well divide its proponents into two groups: the progressive legalizers and the progressive prohibitionists. Both generally agree that drug prohibition *per se* is responsible for much of what people commonly identify as part and parcel of the drug problem. Both agree on the need to assess drug policy options in terms of their costs and benefits, and both tend to believe that the optimal drug policy is one that minimizes both the negative consequences of drug use and the negative consequences of drug control policies. The progressive prohibitionists largely acknowledge that casual drug use is not a problem in and of itself, and the legalizers grant that some policies designed to reduce overall levels of drug use may be effective in reducing the overall negative consequences of use. There is a shared recognition that many dimensions of the 'war on drugs' represent a form of overkill, that more modest criminal justice measures can accomplish the same objectives as successfully as the harsher measures, and that a more vigorous adherence to public health precepts and objectives will result in a superior mix of drug control policies. Both further agree that a dramatic expansion in the availability of drugs in society will likely increase the cumulative consumption of drugs. And both agree that it is important to draw distinctions among different drugs, and among different formulations of the same drugs, in designing drug control policies. Stated otherwise, few in either camp believe that marijuana, or coca tea, should be treated the same as crack cocaine.

This common ground, it should be stressed, is fundamentally at odds with the views expressed by the more conservative and reactionary prohibitionists. Articulated most vigorously by President Bush's first 'drug tsar', William Bennett, this perspective has demonstrated no interest whatsoever in analyses of costs and benefits, nor in the need to minimize the negative consequences of drug control policies. Casual use of illicit drugs has been depicted as an immoral form of activity as well as a dangerous source of contagion requiring the treatment of users (Office of National Drug Control Policy, 1989, p. 11). Social science research and public health precepts are of value only insofar as they conform with their ideologically based assumptions and policies. There is, in short, no room for dispassionate dialogue concerning any policy alternatives that do not appear 'tougher' than what has been tried before (Zimring and Hawkins, 1992, pp. 4–21). Combining a penchant for punitive sanctions with a view of drug use best described as 'pharmacological Calvinism' (Klerman, 1972), the reactionary prohibitionists have insisted that the only legitimate objective of drug control policy must be the elimination of illicit drug use.

The common ground is also at odds, albeit not quite so fundamentally, with the 'conservative' libertarian perspective on drug control (Boaz, 1990; Friedman, 1991; Szasz, 1992). For those libertarians who believe as an absolute matter of principle in the sanctity of individual sovereignty over property and the freedom of contract, no governmental controls on the commerce in drugs are acceptable no matter what the consequences. Other libertarians are more utilitarian in their thinking insofar as they place their faith in the magic of the free market and assume that the dual policy objectives would best be accomplished in the absence of governmental interventions. Less committed libertarians start from the same assumptions about the magic of the free market but acknowledge that modest governmental controls, in particular truth-in-advertising and labeling requirements, may be necessary to correct for the excesses and abuses that the free market invites. All of these libertarians tend to support as well the more civil libertarian commitments to individual privacy and freedom in the choice of one's lifestyle, although they insist that freedom of contract includes the freedom of employers to insist upon drug testing as a condition of employment. Civil libertarians, by contrast, tend to regard the freedom of contract with less deference than the right to privacy. They are more apt to speak of a right to consume drugs (Richards, 1982). And they are far more likely to integrate considerations of social justice and public health into their principles and policy calculations.

Putting aside the perspectives of the reactionary prohibitionists and the hardcore libertarians, the principal differences among the progressive legalizers and the progressive prohibitionists are of two sorts. The more obvious difference reflects disagreements as to the weight that should be accorded values such as individual liberty, privacy and tolerance in calculating the costs and benefits of different drug control policies (Bakalar and Grinspoon, 1984; Macklin, 1984; Murray, Gaylin and Macklin, 1984; Husak, 1992). Most legalizers weight these values heavily, with the more committed civil libertarians regarding them as absolutes that cannot be compromised and other progressive legalizers perceiving them as highly important but not inherently immune to some restraints. At the very least, most legalizers insist, the possession of modest amounts of drugs for personal consumption should not be the subject of criminal laws. The progressive prohibitionists are sympathetic to such values but accord them much less weight, both because they perceive them as undermining efforts to reduce drug abuse and because they are more willing to defer to majority opinion in defining and weighting them. Confronted with potential trade-offs between levels of drug abuse and levels of coercion directed at drug users and sellers, most legalizers are willing to concede modest increases in drug abuse levels in return for reductions in the numbers of those punished for using and selling drugs. Progressive prohibitionists, by contrast, are far more willing to limit individual liberty to the extent they perceive a potential gain in public health.

The two perspectives also diverge in their assessments of the vulnerability of modern societies to the substantial increases in drug availability that would follow from any of the more far reaching drug legalization schemes. Most prohibitionists can envision the possibility of a fifty-fold increase in the number of people dependent upon cocaine, and conclude that the future of the nation might well be at stake if cocaine were made as available as alcohol. As John Kaplan wrote in 1988, 'It is true that if the number of those dependent upon cocaine merely doubled, we would arguably be well ahead of the game, considering the large costs imposed by treating those users as criminals. But what if there were a fifty-fold increase in the number of those dependent on cocaine? We simply cannot guarantee that such a situation would not come to pass; since we cannot do so, it is the height of irresponsibility to advocate risking the future of the nation' (Kaplan, 1988). Avram Goldstein and Harold Kalant assert more confidently: 'There is no reason to doubt that the increased costs to society [of drug legalization] would rival those now attributable to alcohol' (Goldstein and Kalant, 1990). Most legalizers, by contrast, regard such estimates and predictions as the unsubstantiated folly of doom-sayers. Both legalizers and progressive prohibitionists agree that substantial research is required to better estimate this vulnerability, but the wide disparities are, I suspect, primarily a reflection of visceral fears, beliefs and instincts regarding individual and collective human nature in the context of their societies. Whereas most legalizers perceive, both instinctually and intellectually, ample evidence of a fundamental societal resilience, most progressive prohibitionists share with their more reactionary allies a fundamental pessimism regarding the susceptibility of their societies to a dramatic liberalization of drug availability.

The roots of this viscerally based debate can be found in a related difference of opinions regarding the balance of power between psychoactive drugs and the human will. Prohibitionists typically see the balance favoring the former, with its potential to disrupt and destroy the lives of consumers. Legalizers, by contrast, emphasize the latter, with its assumption that the balance of basic human desires in most people effectively limits the destructive potential of drugs. For most prohibitionists, the relevant evidence includes the worst case examples of drug addiction and other abuse, the experiments on captive rats, monkeys and other non-human animals to determine the addictive liability of different drugs, and the biological evidence of withdrawal symptoms in human beings following sustained consumption of particular drugs. Most legalizers, by contrast, focus on the less dramatic but more abundant evidence of casual and controlled drug use, insist that the 'set and setting' of drug use are at least as important as the drug itself in determining whether a person becomes a drug abuser, and see the animal studies and biological evidence as less significant than the abundant historical, cross-cultural and contemporaneous evidence of individual and societal resilience *vis-à-vis* all psychoactive drugs. ('Set is a person's expectations of what a drug will do to him, considered in the context of his whole personality. Setting is the environment, both physical and social, in which a drug is taken' (Weil, 1972; Zinberg, 1984). Many prohibitionists seem to see some psychoactive drugs as possessed of powers akin to those of the Sirens whose alluring voices no man could resist. Most legalizers, by contrast, perceive such a notion as absurd. They find more persuasive the substantial evidence that most people (including children), given sufficient information, are unlikely to use a drug in the first place, that most of those who do try a particular drug tend either to stop shortly thereafter or to use it in moderation, and that even most of those who become addicted to a drug or otherwise misuse it ultimately moderate or stop their use.

These viscerally based differences, however, still leave abundant room for common ground on how drug control policies can be reformed in the short term. For even though the progressive prohibitionists share with their more reactionary allies a deep seated fear of greater drug availability, they lack the reactionaries' political and moral commitments to repressive policies. And even though most legalizers feel substantial revulsion for the more punitive prohibitionist measures, they recognize both the inevitability of, and the need for, some criminal justice accompaniments to any regulatory regime. The public health model, with its emphasis on reducing morbidity and mortality, appears to provide something of an ideologically neutral set of guidelines and parameters for working out a preferable set of drug policies, although 'legalizers' are wary of the totalitarian potential of a public health model taken to its logical extreme. 'Harm reduction' thus provides both a language and models for directing the joint efforts of progressive legalizers and prohibitionists.

There is also a shared assumption, from which only the most libertarian of the legalizers dissent, that government does have an important role to play in shaping and improving the lives of its citizens. Where all sides differ is in their view of the appropriate means by which government should pursue this role, with the progressive prohibitionists viewing criminal justice and other coercive mechanisms as perfectly acceptable and often efficient means and the progressive legalizers favoring less coercive measures ranging from education and voluntary treatment programs to broader provision of social services. There also is something of a consensus that the top priority of drug control programs should be to minimize the harm that drug users do to others, with the secondary priority involving the more traditional public health objectives of minimizing the harm that drug users, and especially children, do to themselves. But underlying even this consensus are differing assumptions regarding the appropriate reach of social control measures designed to detect and curtail the illicit use of drugs. Thus even among those who identify themselves as proponents of a 'public health' approach to the drug problem, there are some who sympathize deeply with the legalizers but prefer to keep their more ideological, liberty-based values out of their analyses, and others who see criminal justice sanctions and civil commitment laws as useful means with which to coerce drug users into treatment programs (Gostin, 1991).

The fact that legalizers and progressive prohibitionists have so much in common is significant for a number of reasons. First, it suggests that there is a basic framework of analysis, predicated upon systematic assessment of costs and benefits, that is regarded as intellectually legitimate by all serious analysts of drug control policy. The fact that evaluation of costs and benefits varies greatly depending upon one's ethical values and ideological assumptions does not negate this. Second, it suggests that the current framework and direction of drug prohibition policies in the United States and those countries that have followed closely in its footsteps is fundamentally at odds with any conceivable policy predicated upon either public health precepts or notions of 'harm reduction'. Indeed, the only way to explain and justify many current policies is by reference to the fears, prejudices and primitive moralisms of those who have transformed drug control policy into a modern version of an authoritarian crusade. Third, it suggests that the debates *among* the legalizers over the design and evaluation of alternative drug control policies may well be of interest to many who share neither all of the legalizers' values nor their visceral confidences.

References

Bakalar, J. B. and Grinspoon L. (1984). *Drug Control in a Free Society*. New York: Cambridge University Press.

Boaz, (1990). The consequences of prohibition. In Boaz, (Ed.). *The Crisis in Drug Prohibition*, pp. 1–8. Washington, DC: CATO Institute.

Dorn, N. (1992). Clarifying policy options on drug trafficking: Harm minimization is distinct from legalization. In P. O'Hare, R. Newcombe, A. Matthews, E. C. Buning and E. Drucker (Eds). *The Reduction of Drug Related Harm*, pp. 108–121. London: Routledge.

Friedman, M. (1991). Speech to the Fifth International Conference on Drug Policy Reform, Washington, DC.

Goldstein, A. and Kalant H. (1990). Drug policy: Striking the right balance. *Science*, 249, 1513–1521.

Gostin, L.O. (1991). Compulsory treatment for drug-dependent persons: Justifications for a Public Health approach to drug dependency. *Milbank Quarterly*, 69 , 561–593.

Hamowy, R., (Ed.). (1987). *Dealing with Drugs: Consequences of Government Control*. Lexington, MA: Lexington Books.

Husak, D. (1992). *Drugs and Rights*. New York: Cambridge University Press.

Kaplan, J. (1988). Taking drugs seriously. *The Public Interest*, 92, 32–50.

Kleiman, M. A. R. and Saiger, A. J. (1990). Drug legalization: The importance of asking the right question. *Hofstra Law Review*, 18, 527–566.

Klerman, G. L. (1972). Psychotropic hedonism vs. Pharmacological calvinism. *Hastings Center Report*, 2, 1–3.

Krauss, M. B. and Lazear, E. P. (Eds) (1991). *Searching for Alternatives: Drug-control Policy in the United States*. Stanford,California: Hoover Institution Press.

Macklin, R. (1984). Drugs, models, and moral principles. In T.H. Murray, W. Gaylin and R. Macklin (Eds), *Feeling Good and Doing Better: Ethics and Nontherapeutic Drug Use*, pp. 187–213. Clifton, NJ: Humana Press.

Miller, R. L. (1991). *The Case for Legalizing Drugs*. New York: Praeger.

Murray, T. H., Gaylin, W. and Macklin, R. (Eds). (1984). *Feeling Good and Doing Better: Ethics and Nontherapeutic Drug Use*. Clifton, NJ: Humana Press.

Nadelmann, E. A. (1988a). US drug policy: A bad export. *Foreign Policy*, 70, 1–39.

Nadelmann, E. A. (1988b). The case for legalization. *The Public Interest*, 9, 3–31.

Nadelmann, E. A. (1989). Drug prohibition in the United States: Costs, consequences and alternatives. *Science*, 245, 939–947.

Nadelmann, E. A. (1992). Thinking seriously about alternatives to drug prohibition. *Daedalus*, 121, 85–132.

Office of National Drug Control Policy, Executive Office of the President (1989). *National Drug Control Strategy*. Washington, DC: US Government Printing Office.

O'Hare, P., Newcombe, R., Matthews, A., Buning, E. C. and Drucker, E. (Eds). (1992). *The Reduction of Drug Related Harm*. London: Routledge.

Ostrowski, J. (1990). The moral and practical case for drug legalization. *Hofstra Law Review*, 18, 607–702.

Pearson, G. (1992), Drugs and criminal justice: A harm reduction perspective. In P. O'Hare, R. Newcombe, A. Matthews, E. C. Buning and E. Drucker (Eds). *The Reduction of Drug Related Harm*, pp.15–29. London: Routledge.

Richards, D. A. J. (1982). *Sex, Drugs, Death, and the Law: An Essay on Human Rights and Overcriminalization*, pp. 157–214. Totowa, New Jersey: Rowman and Littlefield.

Strang, J. and Stimson, G. V. (Eds) (1990). *AIDS and Drug Misuse: The Challenge for Policy and Practice in the 1990s*. New York: Routledge.

Szasz, T. (1992). *Our Right to Drugs: The Case for a Free Market*. New York: Praeger.

Trebach, A. S. (1987). *The Great Drug War*. New York: Macmillan.

Trebach, A. S. and Zeese, K. B. (Eds) (1990a). *Drug Prohibition and the Conscience of Nations*. Washington, DC: Drug Policy Foundation.

Trebach, A. S. and Zeese, K. B. (Eds) (1990b). *The Great Issues of Drug Policy*. Washington, DC: Drug Policy Foundation.

Trebach, A. S. and Zeese, K. B. (Eds) (1991). *New Frontiers in Drug Policy*. Washington, DC: Drug Policy Foundation.

Van de Wijngaart, G. F. (1988). A social history of drug use in the Netherlands: Policy outcomes and implications. *Journal of Drug Issues*, **18**, 481–495.

Velleman, R. and Rigby, J. (1990). Harm-minimisation: Old wine in new bottles? *International Journal on Drug Policy*, **1**, 24–27.

Weil, A. (1972, revised edition 1986). *The Natural Mind: An Investigation of Drugs and the Higher Consciousness*, p.29. Boston: Houghton Mifflin.

Wisotsky, S. (1986). *Breaking the Impasse in the War on Drugs*. Westport, Connecticut: Greenwood Press.

Zimring, F. E. and Hawkins, G. (1992). *The Search for Rational Drug Control*, pp.82–110. New York: Cambridge University Press.

Zinberg, N. E. (1984). *Drug, Set, and Setting: The Basis for Controlled Intoxicant Use*. New Haven, Connecticut: Yale University Press.

Part II
Perspectives on Harm Reduction

Chapter 4
Reduction of Alcohol- and Drug-related Harm in Australia: A Goverment Minister's Perspective

PETER STAPLES

The spread of HIV infection into the general community through the drug injecting population provided the impetus for many nations to re-assess their drug policies and consider harm reduction. Australia was no exception. Although the reduction of drug-related harm was initially identified with the problems of HIV/AIDS and illicit drugs, particularly injected illicit drugs, there are many other aspects to the reduction of drug-related harm and a particular need to increase the emphasis on legal drugs. In the 1980s, the Australian Government began for the first time to consider ways to reduce the harm caused by *all* drugs.

Drugs such as tobacco and alcohol have been estimated conserva-tively to cost the Australian community in the vicinity of A$13 billion in 1988 (Collins and Lapsley, 1991). In comparison, illicit drugs were esti-mated to cost at least A$1.4 billion. These estimates, based on research by senior economists commissioned by the Commonwealth Department of Health, Housing and Community Services, included costs incurred in the treatment of drug-related illness, accidents result-ing from drug use and misuse, property crime and damage, and law enforcement measures. While this research did acknowledge the diffi-culty of assessing all of the costs of illicit drug use and misuse, it has helped me to have a clearer picture than we otherwise would of the costs attributable to illicit drugs.

The health, social and economic adverse consequences of drug use in Australia are substantial but there are grounds for some optimism. For instance, the proportion of males who smoke has fallen from 72% in 1945 to 30% in 1989. The proportion of females who smoke rose from 26% in 1945 to 31% in 1980 and then declined to 27% in 1989. Despite these trends approximately 19 000 people die annually in Australia as a consequence of tobacco consumption, representing 72% of all drug-related deaths and 15% of deaths from all causes. It is horri-fying to think that this is actually more than the number of members of the Australian Armed Forces who died annually in each of the two World Wars! However, population-adjusted, tobacco-related deaths declined in Australia 6% between 1981 and 1990 (Department of Community Services and Health, 1992).

The problems of illicit drug use and abuse, which fall heavily on our youth, are a source of national concern in Australia notwithstanding the magnitude of problems associated with legal drugs. The Australian Government is wholeheartedly committed to reducing the harm associated with the use of illicit drugs as part of our overall objective of attempting to reduce the economic, social and personal costs associated with the use and abuse of all drugs. This requires a degree of objectivity and balance when dealing with drug issues.

As good international citizens, Australia wishes to contribute to international efforts, and especially to developing nations, in formulating policies to reduce the harm associated with drugs. All nations need to find the correct policy mix when dealing with drug problems. It would be presumptuous of developed nations to try to impose their own policy prescriptions on others. Nevertheless, many of the experiences of developed nations may provide insights and practical solutions to the problems faced by developing nations.

The term 'harm reduction' is open to a variety of interpretations. Since its inception in 1985, Australia's National Campaign Against Drug Abuse (NCADA) has specified that its underlying aim was 'to minimise the harmful effects of drugs on Australian Society' (Department of Health, 1985). Although some may consider this aim represents a 'soft option' in dealing with drugs, the Australian Government does not. The Australian Government does not condone the use and misuse of drugs and firmly believes that a harm-reduction approach is realistic. We do not consider that a drug-free society is an achievable goal. Furthermore, the Australian Government believes that our efforts will bear fruit in the long term and engender in our society a responsible attitude to drugs.

The implementation of drug policy in Australia is based on an administrative arrangement between the Commonwealth, six State and two Territory governments. Several major institutions have been created to formulate, implement and monitor policy. The National Campaign Against Drug Abuse is a cooperative arrangement between the Federal, State and Territory governments. A Ministerial Council on Drug Strategy (MCDS), comprising health and law enforcement ministers, oversees the National Campaign. This arrangement helps to provide a co-ordinated and relatively uniform approach to the implementation of drug-related policies and programmes in Australia. Australia has aimed, and we believe achieved, a balanced approach to drugs and a policy mix that recognises the need to maintain supply reduction strategies while adopting demand reduction strategies tailored to our national and regional conditions.

Over A$250 million has been spent on NCADA during the last six years by Commonwealth, State and Territory Governments on a range of approaches to minimise the harm resulting from drugs. This has involved police, customs and health professionals working together to establish, maintain or monitor a variety of activities including education and treatment programmes, media and public information programmes, research programmes and control and enforcement measures. Australia has been party to and actively supports international treaties to curtail the trade in illicit drugs, including the *Single Convention on Narcotic Drugs* (1961: amended 1972) and the *United Nations Convention Against Illicit Drug Traffic in Narcotic Drugs and Psychotrophic Substances* (1988).

Essentially, Australia's approach to drug-related problems is both comprehensive and multi-disciplinary. It is based on the prevention and reduction of demand for illicit drugs, the control of supply, action against illicit trafficking, and treatment and rehabilitation of drug users. The underlying philosophy and aims of the National Campaign have remained largely intact over the last six years. During this time, of course, the world has witnessed the spread of HIV/AIDS. Australia, like many nations, responded to the threat of the spread of HIV/AIDS by re-assessing drug policies and services. The potential for rapid spread of HIV infection as a result of injecting drug use is widely recognised. This reassessment in Australia, however, did not result in a major change in direction. Rather, it reaffirmed the general approach to drug policy described above.

As discussed, harm reduction as an issue has only come to the fore since the advent of AIDS, although harm-reduction approaches to drug problems have a long history and even predate the AIDS epidemic. The importance of HIV/AIDS is that it represents a major risk to public health and therefore requires an immediate and high priority response. There is now unfortunately ample evidence from a number of other countries that HIV/AIDS represents a major threat to the health of injecting drug users. In some southern European countries, injecting drug users represent about two thirds of all AIDS cases. HIV infection is now also very common in drug users in parts of the United States of America. To date, however, Australia has been remarkably successful in preventing the spread of HIV infection among injecting drug users. The harm minimisation approach has been exemplified by the early and widespread establishment of needle and syringe exchange schemes in nearly all states and territories in this country.

Community organisations have been involved in the development and delivery of educational interventions which target drug users. These measures have contributed to the high levels of awareness among injecting drug users of the need to avoid sharing injecting equipment and the importance of cleaning equipment when this is shared. In adopting this strategy, the Australian Government is emphatic that it does not condone the use of illegal drugs. This response recognises that for many dependent drug users abstinence is not an achievable goal, especially in the short term.

Australia actively supports demand reduction strategies for both licit and illicit drugs. At the international level, Australia has been a strong advocate of the increased emphasis that the international community is now starting to place on education and treatment strategies aimed at reducing the demand for drugs. The Federal, State and Territory Governments have implemented numerous programmes aimed at reducing the harm associated with drug use and misuse. These have been described in detail elsewhere (Ministerial Council on Drug Strategy, 1992).

Education is a very important component of the comprehensive strategy to reduce the harm associated with drugs in Australia. 'The Drug Offensive', which is the media arm of the National Campaign Against Drug Abuse, has begun to alter the perceptions Australians have about drugs. For instance, in 1989, 28% of young people saw alcohol consumption as the most important issue facing teenagers compared to 20% the previous year. In a study commissioned by the Drug Offensive, parents rated 'drinking too much alcohol' as the most important issue facing young Australians.

Education is seen as a vital means of dissuading people from taking up drugs as well as challenging them to take responsibility for their behaviour in relation to drugs. The Australian Government recognises that prevention is a very important means of minimising the harm associated with drugs. On the other hand, for those already suffering the ill effects of drug misuse, the National Campaign Against Drug Abuse has supported a variety of treatment and rehabilitation programmes implemented by the States and Territories. These have included, for example, greatly expanded methadone programmes, development of hospital-based services, significant expansion of networks of community and outreach workers, and development of telephone information and referral services. Methadone treatment programmes have undergone increasing diversification and expansion in recent years, with patient numbers increasing from around 2000 in 1985 to about 10 000 by the end of 1991. Methadone treatment is recognised internationally as an appropriate treatment for opioid dependence. The benefits of providing methadone include giving 'breathing space' to dependent heroin users to get their lives in order without the difficulties and dangers of having to obtain and use illicit heroin, reducing involvement in crime, and allowing for greater employment opportunities.

Treatment and rehabilitation services in Australia have been extensively evaluated since 1985. Alcohol and drug treatment services are being directed in favour of the new public health model, with increased emphasis on early and brief interventions relevant to individuals with low level problems and the training of generalist workers. More specialist interventions, however, are considered to be necessary for those with more severe problems.

The Australian Government plans to continue this commitment to harm reduction and has devised a number of new projects. Research recently commissioned determined that community support exists for using the concept of a 'standard drink' to enable members of the community to assess their own alcohol consumption. However, independent research conducted for the Federal Office of Road Safety indicated that the ability of members of the community to measure their own alcohol consumption accurately is limited. Therefore it has been decided to conduct a campaign to educate the community about standard drinks. The Australian Government also plans to educate people about how to use alcohol responsibly, drawing on the understanding that has already been gained for the 'standard drink' through this advertising campaign.

Amphetamine usage has caused considerable concern in recent years due to a sharp increase in amphetamine-related deaths. Hospital admissions, drug seizures and research undertaken to ascertain usage showed a significant increase in recreational and experimental use by young people aged 18–25 years. A proposed national amphetamines campaign aims to reduce the harm associated with amphetamine use and is specifically targeted at this age group to generate and reinforce negative attitudes towards the use of amphetamines, reinforce the intention amongst non-users not to try amphetamines, and to generate and reinforce among novice and moderate users an intention to modify their use of amphetamines.

The Australian Government draws much encouragement from the 8% reduction in population-adjusted deaths due to all drugs between 1981 and 1990 (Department of Community Services and Health, 1992). This includes a 17% reduction for alcohol and a 6% decrease for tobacco. An 85% decrease in deaths due to barbituates was balanced by a 170% increase for deaths due to opiates and 46% for deaths from other illicit drugs. Although most of these trends are in the right direction, the health, social and economic costs of alcohol and other drugs in Australia remain at unacceptably high levels.

References

Collins, D.J. and Lapsley, H.M. (1991). *Estimating the Economic Cost of Drug Abuse in Australia*. Canberra: Department of Community Services and Health.

Department of Community Services and Health (1992). *Statistical Update no. 18.* Canberra: Department of Community Services and Health, Drugs of Dependence Branch.

Department of Health (1985). *National Campaign Against Drug Abuse: Campaign Document Issued Following the Special Premiers' Conference, Canberra, 2 April 1985*. Canberra: Australian Government Printing Service.

Ministerial Council on Drug Strategy (1992). *No Quick Fix: An Evaluation of the National Campaign Against Drug Abuse*. Canberra: Ministerial Council on Drug Strategy.

Chapter 5
Harm Minimisation and Public Health: An Historical Perspective

VIRGINIA BERRIDGE

The advent of AIDS appears to have brought some radical changes in drug policy in Western Europe, in Australia, and in Britain above all. The general view has been established that the danger of the spread of AIDS from drug users into the general population is a greater threat to health than the danger of drug use itself. The words and concepts of harm minimisation and harm reduction are on everyone's lips. For Britain, some commentators have argued that AIDS has changed the direction of drug policy. Fox, Day and Klein (1989), for example, in a cross-national study of AIDS policies in Sweden, Britain and the US:

> The only instance of AIDS overriding established policy objectives has been in the field of drugs... The government had abandoned its previous stance of augmenting its restrictive and punitive policies on drugs now that AIDS had come to be seen as the greater danger.

Others have been more cautious. Gerry Stimson, for example:

> These new ideas appear as a distinct break with earlier ones, but as with many conceptual and practical changes, the possibilities are inherent in earlier ideas and work. It is perhaps a matter of emphasis and direction, rather than any abrupt rupture with the recent past.
>
> *(Stimson, 1990)*

But in general, AIDS has been seen as bringing a kind of new dawn, the 'new public health' approach to drug policy, an integration of drugs into the mainstream of health policy. The decision to expand the needle and syringe exchanges in the UK was, according to one senior civil servant of 'fundamental importance'. This was a new departure for drug policy.

Was this indeed the case? Using British drug policy (on which most attention has focused) as the example, this chapter will focus on two questions, both relating to the 'newness' of drug policy post-AIDS. Firstly, how far has drug policy been radically changed under the impact of AIDS? How far has AIDS been simply a vehicle whereby developments in existing policy have been achieved more quickly than otherwise might have been possible? And, from a longer term perspective, how much is really new at all? How far do recent changes merely exemplify some very long-standing themes and tensions within drug policy?

Let us start with a historical analogy, the impact of war on social policy. Historians have in recent years begun to look more closely at the impact of the Second World War on social and health policy in particular (Webster, 1988). They have questioned the view that war was the only catalyst for radical change, in the British case, the coming of the National Health Service. The wartime national consensus for social change appears to have been less than unanimous; the roots of the NHS can be found not just in wartime change, but in pre-war debates and blueprints for health care. What war did was to enable this to happen more quickly and in rather a different fashion than might otherwise have been the case. War served to overcome vested interests and opposition to change, but essential continuities with the pre-war service remained.

AIDS too, fits into this paradigm. Like war, it evoked a period of political emergency reaction which, in Britain, was at its peak from 1986 to 1987, and which, in the case of drugs, spilled over into 1988 with the government reaction to the Part One report of the Advisory Council on the Misuse of Drugs (ACMD) on *AIDS and Drug Use*. There was the creation of an emergency Cabinet committee on AIDS chaired by the Deputy Prime Minister, William Whitelaw; the 'AIDS week' on television in February 1987 when both television companies joined with government to broadcast programmes on the wartime model; and the Commons emergency debate in November 1986. Many of the actions of central government in this period had a wartime flavour.

The 'Pre-history' of AIDS and Drug Policy

As I have argued elsewhere, the impact of AIDS across a whole range of policy areas cannot be understood unless we understand something of their 'pre-history' (Berridge, 1992). What was happening in genito-urinary medicine, for example, or in health education, prior to AIDS? We can only assess the impact of the disease within that type of framework. Let us look at the immediate pre-history of drug policy. Here it is clear that harm-minimisation was by no means a new policy objective.

Throughout the 1980s there was a growing belief in some circles that this was a more realistic aim than more rigid and medically-based ideas of 'treatment' and 'cure' or 'abstinence'. The concept received its best known public expression in the 1984 ACMD Report on *Prevention* which abandoned the traditional division into primary, secondary and tertiary prevention in favour of two basic criteria: (1) reducing the risk of an individual engaging in drug misuse; (2) reducing the harm associated with drug misuse (DHSS, 1984). Such ideas were commonplace, too, in the increasingly important voluntary sector of drug services. They were accompanied by a tendency, at both a practical and a theoretical level, to downplay the 'medical model' of addiction as a disease requiring specialist treatment. The change in definitions received official sanction in the 1982 ACMD report on *Treatment and Rehabilitation* which declared:

> Most authorities from a range of disciplines would agree that not all individuals with drug problems suffer from a disease of drug dependence...There is no evidence of any uniform personality characteristic or type of person who becomes either an addict or an individual with drug problems.
>
> *(DHSS, 1982)*

Accompanying this change in definitions was an emphasis on a multidisciplinary approach, based on regional and district drug problem teams and local drug advisory committees.

What the early and mid 1980s saw, too, was a distinct 'policy community' forming which held these ideas. There was a shift from the previous primarily medical community to one that was more broadly based, comprising revisionist doctors involved in drug services, researchers, service workers and leaders in the drug voluntary sector, and, most crucially, civil servants with similar objectives within the Department of Health. The change can be characterised through the membership of the Advisory Council on the Misuse of Drugs, the main British expert advisory body on drug policy. In the 1980s it recruited, to a mainly medical membership, representatives of the voluntary agencies, of health education, social science research, the probation service and general practice. This new policy community adhered to the conclusions of the *Treatment and Rehabilitation* report. There were differences over questions of implementation and practice, but one policy objective, that of minimisation of harm from drug use, found general support. However, this remained difficult to enunciate publicly in relation to drug use. It lacked political acceptability. When, in 1981, the Institute for the Study of Drug Dependence published a pamphlet advocating harm minimisation techniques for glue sniffing there was a public and political outcry.

There was a yawning gap between the 'political' and 'policy community' view of drugs. This was because 1980s drug policy, pre-AIDS, had a dual face – a 'political' penal policy with a high public and mass media profile, and an 'in-house' health policy based on a rhetoric of de-medicalisation, the development of community services and harm minimisation. AIDS, like war and the NHS, gave this latter strand of policy political feasibility. A policy that previously could be advanced only slowly, as the unspoken other side of penal policy, 'came out' as a result of AIDS. As a senior medical officer commented:

> AIDS may be the trigger that brings care for drug users into the mainstream for the first time ever...The drug world can come 'in from the cold' through AIDS...it's a golden opportunity to get it right for the first time.*

Research by social scientists was an important legitimating factor – in itself a telling comment on the power of the new policy community and the complex relationship between research and policy in the drugs area. But so, too, was the willingness of Conservative politicians to push for change. It was Norman Fowler (overall minister at the DHSS) and his advocacy of needle exchange which won the crucial battle at the political level. What was in-house policy became a priority for politicians, too. This approach was by no means unanimous within Conservative ranks. Sir Bernard Braine, a long time spokesman on drug policy, commented:

> If dirty, reused needles and syringes are the principal means of spreading infection among drug users, would not a freer supply result in the means of infection being more widely available than is now the case? Is this not the equivalent of trying to control an epidemic of smallpox by issuing vials of smallpox to the population at large?
>
> *(Hansard, 1986)*

However, it was a liberal consensual approach that was established. It was harm minimisation and safe sex approaches that were established, not prohibition or social segregation. One senior Conservative politician saw drug policy post-AIDS as 'increased controlled availability at home and stronger prohibition round the edges'† Pragmatism was the order of the day. The policy impact of AIDS at this level raises some fascinating questions about the reality of the supposed New Right Thatcher revolution in government and stresses the continuity of policy traditions rather than change.

Harm Reduction as a Long-term Trend in Drug Policy

We also need to look further back than the 1980s, for I wish to argue that the reduction of harm broadly defined has been a consistent theme in drug policy in Britain even before that decade. To support my case, I will look at two other periods of 'war time crisis' and policy change in the twentieth century. These are the debates surrounding

---

* DHSS senior medical officer speaking at a conference in June 1989.
† Conservative politician, comment at private meeting, 1989.

drug control in the 1920s; and the emergency response to the drug
epidemic of the 1960s. In the 1920s, a hard line emergency response to
drug use was at its height in the post-war period. Although the numbers of addicts were at their lowest ever level, the Home Office,
inspired by American example, and by its new responsibility for drug
control under the 1920 Dangerous Drugs Act, saw the solution as prohibition, as stamping out addiction via the courts and a penal response.
The story of how the medical profession defended its role and the disease concept of addiction via the Rolleston Committee of 1924–1926
has often been told (Berridge, 1984). From our point of view, what is
significant is the principle enunciated in the 1926 report, justifying the
legitimacy of maintenance prescribing.

> When, therefore, every effort possible in the circumstances has been made, and
> made unsuccessfully, to bring the patient to a condition in which he is indepen-
> dent of the drug, it may...become justifiable in certain cases to order regularly
> the minimum dose which has been found necessary, either in order to avoid
> serious withdrawal symptoms, or to keep the patient in a condition in which he
> can lead a useful life.
>
> *(Rolleston Report, 1926)*

This was a framework in which the minimisation of harm to the individual drug user was paramount, albeit also as a means of allowing the
addict to lead a 'useful', that is economically productive life.

This was a variant of the health and human capital arguments which
were common in the nineteenth century. The public health rationale
for improving the health of the population invariably had an economic
justification. In the 1960s, my other example of the durability of harm
minimisation as a concept in drug policy, the arguments encompassed
this societal dimension more directly. As in the 1980s, the 'epidemic', in
this case of drug addiction itself, led to the language both of infectious
disease, of public health and of national crisis. The 1965 Brain Report
saw addiction as a 'socially infectious condition', a disease which, 'if
allowed to spread unchecked, will become a menace to the community'. The responses of notification and compulsory treatment (the latter
subsequently dropped) were classic public health ones. The rationale
of the clinics was one of harm minimisation; but, as in the 1980s, of the
minimisation of harm to society as much as to the individual drug user.
Clinic doctors had to prescribe opiates to undercut the black market,
but not so much that the market was supplied and new addicts created.
Max Glatt, a psychiatrist who was involved in the debates round the
establishment of the clinics, recalled:

> Most of us were very averse to prescribe what we thought were killer drugs. But
> in the end when we were asked to man the new addiction centres, the argu-
> ments were that if we didn't prescribe, the black market would take over. The
> aim was to take the prescribing of narcotics out of the hands of private and gen-

eral practitioners and put it into the hands of NHS doctors at specially licensed clinics. Whilst one hated what one was doing, one would participate, as it seemed the lesser evil. But it's quite wrong to say (as people do nowadays) that we thought at the time this was the *treatment* for drug addiction. It was just a kind of first aid...

(Glatt, 1991)

Treatment was of minor importance to the minimisation of social harm.

Nineteenth-century Harm Reduction

If one looks even further back, into the nineteenth century, one can see that both formal and informal controls on drugs were justified on this basis. The debates around the need for increased formal control of the sale of opiate drugs in the nineteenth century owed much to the professional aspirations both of doctors and of pharmacists; for the latter, exclusive control of opium suited both professional and economic strategies. But professional control was also justified on the public health grounds of an end to child doping, to opiate overdoses, and the abuses of adulteration and unrestricted sale. The form of control was set at a level which balanced both the needs of the pharmacists' trade and a realistic assessment of what individual consumers needed in order to function. Spencer Walpole, Home Secretary at the time of the debates around the various Poisons Bills of the 1850s and 1860s, summed this position up: 'If you put a difficulty in the way of giving it in small quantities to persons who desire it, you may interfere inconveniently with these requirements as well as with the trade of the chemist' (Hansard, 1859). One technique suggested was that by Professor Alfred Taylor who advised that consumers needing regular doses of opium be issued with a six month certificate which they could use to obtain supplies from chemists in the neighbourhood (Taylor, 1857).

Developing professional control was at one level predicated on a recognition of the need to maintain a balance. As Dr C.R. Francis commented in 1882, on the case of a friend who was a stable addict and led a productive life:

Yielding to the popular prejudice against opium eating, Mr A has repeatedly endeavoured to break it off... Doubtless he would succeed in time, as others have, but *cui bono*? He enjoys excellent health, is able to do a good day's work (mental as well as physical) and is entirely free from a variety of minor troubles having a nervous origin which used to annoy him before he began the opium.

(Francis, 1882)

At the level of informal lay controls, too, which operated in tandem with, and some times in opposition to, the formal professional structures, there was a realistic assessment of the balance of harm. Dr Rayleigh Vicars, struggling to treat a patient in Lincolnshire, found his attempts at treatment hampered by the patient's family and friends, who, convinced that withdrawal was doing more harm than good, good naturedly lent their own stores of laudanum (Rayleigh Vicars, 1893)

Harm Minimisation and the Tensions within Drug Policy

Clearly, then, the reduction or minimisation of harm is not without its history – both immediate and long-term – in drug policy. But to say that, as an historian, is also to be guilty of what some historians would call 'Whiggishness', others 'presentism'. What do I mean by this? I mean plucking historical examples out of the past to prove a particular contemporary case, seeing the past 'through the wrong end of the telescope', by emphasising only those issues which concern us at the moment. In the final section of this chapter, I will try to redeem myself slightly by drawing attention to some more complex tensions in drug policy and how these relate to the issue of harm reduction. So far I have talked about present and past harm minimisation approaches as if they were almost timeless. But any good historian knows that the essence of historical analysis is a sensitivity to particular time bound structures and concepts, interpreting the past on its own terms, not on ours. Ideas of harm minimisation have had their place amid a plethora of conflicting, sometimes interconnecting forces. The classic overarching paradigm in many analyses has been the conflict between penal and medical forms of control. Even on its own, this is too simplistic an approach, as I will argue below. In addition, there are, and have been conflicts between different forms of medical control, between individual curative and community focused approaches, the latter encompassed in the concept of public health. But even that concept itself has not been an unchanging absolute. Public health conjures up a vision of the nineteenth-century battles against disease and poor living conditions, but that environmentalist concern narrowed under the impact of the bacteriological revolution which assigned specific medical causes for disease. Social hygiene, with its emphasis on individual responsibility for health, was the reformulated public health of the early part of this century. The 'new public health' of the 1970s and 1980s with its emphasis on individual lifestyle and prevention has to some degree revived those earlier concerns, although there are also strong efforts to broaden the public health paradigm to encompass questions of inequality and social structure.

'Public health' thus contains within itself the seeds of an individually focused medical approach. The balance of forces between types of approach can alter over time. In the nineteenth-century, the 'public health' focus on child doping or working class industrial opiate use was stimulated by the urban crisis of industrialisation; it gave place to individually focused medical theories of addiction and disease. In the 1960s, Brain's justification of change on public health grounds of the control of potentially epidemic disease shifted imperceptibly in the 1970s into an individually focused, abstinence oriented treatment approach. There has always been an implicit tension in drug policy between preventive and curative approaches, and in other areas of health policy as well.

The tension between penal and medical approaches is also more complex that the simple positing of opposites would make it appear. Let us look as some historical examples of this. The nineteenth-century advocates of inebriety as a disease saw treatment as the more humane alternative to prison, but what they argued for was compulsory incarceration in inebriate asylums, a prison under medical rather than penal control. Likewise in the 1920s, the Rolleston Report's defence of liberal humanitarianism in drug treatment applied only to those middle class addicts whom doctors were likely to treat. Chlorodyne, as a working class tipple, was not even included in the terms of reference to start with; and opiate use in prisons was accorded a distinctly harsher response by the medical experts – compulsory treatment and 'cold turkey' were both appropriate. Most important of all, Rolleston did not mark some autonomous medical 'victory'. Maintenance prescribing operated within a system of domestic and international control, in which the perspectives of the Home Office, the justice ministry, were predominant. How that balance of forces operated could easily alter over time.

AIDS and its aftermath in British drug policy have displayed these tensions in all their complexity. While nominally 'normalising' drug use via harm minimisation, in some respects it appears to have brought a revival of medical involvement, both in practical terms and in conceptualisation of the issue. It has brought doctors back more centrally through the emphasis on prescribing as an option, the focus on the role of the general practitioner and the new emphasis on the general health of drug users. Clinic doctors have begun to be interested in issues such as hepatitis B, although previously these hardly figured in clinic work. The need to attract drug users not normally in contact with services, sanctioned by a range of official reports, has served to elevate the notion of treatment, which has resumed its place as an unchallengeable good. AIDS served to revive other medical arguments around treatment. Prescribing methadone as a 'bait' to attract users into services and hence away from syringe sharing reproduced the arguments of the 1960s, when prescribing was the option to attract addicts and to prevent harm to society. The old 'competitive prescribing' argument revived via AIDS. Increasingly, too, voluntary (non-medical) and statutory (medical) services were being brought into closer relationships and the differences between them blurred, a process hastened by the NHS reforms and which owed much to more general trends in health policy. So far as the power relationships in policy making went, the situation exemplified the long-standing policy influence of the medical profession. Both doctor civil servants and medical expert advisers were of key importance. Without the support of influential and centrally placed doctors, the 'new departures' in policy could not have been sustained. To sum up, then, the 'non-medical' rhetoric of policy post-AIDS disguised some clear tendencies towards sustained or even increased medical input in terms of treatment and services, and revived some earlier medically focused arguments. Whether this can be seen as de- or re-medicalisation depends on perspective.

We can also link these developments to the other set of tensions I mentioned – between individual and community focused interpretations of health. For the 'public health' paradigm of post-AIDS policy as applied to drugs contained within it a strong focus on the individual. The emphasis on health education for individuals, on the drug user as a 'normal' person responsible for her or his own actions, epitomised key elements of the 'new public health'. As with past public health responses, the potential for a shift to an individualistic medical response is present. The conceptual distance is, on present definitions, not a large one.

The conceptual differences between penal and medical approaches have also blurred under the impact of AIDS. The potential impact of HIV among overcrowded prison populations has been the impetus behind the introduction of harm reduction into the probation service, of treatment into prisons, and of penal aspects into the treatment and rehabilitation response. The Prison Medical Service is becoming the Prison Health Service; but offenders can now also be 'sentenced' (via pre-trial diversion) into treatment (Bild, 1992). An historically minded observer could point to the examples of the inebriates acts, to Brain's advocacy of compulsory treatment in the face of epidemic spread of addiction. Timothy Harding has commented that HIV has emphasised the health aspects of the penal response; but it has also emphasised the punitive aspects of the medical.

It would be an unwise historian who attempted to predict what the long term balance of policy might be. History, the underlying theme in this chapter, was absent from the initial policy debates around AIDS and drug use, despite the long tradition of 'using history' to support particular lines in drug policy. However, this time, the achievement of established policy objectives was better served by emphasis on these aims as new ones and their lack of connection with the drug policy past. As this chapter has attempted to show, many aspects of policy change did draw on distinct pre-AIDS continuities. War and crisis – our initial analogy – does indeed lead to change, but long standing themes also reassert themselves. The complex historical tensions within drug policy have been clearly displayed in the wake of AIDS. Whatever the future of that policy, it will not escape from its history.

References

Berridge, V. (1984). Drugs and social policy: The establishment of drug control in Britain, 1900–30. *British Journal of Addiction*, 79, 17–29.

Berridge, V. (1992). The early years of AIDS in the UK 1981–86: Historical perspectives. In P. Slack and T. Ranger (Eds), *Epidemics and Ideas*. Oxford: Oxford University Press.

Bild, M. (1992). Probation, harm reduction and drug services. *Druglink*, 7, 10–12.

DHSS (1982). *Treatment and Rehabilitation: Report of the Advisory Council on the Misuse of Drugs*. London: HMSO.

DHSS (1984). *Prevention: Report of the Advisory Council on the Misuse of Drugs*. London: HMSO.

DHSS (1988) *AIDs and Drug Use, Part I: Report of the Advisory Council on the Misuse of Drugs*. London: HMSO.

Fox, D.M., Day, P. and Klein, R. (1989). The power of professionalism: AIDS in Britain, Sweden and the United States. *Daedalus*, 118, 93–112.

Francis, C. R. (1882). On the value and use of opium. *Medical Times and Gazette*, 1, 87–89, 116–117.

Glatt, M. (1991). Interview in G. Edwards (Ed.), *Addictions: Personal Influences and Scientific Movements*. New Brunswick: Transaction.

Hansard (1859). *Parliamentary Debates*, 3rd Series 152 col. 209.

Hansard (1986). *Parliamentary Debates*, 93 cols. 599–66.

Rayleigh Vicars, G. (1893). Laudanum drinking in Lincolnshire. *St George's Hospital Gazette*, 1, 24–26.

Rolleston Report (1926). *Report of the Departmental Committee on Morphine and Heroin Addiction*. London: HMSO.

Stimson, G. (1990). AIDS and HIV: The challenge for British drug services. *British Journal of Addiction*, 85, 329–339.

Taylor, A. (1857). *Evidence to the Select Committee of the House of Lords on the Sale of Poisons etc. Bill*. Parliamentary Papers XII.

Webster, C. (1988). *The Health Services Since the War. Vol.I: Problems of Health Care. The National Health Service before 1957*. London: HMSO.

Chapter 6
Achieving a Reduction in Drug-related Harm through Education

JULIAN COHEN

In recent years the UK, like many other countries, has experienced an increase in illicit drug use among young people. Despite this trend very little research has been devoted to examining patterns of use amongst the younger age range. The evidence available is mainly from relatively small scale local research. In my own work area, Tameside in Greater Manchester, we conducted a survey of 15-year-olds in 1988 (Cohen, 1989). We found that almost one third of respondents said they had used an illicit drug or solvents and that 10% were regular users, most commonly of cannabis. These results were similar to those obtained from other surveys elsewhere in the UK (Newcombe and O'Hare, 1987; Diamond, 1988; Parker, Bakx, and Newcombe, 1988; Swadi, 1988). Since 1988 smaller scale surveys and anecdotal evidence in Tameside have indicated that:

1. There has been an increase in the number of young people experimenting with and regularly using illicit drugs.
2. A broader range of substances are available to young people. In particular there has been an increase in the use of cannabis, amphetamine and LSD and the introduction of Ecstasy.
3. The average age of first use is falling.

Colleagues elsewhere in the UK report similar trends such that in some areas and groups illicit drug use is replacing the use of alcohol as a central recreational activity. Research has shown that numbers using and frequency of use increases in the post-16 age range (ISDD, 1990) and that growing drug use amongst young people is a long term phenomenon spanning the 1960s to the late 1980s (Wright and Pearl, 1990). The indications are that this trend will continue into the 1990s.

The Response to Young People's Drug Use: Primary Prevention

As in other Western countries, the main UK response to increasing levels of illicit drug use among young people has been the development of school and mass media programmes based on primary prevention, or in the new parlance 'demand reduction'. The message has been 'Say no to drugs' and abstinence has been regarded as the only legitimate goal.

Primary prevention drugs education has developed over the years. A number of different approaches can be identified:

1. The shock/scare approach as exemplified in films like 'Better Dead', the talk by the ex-junky emphasising the horrors of drug use or the UK government TV and billboard campaigns against drugs.
2. The information approach whereby young people are given the 'facts' about drugs (and especially the dangers) on the assumption that they will decide not to use drugs if they know the 'facts'.
3. The attitudes/values approach whereby the attempt is made to develop 'personal responsibility' and 'strong moral beliefs' and the attractions of a 'drug-free lifestyle' are emphasised.
4. Teaching refusal skills whereby young people are regarded as easy prey to peer pressure to use drugs and in need of developing the skills to 'Say no'.
5. Teaching decision-making skills – a more sophisticated version of 4, in which talk of drugs is not so upfront and it is assumed that young people lack the generic skills to make rational decisions and that if they learn these skills they will decide not to use drugs.
6. Alternative highs whereby the attempt is made to replace the highs and excitement of drug use with other forms of risk taking, such as pot-holing, absailing, etc., on the assumption that young people will then not need drugs.
7. Enhancing self-esteem whereby the focus is on the individual person rather than drugs *per se*, on the assumption that it is only, or mainly, young people with low self-esteem who use drugs.
8. Peer education whereby if young people will not listen to adults telling them not to use drugs, it is assumed they might listen to people of a similar age to themselves giving the same message.

The above list is roughly chronological. As one approach has been deemed ineffective, inappropriate or even counter-productive, a new way of selling the anti-drugs message has been dreamt up. Peer education is the most recent fashion in primary prevention drugs education in the UK. However, the old approaches, and especially the shock/scare approach, are still alive and well. In the most recent moral panic over young people's drug use, we are currently witnessing more shock/scare media campaigns, theatre productions in schools based on fear arousal and a resurgence of police involvement in school-based drugs education. In the drugs education world old habits die hard!

The Critique of Primary Prevention

The first point to emphasise is very simple but one that many people refuse to accept despite the evidence. Primary prevention does not work. A host of evaluative studies have shown that all kinds of primary prevention education programmes and media campaigns have failed to prevent or reduce illicit drug use amongst young people (Kinder, Pape and Walfish, 1980; Schaps et al., 1981; Sheppard, 1985; Bagnall and Plant, 1987; De Haes, 1987; Coggans et al.,1990; Dorn and Murji, 1992). Some studies have even concluded that shock/scare and information approaches can glamorise and encourage drug use amongst young people (De Haes and Shuurman, 1975; Schaps et al., 1981). At the macro level, the Western world has devoted huge resources to primary prevention programmes whilst, at the same time, drug use has increased amongst young people. A critical analysis of primary prevention suggests that it is based on untenable assumptions about young people's drug use and that it will continue to be ineffective in whatever form it takes.

Primary prevention assumes that young people's drug use is abnormal, even pathological, behaviour and that young people who use drugs must somehow be lacking in knowledge, skills or self-esteem. The fact that drug use is functional, often has immediate benefits and is mostly experienced as pleasurable, with only a small minority experiencing significant problems, is ignored (Moore and Saunders, 1991). The widely held assumption that young drug users are personally or socially inadequate is not supported by the evidence (Segal et al., 1980; Bentler, 1987; Pearson, Gilman and McIver, 1987; Schedler and Block, 1990). Indeed, the most recent UK evaluation of the impact of drugs education on young people stressed that positive health practices and high self-esteem do not preclude the use of drugs and that peer leaders are often the first to experiment with drugs and try out new experiences (Coggans et al., 1991). Low-self esteem may be related to chaotic, problematic drug use but does not delineate between users and non-users *per se*.

Primary prevention is based on individualism and victim blaming (Wibberley and Whitelaw, 1990). It drives a wedge between 'users' and 'abstainers' and focuses on the need for individuals to resist 'peer pressure' to use drugs. Peer pressure is seen as a negative, threatening force despite the fact that peer groups are so important for, and usually experienced positively by, young people. As Glassner and Loughlin

(1987) emphasised, following their study of young drug users, 'peer pressure' is used as a way of negatively stereotyping young people and rarely used to provide explanations of adult behaviour.

Primary prevention inevitably paints a bleak picture of drug use to the extent that misleading assertions are often made, stereotypes are perpetuated and dangers are exaggerated. Sometimes this is deliberately the case – 'prophylactic lies' in the words of Trebach (1987). The reality of young people's drug use often contradicts the information and messages they are given in school or through the media. The result is that many young people do not trust such information sources and that dialogue between young people who use drugs, or are contemplating use, and adults is minimal. For example, in a survey carried out in my locality, 15-year-olds (just under a third of whom said they had used illicit drugs or solvents) were asked who they felt they would be able to approach if they, or a friend, had problems with drugs (Cohen, 1989). Only 41% said they could approach their parents, 33% a youth worker, 31% a teacher in their school, 22% their form teacher and 10% their headteacher. A danger of primary prevention is that it pushes drug use underground and results in 'deviancy amplification' – something the UK sociologist Jock Young warned against in his study of drug use as long ago as the early 1970s (Young, 1971). A further danger is that in not having anything of relevance to say to the ever-growing number of young people who choose to use drugs, primary prevention is itself contributing to drug-related harm.

Harm-reduction Drugs Education (HRDE)

In the wake of the ineffectiveness of primary prevention to address the realities of young people's drug use and alongside the development of a harm-reduction practice in the treatment field, especially around HIV and injecting drug use, a new harm-reduction approach to drugs education has been developed in the UK (Kay, 1986; Newcombe, 1987; Clements, Cohen and O'Hare, 1988). HRDE is distinct from, and an alternative to, primary prevention. In the words of Newcombe (1987), harm reduction is:

> A social policy which prioritizes the aim of decreasing the negative effects of drug use. Harm reduction is becoming the major alternative drugs policy to abstentionism, which prioritizes the aim of decreasing the prevalence or incidence of drug use. Harm reduction has its main roots in the scientific public health model, with deeper roots in humanitarianism and libertarianism. It therefore contrasts with abstentionism, which is rooted more in the punitive law enforcement model, and in medical and religious paternalism.

In contrast to primary prevention, HRDE views drug use as a normal part of adolescent behaviour. Experiencing new sensations and states of consciousness, experimenting and taking risks, as well as doing things adults tell you not to do, can all be important and positive aspects of growing up, defining identity and establishing independence. As with criminal activity in general, many young people moderate or give up use of illicit drugs once they become burdened with the social and economic constraints of adulthood and then take on more accepted licit drug-using practices. In the words of Glassner and Loughlin (1987) there is a move from being 'burnouts to straights'. Responding positively to adolescent drug use can be regarded as a holding operation in which the goal is to reduce the number and severity of casualties. As Davies and Coggans (1991) have recently written in their book on adolescent drug use: 'If we cannot persuade our drug users to stop immediately, we can at least keep them as healthy as possible until such time as they decide to do so'.

HRDE is secondary rather than primary prevention on the understanding that we cannot prevent drug use *per se* and that attempts to do so may be counterproductive. It is education about rather than against drugs (O'Hare, 1988). It is non-judgemental and neither condones or condemns drug use but accepts that it does, and will continue to, occur. As such it is consumer education. A key aim is to develop an open and honest dialogue with young people. A key principle is that the right of young people to make their own decisions regarding drug use is respected.

The benefits, as well as the risks, of drug use need to be considered within the context that use actually takes place. The effects, and potential risks, of drug use are dependent on drug, set and setting factors (Zinberg, 1984). What is taken, how, how much, how often, when, where, why, who with etc. are all important in determining outcomes. As Dorn (1987) has noted, it is particularly young novice drug users who are 'confused about how much to take, where to take it, how to handle the effects, how to think about the experience in retrospect, how to deal with other people's real or imagined reaction, and so on'. Young people in my locality experience some of the main harms from drug use as conflict with parents and authority, disturbing experiences and accidents whilst under the influence, ill-considered sexual activity whilst under the influence (including unwanted pregnancy and HIV transmission), getting a criminal record, and the danger of losing consciousness and overdose.

Reducing these potential harms involves manipulating drug, set and setting factors. These factors are influenced by social and economic policy but can also be affected by drug education. To be able to manipulate drug, set and setting factors young people need accurate information about different drugs and their properties and effects, reducing risks, the law and legal rights and where to get help if needed. (More recently, some drug agencies have woken up to the fact that their service provision has not met the needs of the younger drug users). They also need to develop a wide range of skills in assessment, communication, assertiveness, conflict resolution, decision making and safer use. Whilst information is crucial, it is of limited use unless young people have developed the skills with which to act upon it.

As well as making decisions about their own use, young people play a crucial role with regard to their peers by passing on information and tips, and looking out for and helping each other. Rather than encouraging young people to 'resist peer pressure' and perpetuating negative stereotypes, HRDE aims to foster 'positive peer support', debunk stereotypes, develop more accepting attitudes towards drug users and helping skills. These are not fancy theoretical ideas but have lifesaving practical application. It has been common in my locality for young people who use certain drugs chaotically to be stereotyped and rejected by their peers, increasing their isolation and placing them at greater risk. Even more alarming have been a number of instances where young people have panicked and run away when peers have lost consciousness. In some situations the ability to perform first aid would have saved lives.

The exact form HRDE takes in practice will depend on the local situation and individual and group needs. The 'educator' needs to know their group well, have established a trusting relationship with them and negotiate more detailed content and method with them. The teacher, lecturer or youth worker is thus a facilitator. HRDE encompasses the new developments in Personal, Social and Health Education, recognising the need for groupwork methods and integration of drugs education into the school, college or youth service curriculum (Clements et al., 1988).

It is important to emphasise that HRDE is appropriate to current users and non-users. Apart from the problems associated with targeting users (how do we know?, who chooses?, on what basis?, does it become a self-fulfilling prophecy?), we need to recognise that many current non-users may later go on to use and that non-users play an important role in understanding and supporting users.

Materials for Harm-reduction Drugs Education

Until recently all the major drugs education packages in the UK have been based on primary prevention. To remedy this situation, three UK drug education practitioners wrote *Taking Drugs Seriously* (Clements, Cohen and Kay, 1991). This package is designed to be used mainly in schools, colleges and youth projects with the 12 years plus age range. It contains guidance for the facilitator and groupwork exercises in eight main sections:

1. Facts about drugs – which gives accurate information and focuses on benefits as well as risks.
2. Personal drug use – in which risk-taking is examined in a non-judgemental manner.
3. Attitudes – in which stereotypes are challenged.
4 Harm reduction – in which drug, set and setting factors are highlighted.
5 The law and drugs – which looks at laws and rules, legal rights and handling conflict.
6. Giving and receiving help – which focuses on skills to help oneself and to help others.
7. Community action – which looks at responses to drug use in the locality and nationally.
8. Parents and Community Workshop – to help educate parents and other adults

An accompanying package, *Don't Panic – Responding to Incidents of Young People's Drug Use* (Cohen and Kay, 1992), has also been published. This is an information, individual learning and training package aimed at all professionals and establishments who work with young people. It encourages calm and considered responses to the increasing number of incidents of drug use coming to the attention of schools, colleges, youth clubs etc. This is an important part of HRDE because caring rather than punitive responses increase the likelihood that young people will seek help, if needed, at an early stage, and trust and open dialogue in the 'taught' curriculum are unlikely to develop if establishments over-react to actual incidents of use.

The Experience of Developing Harm-reduction Drugs Education in Schools and Youth Projects in Tameside

In Tameside the following development strategy has been adopted:

1. Training of teachers and youth workers.
2. Production and dissemination of curriculum materials, drugs information materials and guidance documents.
3. Support for staff regarding curriculum and pastoral matters.
4. Workshops for parents and school governors.

Although senior managers have been kept informed and participated in some parts of the programme, the main target groups have been teachers and youth workers who specialise in Personal, Social and Health Education (PSHE). Participation has been voluntary. All 11–16 schools and all youth projects have had some involvement but some have been much more involved than others. In particular, some schools have shown little interest in developing drugs education at all, let alone HRDE.

The strategy has been initiated at a time when there have been many changes in education, particularly in schools. Morale is very low amongst teachers and resources are often stretched to the limit. The introduction of the National Curriculum has often resulted in PSHE and drugs education becoming an even lower priority for schools. Local Management of Schools has increased competition between schools for students and reinforced concerns amongst some heads that giving drugs education, especially HRDE, a high profile will make parents think there is a drug problem in their school. Many teachers feel that HRDE will be seen as 'condoning' drug use and that they must make it clear to students that they 'condemn' it. The easy options are for schools to avoid drugs education altogether, stick to discussion of legal drugs or revert to high profile 'anti-drugs' events and punitive measures against students who are using drugs.

Despite the pressures on schools, some teachers have not taken the easy options and have been involved in a sometimes heated debate about HRDE. Some staff, particularly older and more senior teachers, have remained committed to primary prevention. Another group have been convinced of the arguments for HRDE but have not felt able to put it into practice in their schools. A third group have been enthusiastic and begun experimenting with HRDE in their teaching and pastoral work.

These pioneering teachers tend to have very good relationships with their students, be non-judgemental about drug use and be very confident in their role. To date they have worked in relatively covert ways. They have sometimes experienced problems with senior managers, including vetting of materials and in one case a directive to teach in an 'anti-drugs' manner. Some of the other issues they have highlighted include:

1. The facilitator needs to be very confident and skilful, especially as HRDE tends to increase personal disclosures about drug use and questioning of staff about their own use.
2. HRDE is difficult to integrate into short lessons. Important issues and discussions are too often prematurely curtailed.
3. Young people can be resistant to HRDE in that they expect 'anti-drugs' messages in school and do not trust teachers enough to talk openly.
4. Young people can also be resistant to HRDE because they have been inundated with drug stereotypes through the media etc. Even young people who use drugs may fail to connect their images and ideas about drug use with their own use. Drugs are seen as something

only other people use. Breaking down stereotypes is thus often a first step in HRDE.

5. Parental resistance is rare and too often used by teachers as a way of legitimising their own doubts. HRDE, with its focus on reducing harm, safety and helping others does not necessarily come across as being 'soft on drugs'. In workshops for parents and school governors HRDE has gained a lot of support.

6. Work by individual teachers is important but limited. To be really effective HRDE needs to become part of a whole school approach to PSHE.

In the youth service there is less of a power differential between staff and young people. It is more informal, attendance is voluntary and there is more open discussion of real life experiences, including drug use. Most of our youth workers have been convinced of the appropriateness of HRDE and senior management have supported it. A range of harm-reduction practice has been developed in youth clubs and through detached work, including one-to-one work, joint working with the Community Drugs Team with young injectors, use of harm-reduction leaflets and drugs education programmes with groups.

Whilst the development of HRDE has been smoother in the youth service, impact is limited by the fact that only a small percentage of young people use it. We have also found that there is a danger of over-keen staff foisting HRDE on groups who are not interested. Youth workers need to know their groups well and choose the right time, format and setting to develop HRDE. Some workers have been very successful at doing this. A number of projects have run *Taking Drugs Seriously* evening or weekend courses and been inundated with young people attending on a regular basis to the extent that there are waiting lists for future courses. In addition, some of our youth workers have begun developing HRDE in schools

Youth workers experience some of the same difficulties with HRDE as teachers but have fewer constraints. Their work has resulted in a lot more open discussion about drugs among young people in the area. One effect has been open use of drugs in front of staff. This has raised issues for detached workers in particular but also necessitated negotiating clear rules in a number of our youth centres.

In Tameside we have only begun to develop HRDE and some of the results are encouraging. Some young people have access to a relevant and useful educational experience that stands them in good stead for their current and future drug-using career. However, we have a long way to go and are currently considering a number of new initiatives including:

1. Further training and projects involving teachers and youth workers working together.

2. Direct involvement of young people in developing HRDE using peer education.
3. New teaching and information materials.
4. More work influencing senior managers and decision makers.
5. Revised and updated guidelines.
6. Whole school developments involving teachers, students, parents, governors and youth workers working together.
7. An evaluation project examining staff and young peoples' experiences of drugs education.

Conclusion

I have attempted to show in this chapter that an effective response to increased drug use among young people necessitates the development of a new harm-reduction drugs education practice. I have described the components of HRDE and attempts to introduce it in schools and youth projects in one locality. However, the future of HRDE needs to be considered in a wider context.

We need more resources devoted to the development of HRDE, more examples of practice within the education system, through the media and in more informal ways, and research into the outcomes. One would expect HRDE to be more successful in achieving its aims than primary prevention is in promoting abstinence because much smaller behaviour changes are involved that do not attempt to completely deny the potential benefits of drug use. However, proper evaluation is crucial. The issue also arises as to whether HRDE could increase experimentation while at the same time reducing harm, and whether this is an acceptable outcome (Newcombe, 1992). Harm reductionists should find this possibility acceptable although there is, as yet, no evidence that increased experimentation will result.

Whilst there are beginning to be more examples of HRDE, development is chronically under-resourced compared to primary prevention. In the UK there is currently a resurgence in primary prevention drugs education. This has included 20 new prevention projects funded through the Home Office, a national schools competition, touring theatre groups, a touring anti-drugs video extravaganza sponsored by Pepsi-Cola and a national 'Drugs Prevention Week'. The advocates of primary prevention hold the main purse strings and are very much committed to more of the same. They have us in a Catch 22. They want evidence that HRDE works and that it will not increase drug use before they agree to fund it. If only they applied the same criteria to their beloved primary prevention!

Harm reduction has almost become the norm in the drug treatment field in the UK but many people who will happily endorse harm reduction for adults become a bit nervous when it comes to applying the same principles to the younger age range. Too often drug workers steer clear of HRDE for young people and too often drugs education is side-lined at national and international gatherings of harm-reduction practitioners. This may have something to do with the ambivalent position of adolescents in our society and over-protective and patronising attitudes towards them. It may also have to do with fear that taking harm reduction into schools and youth projects and directly challenging primary prevention would threaten the progress that has been made in the treatment field.

Developing HRDE will take persistence and courage. To move forward and establish an effective practice to reduce drug-related harm amongst young people, educationalists and drug specialists need to work together at national and international levels.

References

Bagnall, G. and Plant, M. (1987). Education on drugs and alcohol: past disappointments and future challenges. *Health Education Research*, **2**, 417–422.

Bentler, P.M. (1987). Drug use and personality in adolescence and young adulthood. *Child Development*, **58**, 65–79.

Clements, I., Cohen, J. and Kay, J. (1991). *Taking Drugs Seriously: A Manual of Harm Reduction Education on Drugs*. Liverpool: Healthwise.

Clements, I., Cohen, J. and O'Hare, P. (1988). Beyond just say no. *Druglink*, *May/June*, 8–9

Coggans, N., Shewan, D., Henderson, M. and Davies, J.B. (1991). Could do better: An evaluation of drug education. *Druglink*, September/October, 14–15.

Coggans, N., Shewan, D., Henderson, M., Davies, J.D., and O'Hagan, F.J. (1990). *National Evaluation of Drug Education in Scotland: Final Report*. Edinburgh: Scottish Education Office.

Cohen, J. (1989). *Drug Use Amongst Young People in Tameside*. Tameside: MBC.

Cohen, J. and Kay, J. (1992). *Don't Panic: Responding to Incidents of Young People's Drug Use*. Liverpool: Healthwise.

Davies, J. and Coggans, N. (1991). *The Facts About Adolescent Drug Abuse*. London: Cassell.

De Haes, W. (1987). Looking for effective drug education programmes: Fifteen years exploration of the effects of different drug education programmes. *Health Education Research*, **2**, 433–450.

De Haes, W. and Schuurman, J. (1975). Results of an evaluation study on three drug education models. *International Journal of Health Education*, **18**, (suppl.).

Diamond, I. (1988). The incidence of drug and solvent misuse among southern English normal comprehensive school children. *Public Health*, **102**, 107–114.

Dorn, N. (1987). Minimisation of harm: A U-curve theory. *Druglink*, March/April, 14–15.

Dorn, N. and Murji, K. (1992). *Drug Prevention: A Review of the English Language Literature*. London: ISDD.

Glassner, B. and Loughlin, J. (1987). *Drugs in Adolescent Worlds*. London: Macmillan.

ISDD (1990). *Drug Misuse in Britain 1990: National Audit of Drug Misuse Statistics*, London: ISSD.

Kay, J.L. (1986). Prevention Charter. *Druglink*, July, 10–11.

Kinder, B.N., Pape, N.E. and Walfish, S. (1980). Drug and alcohol education programs: A review of outcome studies. *International Journal of the Addictions*, **15**, 1035–1054.

Moore, D. and Saunders, B. (1991). Youthful drug use and the prevention of problems. *International Journal of Drug Policy*, **2**, 29–33.

Newcombe, R. (1987). High time for harm reduction. *Druglink*, January/February, 10–11.

Newcombe, R. (1992). The reduction of drug-related harm: A conceptual framework for theory, practice and research. In P. O'Hare, R. Newcombe, A. Matthews, E. C. Buning and E. Drucker. (Eds), *The Reduction of Drug-related Harm*. London: Routledge.

Newcombe, R. and O'Hare, P. (1987). *A Survey of Drug Use Amongst Young People in South Sefton*. South Sefton Health Authority.

O'Hare, P. (1988). Drug education : A basis for reform. Paper presented at the International Conference on Drug Policy Reform, Maryland: USA.

Parker, H., Bakx, K. and Newcombe, R. (1988). *Living with Heroin*. Milton Keynes: Open University Books.

Pearson, G., Gilman, M. and McIver, S. (1987). *Young People and Heroin*. Aldershot: Gower.

Schaps, E., Di Bartolo, R., Moskowitz, J.M., Palley, C. and Chugrin, S. (1981). A review of 127 drug abuse prevention program evaluations. *Journal of Drug Issues*, **11**, 17–43.

Schedler, J. and Block, J. (1990). Adolescent drug use and psychological health: A longitudinal inquiry. *American Psychologist*, **45**, 612–630.

Segal, B, Huba, G.J. and Singer, J. L. (1980). *Drugs, Day Dreaming and Personality: A Study of College Youth*. New Jersey: Erlbaum.

Sheppard, M.A. (1985). Drug Education: Why we have so little impact. *Journal of Drug Education*, **15**, 1–5.

Swadi, H. (1988). Drug and substance use among 3333 London adolescents. *British Journal of Addiction*, **83**, 935–942.

Trebach, A. (1987). *The Great Drug War*. New York: Macmillan.

Wibberley, C. and Whitelaw, S. (1990). Health promotion, drugs and the moral high ground. *International Journal of Drug Policy*, **2**, 11–14.

Wright, J.D. and Pearl, L. (1990). Knowledge and experience of young people regarding drug abuse 1969–1989. *British Medical Journal*, **300**, 99–103.

Young, J. (1971). *The Drug Takers: The Social Meaning of Drug Use*. London: Paladin.

Zinberg, N. (1984). *Drug, Set and Setting: The Basis for Controlled Intoxicant Use*. New Haven: Yale University Press.

Chapter 7
Rituals of Regulation: Controlled and Uncontrolled Drug Use in Natural Settings

JEAN-PAUL G. GRUND, CHARLES D. KAPLAN and
MARTEN DE VRIES

Similar to other recreational behaviours (such as sports, eating, sex, watching television, gambling), drug use produces sensations of pleasure and the relief of painful and distressing states. These behaviours can potentially become the paramount source of sensation, overruling the significance of other aspects of life. When the 'pursuit of pleasure' contradicts established social norms, the behaviour patterns are labelled as deviant or abnormal (Becker, 1973).

However, while carrying specific risks, drug use also contains important cultural values. Therefore, the use of drugs, in itself, is not simply an expression of psychopathology or illness. On the contrary, drug use may also be an expression of normality. From a global historical perspective, drug use of some kind is a norm. Societies differ only in respect of which specific drugs are defined as acceptable. Furthermore, the capacity to experience the pleasurable effects of drug use is not limited to humans.

The psychopharmacologist, Ronald Siegel (1990) documented a wide range of cases in which a variety of species deliberately sought to change their behaviour by ingesting psychoactive substances. In the more complex human context, drug use fulfils important instrumental and symbolic functions, both for the individual and the social group. Most users display fairly well-regulated use patterns. A proportion of users, however, develop severe problems and lose control over drug-taking and other aspects of life. The factor of controlled and uncontrolled use and the variables that differentiate between uncontrolled and controlled users are, in our opinion, key issues for understanding the complex phenomenon of drug addiction. In this chapter, drug taking rituals are examined. When scientifically examining the concept of 'rituals of addiction behaviour', certain problems related to 'addiction' need to be addressed.

Despite efforts to formulate appropriate definitions and classifications of addiction over the last decades, a strong consensus on its nomenclature remains absent (Edwards, Arif and Hodgson, 1981). Moreover, the concept of addiction is generally presented as an isolated individual behaviour. This concept often does not acknowledge the impact of the 'central cultural conceptions of motivation and behaviour' that vary across cultures and affect drug-taking behaviour (Peele, 1985).

Furthermore, the addiction concept is often hampered by value judgements. Methodological limitations traceable to biased samples of addicts usually collected in treatment settings lead to problems of conceptual generalization. Behaviour that is dysfunctional or abnormal from the clinician's perspective can be highly functional from the drug user's perspective (Meier, 1981; Faupel, 1987). Law enforcement personnel and clinicians generally see drug users 'at their worst' (Fiddle, 1967). Studies of clinical populations usually tell us little about the everyday life motivations and behaviours of drug users. Conceptualisation about addiction becomes limited to the selected subpopulation who enter treatment. The resulting concepts apply less to people for whom drug use is only one aspect of their life and/or who do not seek treatment.

For these reasons it is necessary to look beyond the clinical presentation of drug use and study its variety of forms in the natural environment. Studying drug use in its larger socio-cultural context offers a significant opportunity to develop basic knowledge of the lifestyles, behaviours and interactions of drug users. Such knowledge is of practical value for policy, prevention and treatment.

Study, Theory and Methods

Within the subculture of heroin users, we examined the practical aspects and day-to-day management of drug use in the context of both solitary and social rituals. The key theoretical concept utilised to study the behaviours of daily, hard-drug users was 'ritualisation': 'For an event to be a ritual event it must prescribe a sequence of psychomotor acts and this prescribed psychomotor sequence must be invested with a special meaning for the person performing that sequence' (Agar, 1977).

Rituals play an essential role in formally and informally shaping and organising the experiences, behaviours and interactions of the human (and other animal) organisms. As has been extensively documented, both on an individual and a social level, rituals fulfil various meanings and functions dependent upon the participants' beliefs and the situation at hand (Goffman, 1967; Durkheim, 1971). Rituals can be strictly formal and sacred (e.g. a church ceremony) or informal and secular (e.g. greeting). They can be performed by individuals, (e.g. a prayer) or in groups (e.g. a wedding ceremony). Solitary ritual influences the consciousness (and often performance) of the individual, while social ritual impacts on the collective consciousness of the whole group (Wallace, 1966).

Rituals can furthermore have both instrumental and symbolic functions (Radcliffe-Brown, 1952). Drug use and ritual often have a common history. Drug use can be seen to play an important role in specific rituals, varying from the 'mass wine' or 'peyote button' in formal religious rituals to lighting a cigarette in an unfamiliar environment and the 'Thank God It's Friday' (TGIF) social drink. Drug use rituals have distinct symbolic meanings for the individual and formative functions in their social networks. They are necessary constituents of drug subcultures.

The principal research methodology of the project was ethnographic. A wide array of everyday life situations in the subcultures of heroin users was examined. The concept of ritualisation was operationalised in an 'observational protocol' which guided the participant observation at places where people buy and use drugs. The observations were supplemented by informal interviews. Trust, acceptance and credibility are prerequisites for such an approach. The cooperation and involvement of the drug-using community is a precondition for this kind of research. The inclusion of a 'community fieldworker' in the research team was especially valuable in the collection of the data and the analysis, and in preventing stereotypical or incomplete depictions of the drug using community. These methodologies have been extensively discussed elsewhere (Grund, Kaplan and Adriaans, 1991; Grund et al., 1991).

We would like to propose the term 'experimental comparative ethnography' for studies that incorporate these methods in logical research designs. Ethnography provides information, skills and experience required for working with informants or indigenous research 'collaborators'. Above all, ethnography can generate the theoretical framework and testable hypotheses for subsequent quantification. Thus, ethnography provides not only the eyes and ears of the research but also its thriving analytical power. Designs incorporating multiple research sites, sampling strategies and instruments that make sense to the people under study are included in this conception. 'Experimental' has a double meaning in our conceptualisation. One meaning refers to a design in which intervention groups are compared with controls as in other experimental sciences. The other meaning refers to experimentation with new methodologies that refine ethnographic techniques for intensive case-finding and description.

Methodological innovations such as 'experience sampling methodology' (de Vries et al., 1990; Kaplan et al., 1990; Kaplan, 1992), and randomised snowball sampling (Kaplan, Korf and Sterk, 1987) have been utilised in the field sites. Statistical procedures are being

developed that can be applied to matched samples allowing for generalisations beyond specific research sites.

The application of the concept of ritual has resulted in a rather
unique database. Using this database, we have been able to describe
and explain epidemiological phenomena such as the emergence of
cocaine basing and 'gekookte coke' (the Dutch variant of 'crack') in a
specific subpopulation (Grund, Adriaans and Kaplan, 1991). Likewise,
through this database we were able to describe for the first time in the
literature the practice of 'frontloading', a common drug sharing ritual
(Grund et al., 1990; 1991). This ritual had been an unnoticed mode of
HIV transmission. Using the concepts of ritualisation, parameters of
subculture and other socio-economic indicators comparing Rotterdam
and the Bronx, New York, we were able to explain how certain similar
phenomena produced very different (behaviour) outcomes due to their
different socio-political contexts (Grund et al., 1992).

Functionality and Symbolism in Drug-taking Rituals

The practice of frontloading is a good example of the instrumental,
symbolic and socio-political implications of an injecting drug user sharing ritual. When sharing by frontloading, the drug is prepared on one
spoon and then drawn into one syringe (A). From the second syringe
(B) the needle is removed and the plunger is drawn back. By spouting
a part of the solution from syringe A through the hub of syringe B, the
drugs are divided. In this way the drugs can be divided into two or
more equal parts (Grund et al., 1991). While the dangers for HIV transmission of needle sharing were well understood by our research subjects (Grund, Kaplan and Adriaans, 1991), frontloading was still
common practice.

Frontloading had multiple functions. First of all, it had a highly instrumental function in preventing withdrawal. 'Helping' with a 'betermaker-
tje' (a little dose to ameliorate withdrawal) is a common motivation for
drug sharing. The term 'helping' is an everyday expression referring to
the revered rule of aiding a fellow user who is in withdrawal. Likewise
drugs are frequently bought together and subsequently shared by frontloading. Secondly, frontloading served clear symbolic functions, for
example the opening of communication channels. By sharing drugs,
users make new contacts and existing ones are reinforced. The ties
between individual drug users are strengthened, as participation in
shared drug taking activities (e.g. buying and using at the same house
addresses) results over time in a more structured social network.

Finally, frontloading serves important community functions. Drug
use is not the only factor that brings and keeps drug users together.

Drug users engage in many common activities and spend considerable time in social and other conventional activities (Faupel, 1987; Kaplan et al., 1990). Moreover, the relationships of drug users were often much more intense and multiplex than would be suggested by focusing on only drug use behaviour. Drugs were often shared among sexual partners, family or people sharing living arrangements. A significant percentage (23%) of the intravenous drug users (IDUs) were observed to share drugs typically with running mates or dyads. The acquisition and use of drugs is an essential bonding element in these dyadic relationships (Preble and Casey, 1969; Feldman and Biernacki, 1988).

The Control Function of Drug-taking Rituals

A prominent feature of the rituals and rules we studied was that they aimed to control and regulate the drug taking experience in the following ways: (1) maximizing the desired drug effect; (2) controlling drug use levels; (3) balancing the positive and negative effects of the drugs used; and (4) preventing secondary problems. Contrary to popular conceptions, the use of heroin and cocaine are subject to control mechanisms. This is most apparent in the stereotypical behavioural sequences surrounding self-administration of drugs by the individual drug user but is also evident in many observed ritualised interactions.

Let us illustrate some mechanisms of regulation inherent in drug rituals, considering cocaine use in the heroin-using population. The prevalence of cocaine use among Dutch heroin users is estimated at around 70% of the population (Korf and Hogenhout, 1990; Toet, 1990; Grapendaal, Leuw and Nelen, 1991). In our study 96% of the heroin users also took cocaine. In this population, cocaine is used in patterns similar to those originally developed in heroin use, smoking (primarily 'chineseing' or chasing the dragon) and injecting (up to 30%).

From the observations and comments of the users, it is clear that cocaine has taken over heroin's function as the primary source of pleasure. The addition of cocaine to the menu of regular heroin users has not been without problems. Smoking and injecting cocaine results in an intense, short high, often followed by a dysphoric rebound state. To maintain the high and prevent or postpone the crash, the drug is re-administered after short intervals – for example, every 5–20 minutes until the supply is finished. However, frequent smoking or injecting of relatively high doses of cocaine, typical in this population, inevitably leads to a decrease in the positive effects and an increase in the negative effects. As a result, many heroin users experience problems with cocaine use. Craving, escalation, paranoia and depression were all observed. Among heroin users enrolled in Rotterdam methadone programmes, cocaine use (and in particular problematic cocaine use) was associated with a higher prevalence of psychological problems (Toet,

1990). In order to control the undesired effects of cocaine, users frequently resorted to the use of prescription drugs and heroin.

According to many users, heroin in particular plays a crucial role in the process of controlling the negative side effects of cocaine. Countering undesired effects (dysphoria) is a prominent feature of the observed cocaine/heroin patterns. Many users have an intense paradoxical relationship with cocaine. Use patterns can be observed that spawn and boost the desired pleasurable effects while simultaneously self-medicating the negative side-effects of the cocaine. Drug users alternate or combine cocaine and heroin, depending on personal preference, mood and drug availability. In the following fieldnote excerpt, Nadir explained his preference for alternating the two drugs:

> Nadir isn't sure yet what he wants to buy. He says he only wants to buy some heroin 'because cocaine makes me feel so para (paranoid)'. But then suddenly he decides: 'Well okay, I buy a little bit of cocaine too, just one streep', and he buys one stripe of heroin and one stripe of cocaine. 'I always first smoke the cocaine, pure without heroin. When I have finished the cocaine I start to smoke heroin. I must do it like that, otherwise the cocaine drives me crazy'.

This typical chemical mood control requires careful titration of the two substances. In the following fieldnote, Jack explains two main ways to manage the opposite effects of cocaine:

> Feeling the coke flash or not has to do with your spiritual attitude. When you don't want to feel it, you won't feel it. Users that don't feel relaxed won't get stoned nice... When I take a shot of heroin after I took cocaine the speediness is taken away. You can talk relaxed again, you got time to listen to other people. Then I feel myself becoming relaxed. In use there's a lot of suggestion... A cocktail is a shot with two drugs, with different effects. I'll take a cocktail when I don't want to have such a strong coke flash. I always save some heroin to take after the cocktail. The flash from a cocktail is not as intense as from coke only. But everybody has different experiences.

Jack's explanation underlines the importance of the interaction of pharmacological, psychological and social variables in controlling the drug effects. Drug use rituals regulate these variables by standardising and shaping the procedures utilized in the drug taking experience. Cocaine use in the heroin addict population can be described as 'nested' in rituals developed for heroin use. This nesting has altered the function of heroin use to a great extent. When both drugs are used, heroin changes its function and becomes intertwined with cocaine. The function of heroin becomes that of modulating and ameliorating cocaine's disturbing sideeffects. A functional relationship between heroin and cocaine is established; both drugs become integrated in administration rituals which aim to maintain a delicate balance of desired and undesired drug effects.

Our study identified two cocaine/heroin administration rituals. In the most common type, cocaine is used with an approximately equal amount of heroin. In the second pattern, the amount of heroin is maintained at a minimum level while the amount of cocaine is much higher. Our observations and conversations with users suggested that the latter pattern is more prevalent among users involved in dealing. Pat, a dealer in his late 30s, has been using drugs for about 20 years: 'I use about a gram of "bruin" now and a gram of "wit", but when I'm dealing I use much more cocaine.'

There are relevant reasons for using relatively more cocaine:

> When you're a doorman on an address, you're using more 'wit' (cocaine). I can't be sick then (a doorman rarely is, as he's being paid by the dealer to screen visitors). Using more heroin then doesn't make sense. More heroin gives more tolerance. It also makes it harder to stay not sick all day when I don't have a job as doorman. And you don't feel it anyway (more heroin). A doorman has to stay alert.

The higher prevalence of the second cocaine/heroin administration ritual among dealers is, to a large extent, explained by the effects of both drugs in relation to the dealing activities. Cocaine increases alertness and therefore is functional for the job requirements. In contrast, too much heroin is counterproductive because it decreases attention, resulting in reduced control over the dealing setting. Although both types may ultimately lead to some degree of cocaine-related psychosocial problems, the second type is especially risky. Counter-intuitively, although the second type is more common among dealers and their consumption is generally well above the average, they seemed to experience less problems. Cocaine-related symptoms were not observed in stable dealers even though they were using more of the drugs.

Discussion

Our observations suggest that the ability to exercise control over individual drug use is not evenly spread over all kinds of users. Some users such as dealers seem able to use large amounts of cocaine and heroin without or with little of the characteristic cocaine-related problems. But other users, typically the 'down and out' junkies hanging around Rotterdam Central Station, actually use relatively little but seem most susceptible to problems. Therefore, the ability to control or regulate drug use seems not directly related to the amount of drug consumed. This somewhat paradoxical observation has led us to two conclusions.

1. Control and regulation is more than a matter of limiting the amount of drugs. It refers also to the prevention and management of drug-related

problems and should, therefore, be perceived as a multidimensional process.
2. The effectiveness of rituals and rules in exercising control and regulation over drug use is moderated by additional factors which impact on the individual's ability to comply with these rituals and rules.

Our data support Zinberg's theory that the control of drugs is largely established by (sub)culturally defined social sanctions which pattern the way a drug is used. Ultimately, users themselves regulate their use of intoxicants through a peer-based social learning process, in which specific rituals and rules are developed as adaptations to the effects of the interaction between drug, set and setting (Harding and Zinberg, 1977; Zinberg, 1984). It is evident that the use of intoxicants (including 'hard drugs') does not inevitably lead to harmful consequences. Drug use must compete with other commitments and interests in the user's environment. Thus, as Zinberg argued, controlled use of drugs is mainly determined by setting variables. However, Zinberg's theory does not explain the intra-group variations in the ability to effectively utilise these social controls, as was found in our study. Nor does it account for the multidimensional nature of the concept of control. Beside rituals and rules, there are other potential factors which impact upon the effectiveness of these social controls.

Based on our two conclusions, a theoretical model can be proposed that overcomes some of the limitations of Zinberg's explanation. The model postulates an interaction between three factorial clusters: rituals and rules, life structure and drug availability. These clusters form an interactive 'feedback circuit' constantly adapting to external social influences (Figure 7.1).

Rituals and rules determine and constrain the patterns of drug use, preventing an erosion of life structure. A high degree of life structure enables the user to maintain a stable drug availability which is essential for the formation and maintenance of effective rules and rituals. Thus, control over drug consumption and its (unintended) effects is an outcome of a (precarious) balance of a circular reinforcement chain. Elaborating on Zinberg's theory, this model seeks to specify the variables that constitute the social setting which seems to be the critical factor in controlling drug use. The model also utilises the work of Charles Faupel (1987), who underlined the importance of life structure in addict life.

Although the proposed feedback model is circular, it is neither closed nor independent. The three components of the feedback model are each the result of distinctive variables and processes. Drug availability is determined by price, quality and accessibility which are mediated by market factors and governmental regulations. Drug availability has a

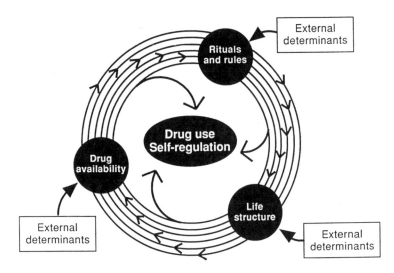

Figure 7.1 Three-cluster feedback model of drug use regulation and control

pivotal impact on the daily lives of drug users. Artificially limiting the availability of drugs may restrict the intake of drugs to a certain degree, but at considerable (psychosocial) expense. Restricting availability not only creates a strong economic incentive for drug trafficking, but also results in a situation in which drugs obtain a strong added meaning, a high subjective importance ushering in a narrowing of focus in the user. Fixation on the drug will lead to a strong limitation of behavioural expressions when the drug is craved and difficult to obtain, and to impulsive indulgence when a dose becomes available.

The rituals and rules around the drug become less directed at control and safety in the sense of health, and more at safeguarding, covering and facilitating drug use and the related activities itself (e.g. drug sales) (Carlson, 1977). In contrast, the absence of uncertainty as to the whereabouts of the next dose liberates the user from recurrent obsessive worries about obtaining the drugs and the necessity to chase them. Sufficient availability thus creates a situation in which rituals and rules can develop which restrain drug use and induce stable use patterns (Figure 7.2).

Rituals and rules are the product of culturally defined social learning processes. These can be rooted in mainstream culture as is the case with alcohol. The rituals and rules that sanction controlled alcohol use are mainly determined by inter-generational, family-centred socialisation processes which offer socially acceptable models of alcohol use and reinforce moderate use. Rituals and rules surrounding illegal drug use largely depend upon subcultural or peer group socialisation characterised by more idiosyncratic and rigid rituals and rules (Figure 7.3).

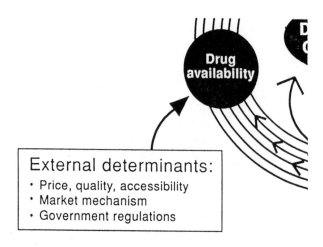

Figure 7.2 External determinants of drug availability

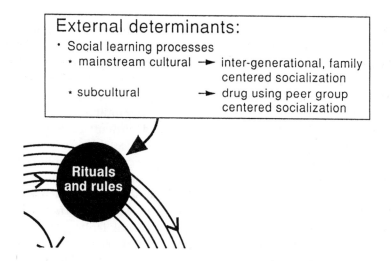

Figure 7.3 External determinants of rituals and rules

The shape and degree of life structure are the product of regular activities, connections, obligations and ambitions which may or may not be drug-related. General socio-economic conditions, actual living conditions, personality structure, psychosocial problems and cultural factors further determine life structure (Figure 7.4).

The model is useful for explaining our paradoxical results. Thus, the greater ability to exercise control over their drug use by dealers is explained by an interaction between drug availability, rituals and rules,

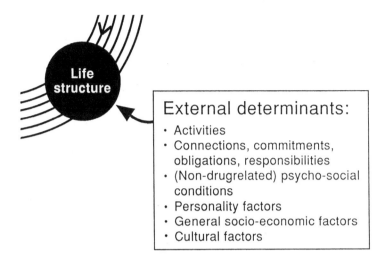

Figure 7.4 External determinants of life structure

and life structure. The high drug availability of dealers is evident. Not so self-evident is that daily involvement in drug dealing requires a necessary degree of life structure. Consumer-level dealing can be compared with a legal small retail business. Successful dealing is primarily a matter of good shopkeeping. Similar economic demands and rules must be obeyed. Dealing provides a structured activity related to customers and suppliers. This activity engenders demanding connections, commitments, obligations, responsibilities and expectancies. Thus, to maintain dealing activities successfully, the dealing user must regulate her/his personal use so that it does not interfere with 'taking care of business' (Preble and Casey, 1969.

Such rituals and rules can only develop under the condition of sufficient drug availability. Likewise, the model can explain the occurrence of frontloading. We can see that this ritual is related to availability. Drugs are scarce and expensive, but cheaper when bought in bulk. This scarcity induces a sharing technique which becomes an established ritual pattern and a subcultural rule, simultaneously uniting individuals and reinforcing network (or life) structures developed around drug use. These life structures then interact with availability forming a feedback circuit.

Although the feedback model is based upon a study of heroin users, it can probably also be utilised in studying the use of other drugs and non-heroin using populations. Thus, one future research question would concern how users regulate the powerful psycho-stimulants, cocaine and MDMA (Ecstasy). Of 1537 client contacts (alcohol 747; drugs 790) registered in 1990 at the Rotterdam Consultation Bureau for Alcohol and Drugs (CAD), only 66 cases concerned people whose primary drug was cocaine. Forty-two of these were new contacts. Cocaine was mostly part of a multiple drug use pattern (heroin users are excluded) (J. Verveen, personal communication, 1992).

A similar picture holds for Amsterdam (J. Jamin, personal communication, 1992). In both cities requests for information about MDMA are frequent. In Rotterdam, the number of Ecstasy-related treatment applications is estimated at one a month or less (B. van Ieperen, personal communication, 1992). No Ecstasy-related treatment applications in Amsterdam were found in a study by Adelaars (1991). This does not mean that the use of cocaine and Ecstasy is completely without problems. For example, most subjects in a recent cocaine study by Cohen (1989) reported experiences with craving and other negative effects of cocaine. A recent Ecstasy study by Korf, Blanken and Nabben (1991) reports similar findings; many of their subjects experienced a range of unpleasant effects during or after MDMA use. In both Cohen's cocaine study and the Ecstasy studies by Adelaars and Korf et al., these unpleasant effects are generally related to periods of high use levels. A consistent finding in all three studies is that when people experience problems with the use of cocaine or Ecstasy, they decrease or (periodically) discontinue their use. All three studies described elaborate self-regulation strategies.

These studies indicate that users' initial enthusiasm for a drug is generally tempered to realistic proportions as use patterns are subjected to social controls. The control procedures of regular users of cocaine and heroin described in this chapter are expressions of the same processes, albeit under conditions of more limited options. The feedback model proposed in this chapter needs further refinement through studies of multiple drug-using populations and should add to our understanding of the complex processes involved in human drug-taking rituals and their relationship to public health issues.

References

Adelaars, A. (1991). *Ecstasy: De Opkomst van een Bewustzijnsveranderend Middel*. Amsterdam: De Knipscheer.

Agar, M.H. (1977). Into that whole ritual thing: Ritualistic drug use among urban American heroin addicts. In B.M. Du Toit (Ed.), *Drugs, Rituals and Altered States of Consciousness*. Rotterdam: Balkema.

Becker, H.S. (1973). *Outsiders: Studies in the Sociology of Deviance*. New York: The Free Press.

Carlson, K.A. (1977). Identifying the stranger: An analysis of behavioural rules for sales of heroin. In B.M. Du Toit (Ed.), *Drugs, Rituals and Altered States of Consciousness*. Rotterdam: Balkema.

Cohen, P. (1989). *Cocaine Use in Amsterdam in Non-deviant Subcultures*. Amsterdam: University of Amsterdam.

deVries, M.W., Kaplan, C.D., Dijkman-Caes, C.I.M. and Blanche, P. (1990). The experience of drug craving in daily life. In J.J. Platt, C.D. Kaplan and P.J. McKim (Eds), *The Effectiveness of Drug Abuse Treatment*. Malabar, Florida: Robert E. Krieger Publishing Company.

Durkheim, E. (1971). *The Elementary Forms of the Religious Life*. London: George Allen and Unwin.

Edwards, G., Arif, A., and Hodgson, R. (1981). Nomenclature and classification of drug- and alcohol-related problems: A WHO Memorandum. *Bulletin of the World Health Organization*, 59, 225–242.

Faupel, C.D. (1987). Drug availability, life structure and situational ethics of heroin addicts. *Urban Life*, 15, 395–419.

Feldman, H.W. and Biernacki, P. (1988). The ethnography of needle sharing among intravenous drug users and implications for public policies and intervention strategies. In R.J. Battjes and R.W. Pickins (Eds), *Needle Sharing Among Intravenous Drug Abusers: National and International Perspectives*. Washington, DC: National Institute on Drug Abuse.

Fiddle, S. (1967). *Portraits from a Shooting Gallery*. New York: Harper and Row.

Goffman, E. (1967). *Interaction Ritual: Essays on Face to Face Behavior*. New York: Pantheon Books.

Grapendaal, M., Leuw, E. and Nelen, J.M. (1991). *De Economie van het Drugsbestaan: Criminaliteit als Expressie van Levensstijl en Loopbaan*. Arnhem: Gouda Quint.

Grund, J-P.C., Adriaans, N.F.P. and Kaplan, C.D. (1991). Changing cocaine smoking rituals in the Dutch heroin addict population. *British Journal of Addiction*, 86, 439–448.

Grund, J-P.C., Kaplan, C.D. and Adriaans, N.F.P. (1991). Needle sharing in the Netherlands: An ethnographic analysis. *American Journal of Public Health*, 81, 1602–1607.

Grund, J-P.C., Kaplan, C.D., Adriaans, N.F.P. and Blanken, P. (1991). Drug sharing and HIV transmission risks: The practice of 'frontloading' in the Dutch injecting drug user population. *Journal of Psychoactive Drugs*, 23, 1–10.

Grund, J-P.C., Kaplan, C.D., Adriaans, N.F.P. Blanken, P. and Huisman, J. (1990). The limitations of the concept of needle sharing: the practice of frontloading. *AIDS*, 4, 702–703.

Grund, J-P.C., Stern, L.S., Kaplan, C.D., Adriaans, N.F.P. and Drucker, E. (1992). Drug use contexts and HIV-consequences: The effect of drug policy on patterns of everyday drug use in Rotterdam and the Bronx. *British Journal of Addiction*, 87, 381–392.

Harding, W.M. and Zinberg, N.E. (1977). The effectiveness of the subculture in developing rituals and social sanctions for controlled drug use. In B.M. Du Toit.(Ed.). *Drugs, Rituals and Altered States of Consciousness*. Rotterdam: Balkema.

Kaplan, C.D. (1992). Drug craving and drug use in the daily life of heroin addicts. In M.W. deVries (Ed.), *The Experience of Psychopathology: Investigating Mental Disorders in their Natural Settings*. Cambridge, UK: Cambridge University Press.

Kaplan, C.D., de Vries, M.W., Grund, J-P.C. and Adriaans, N.F.P. (1990). Protective factors: Dutch intervention, health determinants and the reorganization of addict life. In H. Ghodse, C.D. Kaplan and R.D. Mann (Eds), *Drug Misuse and Dependence*. London: Parthenon.

Kaplan, C.D., Korf, D. and Sterk, C. (1987). Temporal and social contexts of heroin-using populations: An illustration of the snowball sampling technique. *Journal of Nervous and Mental Disease*, 566–575.

Korf, D.J., Blanken, P. and Nabben, T. (1991). *Een Nieuwe Wonderpil? Verspreiding, Effecten en Risico's van Ecstasygebruik in Amsterdam*. Amsterdam: Jellinek Centrum.

Korf, D.J. and Hogenhout, H.P.H.(1990). *Zoden aan de Dijk: Heroinegebruikers en hun Ervaringen met en Waardering van de Amsterdamse Drughulpverlening*. Amsterdam: Instituut voor Sociale Geografie, Universiteit van Amsterdam.

Meier, R.F. (1981). Norms and the study of deviance: A proposed research strategy. *Deviant Behaviour*, 3, 1–25.

Peele, S. (1985). *The Meaning of Addiction: Compulsive Experience and its Interpretation*. Lexington, MA: Lexington Books.

Preble, E. and Casey, J.J. (1969). Taking care of business: the heroin user's life on the street. *International Journal of Addiction*, 1, 1–24.

Radcliffe-Brown, A.R. (1952). *Structure and Function in Primitive Society*. London: Cohen and West.

Siegel, R.K.(1990). *Intoxication: Life in Pursuit of Artificial Paradise*. New York: Pocket Books.

Toet, J. (1990). *Het RODIS Nader Bekeken: Cocainegebruikers, Marokkanen en nieuwkomers in de Rotterdamse Drugshulpverlening Rapport 1990*. Rotterdam: GGD-Rotterdam e.o., Afdeling Epidemiologie.

Vatz, R.E. and Weinberg, L.S. (1983). *Thomas Szasz: Primary Values and Major Contentions*. New York: Prometheus Books.

Wallace, A.F.C. (1966). *Religion: An Anthropological View*. New York: Random House.

Zinberg, N.E. (1984). *Drug, Set, and Setting: The Basis for Controlled Intoxicant Use*. New Haven: Yale University Press.

Part III
Harm-reduction Policies

Chapter 8
Impediments to the Global Adoption of Harm-reduction Policies

DAVID HAWKS

The task of reflecting on the impediments to the global adoption of harm-reduction policies is a daunting prospect. I can lay no special claim to such insight and some may even argue that my location in one of the most isolated cities in the world invalidates my claim to even attempt such an undertaking. What I have done therefore is the only thing open to me: to reflect on what appear to be some of the ideological, philosophical and ethical influences bearing on the adoption of harm-reduction policies. To the extent that these influences are pervasive, and I believe them to be, I have addressed the second requirement of my task which is to refer to the global situation.

In attempting to identify these influences I am not necessarily siding with them or arguing that they will prevail. I am merely arguing that they effect the adoption of harm-reduction approaches to the prevention of drug-related harm. If we are to understand the opposition to the adoption of such policies, we need to understand the values inherent, but often unrecognised, in such opposition.

The advent of AIDS has brought into sharper focus a number of dilemmas that have always been present in the field of public health. To what extent can the rights of individuals be subjugated to the benefit of the majority without doing irreparable harm to the civil rights of that majority? What limits, if any, should be imposed on governments wishing to influence the lifestyle of their populations? When does a pragmatic solution become the abdication of a principle?

If these questions have not always been confronted in the past it is because, at least in modern times, the need to do so has been less pressing. With the introduction of HIV/AIDS the need *has* become pressing, even if the answers are no more forthcoming.

In this paper I will attempt to identify some of the major impediments to the adoption of harm-minimisation policies in the drugs arena. By its very nature such an exercise is subjective; there are no data that bear on the issues and therefore I am happy to acknowledge the extent to which my own values have influenced my judgement on these matters.

The Loss of Idealism

Perhaps the most profound impediment to the adoption of harm-reduction principles in the drugs area is the 'loss of idealism' which it is claimed such adoption signifies. To accept a need for harm reduction is, at least superficially, to give up on harm elimination – it is to accept the inevitability of harm, however desirable its minimisation. Although, when carried to its ultimate conclusion, harm reduction may amount to harm elimination, if one has subscribed to the belief that society can be rid of such harm, to collude with its minimisation is bound to seem like a compromise. The American policy of zero tolerance, itself aiming at a drug-free society (though legal drugs are not included in this pre-scription) is perhaps the most obvious example of a policy which by definition excludes all compromises, including accepting the aim of harm minimisation.

The policies of harm elimination and harm reduction, as I have already observed, are only superficially opposed. To seek to minimise harm does not preclude eliminating all such harm; it only provides for something less. The important question is whether we accept the desir-ability of something less or consider elimination the only measure of success. While those who favour harm reduction as a policy might hope to reduce all harm to a minimum, equally clearly they accept any reduc-tion in harm as desirable.

A particular version of the 'loss of idealism' argument is currently being played out in response to the 'It's alright to say no' sex education campaign being pursued in Western Australia. Essentially the propo-nents of this campaign argue that any attempt to render sex safe will be interpreted as an inducement to such behaviour. A subsidiary argument is the view that no sex, even 'protected sex', is inherently safe.

Countering this view is the argument, supported by empirical find-ings, that a majority of juveniles over the age of 16 are already engaging in sexual behaviour which, unless it is rendered 'safe', places them at risk of sexually transmitted diseasea, including HIV. To advise such peo-ple to say 'No' is to shut the door after the horse has bolted, however much one might have wished that the horse remained in the stable, at least until marriage.

Behind these arguments there is, one suspects, a different view of sexual behaviour, with the one party arguing that sex is an integral part of a married relationship in which it is complemented by a concern for the partner in all areas of their being, while the other adopts the more pragmatic view that people, assured of the possibility of contraception and of 'safe sex', will inevitably regard sexual behaviour as analogous to other behaviour, albeit of a more intimate kind, to be shared with whomever one chooses. Not surprisingly such people will regard the provision of information about safe sex and the ready provision of the means of safe sex as their reasonable due, in much the same way as they would expect the government to assure them of the safety of the water supply.

Collusion with Continued Use

Behind a reluctance to embrace harm-reduction principles is, I suspect, a fear that to do so is to collude with continued drug use. After all, if we talk of minimisation rather than elimination we clearly accept the inevitability, perhaps even the desirability, of continued drug use. In doing so it could be argued that we remove, or at least diminish, the motivation to give up drugs, or at least resist initiation to them. We abandon that particular form of idealism which argues that life should be lived without recourse to drugs, at least illicit drugs.

The majority of the population, even the youthful population, are not regular users of illicit drugs. Although society's refusal to collude with drug use which it defines as illegal will not be the only deterrent to their use, and clearly it is not a wholly successful deterrent, it could be argued that to remove it by employing harm-reduction strategies is to invite more drug use.

Unwillingness to Acknowledge the Demand for Drugs

An impediment of another kind to the adoption, or at least the success, of harm-reduction policies in the drugs arena is the failure to fully countenance the implications of a supply/demand approach to drug use. While the interdiction of supply will always remain a component of any successful approach to the minimisation of that harm associated with drugs, it is, for all of its difficulties, the easiest component to implement.

It can only be a component because attempts to prevent the supply of drugs in the face of demand for them can never be wholly successful, except perhaps in situations whose repressiveness is judged to be intolerable for other reasons. Addressing the demand for drugs will mean acknowledging that drugs are used for a variety of purposes, not always out of an ignorance as to their effects or as an expression of 'pathologies' in the user. Minimising the harm associated with such use will mean, in part, minimising the motivation for use, or failing that, minimising the danger inherent in that use.

Although undoubtedly some drug use is an expression of deprivation of one sort or another, whether material or emotional, some drug
use is celebratory and pursued for recreational or spiritual ends; it cannot be construed as having pathological overtones, however problematic it may be for society.

Addressing the demand for drugs as one aspect of a supply/demand
approach to drug use will mean addressing the complexity and the pro-
fundity of the issues raised by the question 'Why do people use drugs?'.
A proper application of the supply/demand approach to the minimisation of drug-related harm will require that we consider what it is about
the contemporary condition of men and women which encourages and
sustains drug use. At a superficial, but nonetheless important level, this
will mean asking what it is about a person's perceived reality which
prompts them to want to change that reality in ways which, at times,
are not only harmful to society but to themselves as well. At a relatively
superficial (but important) level, this will mean ensuring that young
people have employment available to them and that they have the
means of ensuring their own shelter and safety. The lessons of history
suggest however that drug use is not always, or only, an expression of
material deprivation. It may reflect a deprivation or poverty of a more
profound kind – a lack of meaning and of meaningful relationships, or
a means of acquiring such, as much as a lack of shelter or of occupation.

A government that wishes to pursue a campaign against drug abuse
which can claim to be based on the principle of harm minimisation
cannot morally, on the one hand, pursue policies designed to curb the
supply of drugs, while neglecting those circumstances that promote
demand for them. Nor can it construe that demand as merely reflecting
an ignorance of the effects of drugs to be addressed by education.

In many instances drugs are taken, not because people do not know
what their effects will be, *but precisely because they do*. Finding alternative ways of achieving these desired effects where appropriate is a
task, not only for the whole of government, but one requiring all the
ingenuity of public and private institutions as well.

The Illegitimacy of Risk Taking

Behind an unwillingness to entertain the minimisation of the harm
associated with drug taking, rather than the elimination of such harm,
is an unwillingness to acknowledge the legitimacy of risk taking in this
arena of living, as distinct from most others.

Although it can be argued that in a modern welfare-orientated society practically no individual action is without societal consequence
(Hawks, 1975), clearly no society can expect to prevent all behaviour

having actual or potential adverse implications for it. Even if this were practically possible, it would be philosophically unacceptable.

While much private behaviour is regulated so as to minimise its adverse public consequences, societies nonetheless tolerate a degree of risk taking and even provide financially for the realisation of some of those risks. Not all lone sailors are discouraged from crossing the Tasman Sea, nor are all pot-holers turned back at the entrance to caves. Indeed, risk taking and succeeding is one of the grounds on which we accord people esteem, as illustrated by the status we usually accord entrepreneurs whose failures also often rebound on the public purse. Risk taking by consuming illicit drugs is, however, construed differently, despite our tolerance of the risks inherent in consuming legal drugs. To teach people using illicit drugs how to avoid the harm associated with their use might be seen as, not only to collude with their continued use, but even to accede to the legitimacy of their continued use. It is to allow them to do a 'bad' thing without adverse consequences, even to allow them to maximise their enjoyment of that 'bad' thing.

Related to our unwillingness to acknowledge the legitimacy of risk taking in the illicit drug arena is a reluctance to consult the users of such drugs as to what they want. It has been stated that the principal benefit observed by injecting drug users from the legal provision of heroin for injecting is the provision of a drug of a known quantity and purity. Behind our unwillingness to entertain this option there is likely to be a feeling that users are not deserving of this indulgence – that the risks inherent in taking a drug of uncertain quantity and purity are part of the appropriate danger associated with such behaviour. To reduce the danger is to reinforce the behaviour in a way which would be considered undesirable.

Distrust of Paternalism

Another factor of an entirely different kind which has mitigated against the adoption of harm-reduction principles is what I will call a distrust of paternalism which has expressed itself in a variety of forms – an increasing tendency toward decentralisation, the devolution of power and a move to smaller government. Whether such moves are themselves predicated on the assessment that smaller government is less expensive government or reflects some greater embrace of liberal tendencies, I will leave others to debate. What is clear is that there is an increasing distrust of central control and of further regulation – manifested in Australia by the reaction to the proposal to introduce the Australia Card and giving rise to the expression 'the nanny state'.

Now, it needs to be recognised that much public health is paternalistic; it decides things for us, supposedly for our collective good. It puts

thiamin in our bread, fluoride in our water, regulates the sale of alcohol and tobacco, and renders illegal the use of certain drugs. At the
same time as there accumulates evidence of the effectiveness of some
such measures, there is a growing distrust of their implementation and
the naive assertion that it is sufficient for people to be provided with
information for them to make 'good' decisions – that the state has no
role in making such decisions for them.

Many of the measures recommended by a harm-reduction approach
to drug use require the intervention of the state, whether it is to supply
needles and syringes, free methadone and condoms or regulate the
advertisement of alcohol and tobacco. Objections to the nannyism of
the state or its 'wowserism' inevitability undermine such interventions.

Veracity of the Market-place

There often lies behind such objections an optimistic belief in the
veracity of the free market place – a belief that the market, and particularly its practitioners, will behave in a way which maximises benefit to
the whole of society and not just to the practitioners themselves. It
would seem to me that in Australia there has been more than enough
proof of late of the spuriousness of such arguments. Left to its own
devices the market-place would seem always to seek to maximize its
own profitability, which may incidentally and then only occasionally
coincide with the welfare of the whole of society.

Such trends can also be observed in the international arena. Pressure placed on the Philippines and Japan by the US Government to
import tobacco products is one example of economic considerations
taking precedence over public health principles, whereas the harmoni-
sation of alcohol taxes in the European Community offers another
example of economic principles (the removal of tariff barriers) being
pursued without considering of the implications for the health of the
populations concerned (although this policy has been modified to give
greater consideration to the health concerns of member countries).

Closer to home, the wine industry's insistence that nothing should
be allowed to adversely effect the international competitiveness of Australian wine exports is evidence of the parochial nature of our thinking
and our willingness to compromise the health of others for our own
economic advantage.

Deservedness of Damnation

Although it is no longer acceptable for scientists to be publicly associated
with the eugenics movement, one does not have to look too far in drug
policies to see evidence of its influence. The notion that AIDS, for
example, provides a useful culling function, while never an explicit
premise, is not too far hidden in some countries' responses to this threat.

If AIDS mainly affects the homosexual, bisexual and intravenous drug users, so much the better, it might be covertly but never overtly argued, especially if these groups are disproportionately black or Hispanic. If, as is reported, Africa has been ravaged by AIDS there were in any case too many people in Africa who were too often supplicants for Western economic assistance.

The moral righteousness of the monogamous majority certainly constitutes an impediment to the adoption of harm-reduction principles, if only because of a reluctance to allow that such 'deviant' populations should escape their proper damnation – a view that will only be modified as members of that majority are themselves infected.

The Limited Value Placed on Health

It is a paradox in the way we seek to minimise the problems associated with legal drugs that we willingly employ those means we know to be relatively ineffective, while ignoring those interventions we know to be the most effective (Saunders, 1989).

To understand this paradox we need to appreciate the role of vested economic interests in determining government policy. Although those of us who work in the public health sphere are inclined to believe that health is valued above all else, and will be favoured by governments above every other consideration, health clearly has a price which at times governments and individuals are unwilling to pay. This can be clearly illustrated in relation to the sponsorship of sport by alcohol and tobacco interests. Replying to a concern about the identification of sport with alcohol interests, the Australian Minister for Sport recently wrote:

> Government funding and gate takings no longer provide sufficient income for sporting organisations to fund these activities [sporting events], therefore sports sponsorship has become an increasingly important source of funding for Australian sport ... and any action by the government to force the termination of sports sponsorship arrangements would be premature at this time.

(R. Kelly, personal communication, 1991)

In replying in this vein, the Minister appears to be colluding with a view that sport could not exist without such sponsorship*. Equally clearly, however, there are some of us who can remember watching sporting events and also playing sport which was not sponsored by the alcohol industry. Sport pre-existed alcohol sponsorship and is capable of existing without it, albeit on different terms. What we are acknowledging when accepting the sponsorship of sport by alcohol interests is that the highest bidder, the interest for whom such an association is most

---

*It has since been determined that sponsorship of sport by the tobacco industry will be phased out over a period of years except in those instances approved by the Minister for Health, Housing and Community Services.

valuable in promotional terms, should prevail. If players and their managers had to make do with salaries closer to the national average, would we necessarily be the poorer or sport the less watchable?

While we accept, however, that the economic imperative is the only imperative, or the most important imperative, we are hooked into a system which operates in ways that are frequently inimical to health. Similarly, while we allow that one reason for resisting the further regulation of alcohol advertising is the loss of advertising revenue which such regulation would entail, we collude with a system that pays inordinate returns to its practitioners whose *raison d'être* is a consumerism increasingly recognised as being unsustainable. An impediment to the adoption of policies, at least in the area of legal drugs, which would be truly harm reducing is the acceptance of the *status quo* and a belief that progress is necessarily defined in terms of more of the same.

Aside from these more general or macro impediments to the adoption of harm-minimisation principles for drug use, there are a number of more individual considerations which bear on this issue. Among the reasons given by drug injectors for avoiding needle exchanges is the fear of their being identified as drug users, either because they distrust the source of such exchanges or believe them to be under police surveillance. This is likely to be particularly the case in those instances where the user has not previously been in treatment or come to the notice of the police – users for whom access to needles and education is particularly important. Similarly, if the possession of needles and syringes is regarded as a priori evidence of drug use and users harassed until drugs are found, their possession is hardly likely to be regarded by users as harm reducing. Research has demonstrated that being in touch with treatment agencies and/or needle exchanges is important in the adoption of safe using habits. Clearly, for these sources to be viewed sceptically is an impediment to the adoption of safe using behaviours. Similarly, although the provision of needles and syringes has been taken up by many chemists in Australia, users' reports suggest that in some instances the hostility of chemists acts as a barrier.

The legal ambiguity of possessing injecting equipment presents another barrier to the adoption of harm-reducing strategies. Although there is tacit acceptance of the need for injecting users to have access to needles and syringes, their possession is still ambiguously defined in law, as a consequence of which users believe the police to have too much discretion in deciding to prosecute. Even if this perception is rarely borne out, its very existence is likely to mitigate against the adoption of safe and considered behaviours.

Although research consistently shows that those users in touch with treatment agencies are more inclined to adopt safe using practices, treatment itself obviously presents a barrier to some users. Even when abstinence is not the overt aim of treatment, it is frequently implicit in the programme and in the attitudes of treatment staff. Treatment is inevitably viewed as 'controlling' by users, many of whom will not necessarily want to give up drugs so much as use them without adverse consequence. The insistence that all treatment has abstinence as its eventual objective will undoubtedly discourage users who view their use as 'recreational' and for whom the fine tuning of their drug use is their only occasion for seeking help.

In the same way as it has been belatedly recognised that there are drinkers, even drinkers with alcohol-related problems, who merely want to moderate their drinking rather than become abstinent, it may be necessary to acknowledge that there are drug users who merely wish to be advised as to how they might render their drug use less threatening to their health.

Stimson (1992) has observed that among the impediments to the adoption of safer behaviours is not only a lack of inclination but a lack of access, both material and social. Approaching a clinic, needle exchange or other source of advice requires both social skills and material resources which some users lack.

> It should not be forgotten that while individual behaviours are a target for change and individuals need help to change, these behaviours are rooted in structural conditions. It is hard for drug injectors to adopt safer practices without the necessary resources. This goes beyond the provision of the immediate means to change, such as syringes, bleach and condoms. High risk behaviours are inextricably tied up with poverty, low income, inadequate or absent housing and unemployment.
>
> *(Stimson, p.60, 1992)*

Among the more personal impediments to the adoption of harm-minimising behaviours, impediments that are only now being investigated, is the very subtlety of the negotiation of such behaviours. Indeed, the difference in the adoption of safe needle sharing and safe sexual behaviours may reflect not only the differing risks associated with these behaviours but the different subtleties of their negotiation.

Early research carried out in Australia suggested that users did not regard sharing needles and syringes with their lovers as 'sharing', giving rise to the adage that 'if people were truly in love tap water sufficed'. Sharing a needle was accepted as an extension of the intimacy that had already been extended to the partner. How could one be expected to discriminate in regard to this particular behaviour? Research carried out in Western Australia indicates that female users give more prominence to different reasons for sharing needles than their male counterparts, suggesting that the context of user sharing and negotiating safe sex may be different for men and women (Marsh and Loxley, 1991).

The negotiation of safe sex is likely to be especially problematic, if only because the context of sexual behaviour is likely to be more emotionally laden, unrehearsed and tenuous. Even before the advent of AIDS, surveys had demonstrated that men were reluctant to use condoms and women were ambivalent about insisting on their use, not only, one imagines, because of ignorance but because of the fragility of the negotiation of sex.

Compounding these difficulties, to be observed even in a sober state, are the intoxicating effects of drugs and their ability to significantly alter the risk estimations made by people in relation to these behaviours. Similar changes in estimating the riskiness of certain behaviours are also likely to be made by users experiencing withdrawal symptoms when the prospect of a 'hit', even in risky circumstances, is likely to be paramount in their thinking.

Conclusion

In this paper I have attempted to identify some of the more covert considerations influencing the adoption of harm-reduction policies in the drugs arena. I make no special claim for their exhaustiveness or for their universal applicability. It seems to me, however, that they constitute some of the profound impediments to the adoption of such principles, impediments which unless they are openly acknowledged and addressed are likely to bedevil the universal adoption of such principles.

Whereas in some instances the issues at stake may be resolved by empirical testing – whether, for example, the provision of free needles and syringes increases the rapidity with which people progress to injecting use – some are likely to remain a matter of philosophical dispute, the resolution of which will owe more to the power of their advocates than the scientific veracity of their arguments. One might say that in this regard at least 'Nothing is changed, was it ever otherwise?'.

References

Hawks, D.V. (1975). Drug dependence: A case in point. In: E. Vallance (Ed.) *The State, Society and Self Destruction*. London: George Allen and Unwin.

Marsh, A. and Loxley, W. (1991). *Women at Risk of HIV/AIDS: Unsafe Behaviour Among Women Illicit Injecting Drug Users in Perth*. Technical Report, Curtin University of Technology, Perth: National Centre for Research into the Prevention of Drug Abuse.

Saunders, W. (1989). Alcohol and other drugs : the prevention paradox. *Community Health Studies*; 13, 150–155.

Stimson, G. (1992) Drug injecting and HIV infection: new directions for social science research. *International Journal of the Addictions*, 27(2), 147–163.

Chapter 9
Drug Policies and Problems: The Promise and Pitfalls of Cross-national Comparison

ROBERT J. MacCOUN, AARON J. SAIGER, JAMES P. KAHAN and PETER REUTER

This is a brief essay about what cross-national comparisons can tell us about the relationship between drug policies and drug-related problems, and about some of the difficulties involved in making such comparisons. This essay reflects our thinking and experience roughly halfway through a three-year cross-national study comparing drug policies and problem indicators across a number of Western industrialized nations. For reasons we will discuss, it would be premature for us to present preliminary statistical results in this essay; instead, we hope to stimulate curiosity about the experiences of other countries, and sensitivity as to the hazards of causal cross-national inference.

Hypotheticals and Analogies as Ammunition in the Drug Policy Wars

In the United States, our most recent 'war on drugs' has stimulated two intertwined policy debates (Reuter, 1992), with a third just starting to emerge. First, there is the debate between supply-side 'hawks', who emphasize aggressive law enforcement efforts, and demand-side 'doves', who call for more resources for treatment and prevention. Second, there is a recurring debate between advocates of drug prohibition, decriminalization and legalization. The third debate is between use-reduction and harm-reduction advocates; while it has been most active in western Europe, Canada and Australia, its appearance in the USA is relatively recent. Supply siders and demand siders battle on the common ground of use reduction; both stress the reduction of harms through the reduction of use, and many in each camp believe that use is itself an intrinsic harm. Harm-reduction advocates argue that all use does not lead to harm and that some use-reduction interventions do

more harm than good, so that the focus should be on harm, not use
per se.

A characteristic of all three policy debates is that they become crystal
ball battles, as each side attempts to project a future whose kindness
and gentleness depends essentially on the adoption of its preferred
policies. In our experience, the only thing that can be said about such
debates is that the predictions will all be incorrect in one way or another. Each position is based on different intuitions and beliefs about the
base of the problem, which leads to over-reliance on certain indicators
of the future at the cost of ignoring side-effects. Of course, that one
side's incidental effects may be the other side's main effects is a phenomenon that occurs frequently, is rarely recognized, and leads to considerable confusion.

Projecting hypothetical futures is not in and of itself bad, if it is done
with a healthy dose of skepticism, with a wide-ranging consideration of
consequences, and – best of all – with some model of how policy
changes help tranform the present into some version of the future. For
example, the drug policy games developed at RAND (Kahan et al.,
1992) permit exploration of different futures, while attempting to provide the participants with some idea of the consequences of policy in
consistent and quantifiable terms. But without some form of theory or
model to base comparisons, different views can degenerate into matters of taste.

A second rhetorical strategy in drug debates is reasoning by analogy;
it is particularly popular in the legalization debate. For example,
debaters routinely cite America's experience with alcohol prohibition
and its repeal earlier this century, or the British experience with prescription heroin, or the Dutch experience with *de facto* cannabis legalization. Reasoning by analogy is a basic, almost irresistible mode of
human cognition. Unlike hypothetical reasoning, analogical reasoning
is purportedly grounded in experience, and thus ostensibly more
empirical. But psychological research suggests that we tend to adopt
the analogies that come most readily to mind, which may be neither
accurate nor apt. Once an analogy is chosen, it has a powerful influence on one's interpretation of evidence and endorsement of policies.

One indication of the hazards of analogical reasoning in the drug
debate is that both sides tend to draw upon the same analogies, which
would not be expected if the analogies were both precise and proba-
tive. A second problem is that the analogies are seldom more than
crude anecdotes or 'factoids' (isolated but seemingly authoritative

---

* Although the three debates are interrelated, they are only loosely coupled. For example,
one can defend existing drug laws without urging their aggressive enforcement, and one can
call for more treatment or prevention without decrying drug prohibition. Legalizers tend to
be harm-reductionist, but not everyone in the harm-reductionist camp advocates legalization
(see Strang, Chapter 1, this volume).

'facts' that are often incorrect or at least misleading when presented without context). Consider the following exchange between Ira Glasser, the Executive Director of the American Civil Liberties Union, and William von Raab, the former US Commissioner of Customs, on the Public Television show, 'Firing Line' (March 26, 1990):

> *Glasser*: '...the fact is that the Netherlands has a lower rate of marijuana use since they legalized...and there is almost no crime...'

> *von Raab*: 'They have low crime statistics because the petty crime in Amsterdam is so bad...they don't keep them anymore. The next time you walk down the streets in Amsterdam, look on the concrete. You will see a fine dust over all the streets. That is the glass from all the car windows that have been shattered [by] drug addicts...to pay for their food and their lodging because they don't work.'

Glasser asserts as 'fact' two claims that are questionable and even if accepted, open to multiple interpretations. The evidence on trends in Dutch cannabis prevalence is hardly unequivocal, and in fact, little of it was available in English at the time of Glasser's statement.* Current trends in drug-related crime in Amsterdam (e.g. Grapendaal, 1992; Leuw, 1991) do not seem to support a claim that 'there is almost no crime'. But Glasser's statement has enough 'wiggle room' to be unfalsifiable. What kind of crimes count? How much crime is 'almost none'? Compared to when? Compared to where else?

While Glasser's claims are problematic, Von Raab's claims are pure hyperbole. The Dutch Ministry of Justice carefully documents national crime statistics on an annual basis. And three of us have each spent considerable time in Amsterdam without encountering any glass-dusted streets. However, in the absense of firm, readily available documentation of the Dutch drug experience (or alcohol prohibition, or the British experience), advocates have enormous discretion to tailor analogies to suit their particular rhetorical purposes.

Why Make Cross-national Comparisons?

In our critique of hypothetical and analogical reasoning, we should take care to avoid throwing out the baby with the bathwater. Careful and systematic cross-national comparison provides many of the advantages of more casual hypothetical and analogical reasoning, with fewer of the drawbacks. An elementary principle of scientific inference is the need to make comparisons. In order to make scientific comparisons, one needs adequate variation in the independent and dependent variables under study. In some cases, adequate variation is provided by cross-sectional

---

*It should also be noted that, technically, The Netherlands did *not* legalize cannabis, although they adopted formal, written guidelines for policing and prosecution that resulted in *de facto*, if not *de jure*, legalization of small amounts.

comparisons across cities or states, or by longitudinal comparisons, or by quasi-experimental studies of policy interventions. But the range of variation is often quite restricted, particularly on the policy dimensions.

Cross-national comparisons can overcome this limitation by providing much more dramatic variation along the dimensions of interest. A cross-national approach has made important contributions to the epidemiological study of HIV (e.g. Brenner, Hernando-Briongos and Goos, 1991),* tobacco consumption (e.g. Laugesen and Meads, 1991), alcohol consumption (e.g. Smart, 1989) and homicides (e.g. Messner, 1992). In many cases, cross-national research has clarified conflicting or ambiguous intranational research findings (e.g. Messner, 1992, p. 156).

The nations of western Europe and North America have adopted quite varied means to control the use of prohibited psychoactive drugs. Some have adopted what might be called 'tolerant' policies, using criminal sanctions almost exclusively against those who sell drugs and giving most policy emphasis to minimizing the harms the drug dependent do to themselves and the rest of society, as well as preventing initiation through education. Other countries have adopted more punitive policies, using criminal law aggressively against users as well as dealers, with less emphasis on harm reduction and treatment of current users.

This variation should provide an opportunity for nations to learn from each other. Yet systematic comparative descriptions of the drug control experiences of developed nations are hard to find. Few published studies compare the severity and nature of the drug problems of different countries, nor is there much available on how various nations have attempted to control such problems (see Albrecht and Kalmhout, 1989)[†]. Consequently little has been learned from the national experiences.

On the other hand, Klein (1991, p. 279) has argued that 'comparative studies can distort as well as illuminate;...they bring risks as well as benefits'. Klein notes that some comparisons are misleading. For example, some might argue that the United States is too different from other countries to allow meaningful comparisons. There are indications that many of the aspects of the US drug problem are not replicated in the experience of other developed nations. Few countries have the intensity of drug abuse present in the United States of America and few countries have the disproportionate concentration of drugs in a social underclass observed in the United States.

---

* Indeed, some of the highest quality cross-national drug research to date involves epidemiological research on the HIV-IVDU link. See the March 1992 special issue of *British Journal of Addiction* (Vol. 87) on 'AIDS, Drug Misuse, and the Research Agenda'. This probably reflects the fact that many governments have placed a higher priority on AIDS research than on drug research (see Oppenheimer, 1991, pp. 512-521).

† The European office of the World Health Organization has sponsored a study presenting a good deal of comparative data on European nations. The Pompidou Group, a unit of the Council of Europe, is conducting a comparative study of a number of European cities, following its 1987 study of seven cities.

To move from the uniqueness of America's drug problem to a decla-ration that cross-national comparisons are not helpful is too great a leap. For all of the differences, the cultural similarities among the Western developed nations are great; the motivations for drug use are likely similar and the treatment and enforcement options within the realm of policy possibility are within a small range. Although the expe-riences of other countries may not translate directly into recommenda-tions for US policy, they certainly can provide a starting point; policy failures in other countries are warning signals for similar policies in the USA and policy successes in other countries could be the foundation for an American policy.

A Framework for Comparative Drug Policy Research

Discussions of drug policy tend to adopt a *top-down* perspective, in which drug use and its consequences are governed largely by formal drug policies – the written laws and regulations, expenditures for treat-ment and prevention, and so on. This top-down perspective can be misleading because it is simplistic in a number of ways. First, a formal policy can be implemented in very different ways, or might not be implemented at all in any meaningful fashion. Second, policies can exert influence on behavior through multiple parallel mechanisms, some intended and others quite unintended.* Third, the relationship between policies and outcomes is reciprocal; policies themselves are often a reflection of, or a reaction to, problems. The inevitable time lag between problems and policy responses means that in some cases, policies may be adopted in response to a situation that has already changed in ways that may undermine their appropriateness. Finally, the top-down perspective is misleading because it neglects other factors in the broader context that influence both drug policy and drug prob-lems.

Figure 9.1 presents a general analytic framework that places drug policies and outcomes in that broader context. This framework explicit-ly acknowledges the interrelationships among drug policies, drug prob-lems, other social policies, and non-policy social contextual factors. The goal for researchers is to identify the relative strength of each rela-tionship and the conditions under which it does or does not occur.

It is important to be sensitive to social policies that do not directly address drugs but have implications for the consequences of drug use for the user and for society. Consider for example a comparison of

---

* For example, MacCoun (1993) has identified seven different mechanisms by which pro-hibitory drug laws influence drug use, two of which can actually promote rather than discour-aging drug use.

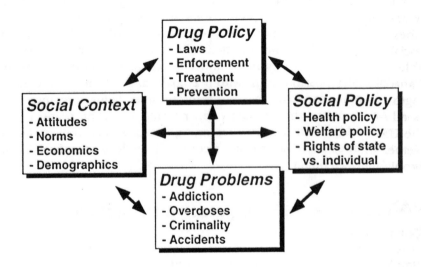

Figure 9.1 Potential complexities in the policy-outcome relationship

heroin addicts in the United States and the Netherlands. When comparing involvement in income-generating crime, it is essential to bear in mind differences in the social welfare policies of the two nations – in particular the availability of state income support for Dutch addicts. Similarly, when comparing addicts' morbidity and mortality in the two countries, one must take into account differences in the availability and quality of publicly subsidized health care.

Similar arguments pertain to social contextual factors such as social attitudes toward drug use, social norms of acceptability of intoxication, and a variety of economic and demographic factors that might influence the prevalence and type of drug use, as well as the consequences of use. Thus, nations differ somewhat in the social characteristics of the addicted population. For example, the involvement of immigrant groups varies substantially in ways that are difficult to explain. In Britain, heroin addiction seems to be rare in migrant populations such as those from the Indian subcontinent and the Caribbean. On the other hand, North African migrants in France have been disproportionately represented in the heroin addict population; the same is true of the small, immigrant population of Surinamese in the Netherlands. In the USA some Hispanic migrant groups (e.g. Puerto Ricans and Mexicans) show high rates of addiction (as evidenced by deaths and emergency room admissions related to cocaine and heroin) while others, notably the Chinese, show very low rates despite strong involvement in trafficking.

One general implication of Figure 9.1 is that our ability to confidently generalize the lessons from one country to another country diminishes as a function of the number and magnitude of differences in social context between the two countries. Thus, we might expect to be able to generalize more between the United States of America and Canada than between the USA and Singapore or Malaysia. By the same logic, the ability to generalize between analogies diminishes with temporal distance. Thus, to anticipate the effects of legalizing marijuana in the USA, we might learn more from contemporary experiences in the Netherlands than from our own experience with the repeal of alcohol prohibition earlier this century.

RAND's Drug Indicator Database

Our project at RAND's Drug Policy Research Center is an attempt to systematically implement this framework for cross-national research. One focus of this research has been the development of a database that describes drug problems and related phenomena for a range of Western countries: the *Drug Indicator Database* (DID). Major features of DID include (as of this writing):

1. Over 500 data indicators in 21 major categories.
2 Data, where available, for 12 nations for 1965–1991.
3 Links between national data and local data for 23 provinces and cities.
4. Complete documentation of data sources.

The choice of indicators included in the database was driven by two factors: interest and utility on the one hand and data availability on the other. In large part, the choice of indicators reflects an 'opportunistic' data-collection strategy: an indicator was included if data were available. (In order to keep DID as inclusive as possible, indicators available only for a few or even one country were included in the database, even though this meant increasing the number of missing elements in the database as a whole.) Currently, the data fall into five broad categories:

1. Prevalence and characteristics of drug users.
2. Drug-related morbidity and mortality.
3. Drug market data, including prices, purity and seizures by government.
4. Criminal justice enforcement and drug treatment indicators.
5. National (and sometime local) sociodemographic data.

Broad categories of data are likely to be added to the database. For example, we are developing data for policy variables that describe drug control laws and the nature of their enforcement, the structure of the criminal justice and treatment systems and policies concerning relevant government activities in areas like health, welfare and education. It is also likely that many of the current database categories will be expanded. For example, we hope to include data on criminal incomes, on the ethnic income and other charcteristics of drug users, treatment clients, and criminals and on the characteristics of drug prevention programs.

In the course of developing DID, we have identified a number of serious methodological obstacles. In the next three sections of this chapter, we briefly describe some of these problems.

Operationalizing Policies

In the early stages of our research, we have characterized national drug policies in terms of a series of dichotomous 'dummy variables'; e.g. is a legal distinction between 'hard' and 'soft' drugs made? Is treatment formally offered in lieu of criminal penalties? As seen in Figure 9.2, we have observed that these criteria roughly array various Western nations along a continuum from more to less tolerant policy, or alternatively, from nations that emphasize 'harm reduction' to nations that emphasize 'use reduction'.*

Although the undimensional harm-reduction/use-reduction array in Figure 9.2 appears to have some face validity, more systematic analysis will require more sophisticated operationalization of drug policies and

	Netherlands	Spain	Italy (pre'90)	UK	Canada	France	Norway	Germany	USA
Legal distinction between hard/soft	■	■	■	☐	☐	☐	☐	☐	☐
Possession for personal use not penalized	■	■	■	☐	☐	☐	☐	☐	☐
Treatment offered in lieu of penal sanction	☐	■	■	☐	☐	■	☐	■	☐
Regular use of methadone in treatment	■	☐	■	■	■	☐	☐	☐	■
Syringes available/retail exchange	■	■	■	■	■	■	■	■	☐

☐ = No   ■ = Yes

Figure 9.2 Classify national policies on a harm-reduction/use-reduction continuum

---

* Note that in the summer of 1990, Italy reintroduced the criminal sanctions that it removed in 1974 but reversed the legislation again in early 1993.

their implementation. It is desirable to move from crude dichotomous policy indicators to more specific ratio-level variables. Specific quantitative policy indicators should allow more sensitive estimation of the policy-outcome link.

Moreover, better policy indicators would allow a more scientific assessment of the dimensional structure of drug policy. The simple unidimensional continuum in Figure 9.2 may be supplanted by a more complex, multidimensional policy space in which, for example, Canada may resemble the Netherlands on some dimensions but the United States of America on others. This multidimensional structure could be identified using exploratory or confirmatory factor analyses of quantitative policy indicators.

Unfortunately, quantifying policy on a cross-national basis is not simple. It is relatively easy to ascertain formal written policies (e.g. Leroy, 1992), but much more difficult to obtain comparable data on actual patterns of law enforcement, prevention and treatment. For example, criminal justice data in the USA are typically reported in terms of arrests, prosecutions and convictions. The United Kingdom, by contrast, reports the number of cautions, compoundings and convictions. 'Cautioning', a written reprimand which does not amount to a criminal conviction, and 'compounding', where police confiscate drugs held by a suspect but take no further action, lack equivalent categories in the USA. Similarly, there are no UK data that describe 'prosecutions' or the number of arrests that end in a determination of innocence.

Measuring Outcomes

Measuring drug use and its consequences is even more difficult. This is not surprising for any secondary data collection effort, especially one based on a multitude of independent data sources developed without reference to one another. The problems are exacerbated in the drug area, however, because of the stigmatized, and (usually) illicit nature of psychoactive drug use, which drives most consumption 'underground'.*

In the USA, the nation for which the most comprehensive data are available, considerable room is present for improvement in data collection programs (Reuter, 1984; Sidney, 1990; Haaga and Reuter, 1991). However, in general, the data collection efforts of European and other Western nations are younger and much more fragmented (Reuband, 1990). As a result, remarkably little is known about several major European drug policy interventions. For example, in the mid 1970s,

* Thus economist Tom Schelling has suggested to us that one advantage of legalizing drugs might be that it would improve the quality of drug-related data collection! A comparison of drug indicator data with indicator data for alcohol and tobacco use certainly supports this claim.

Spain and Italy decriminalized personal possession of psychoactive drugs; yet next to nothing is known about the prevalence of drug use prior to these interventions, or the effects that decriminalization had on the initiation, prevalence, incidence, or consequences of drug use.

Even when suitable outcome data are available, comparing data obtained from diverse sources in different nations can be an adventure. Many governments routinely collect data of various sorts for internal policy purposes, but do not disseminate these data. Thus, the data are sequestered in governmental bureaucracies in their language of origin, instead of being made available in the (largely English language) scientific press. Finding these data is not very difficult, actually, once one gains access to the relevant officials, but gaining such access can be a time-consuming task that is only recommended for the very patient.

Once the data are in hand, translation is necessary. Translation is not restricted to language-to-language transformations, although those are formidable enough. In addition, there is also the need for clarification of meaning. For example, if a table lists drug use and homicides, do the numbers refer to victims or perpetrators? In the USA, crimes are divided into misdemeanors and felonies, which are handled by largely parallel criminal justice systems. These distinctions are not always followed in other countries and even if they are, the dividing point between categories is not always the same. Finally, countries have often idiosyncratic views of what constitutes a worthwhile category for data entry. For example, the Italians have a category called *rapina sotto minaccia siringa*, which has been translated for us as 'kidnapping under threat of a syringe'. It appears that this is some form of assault involving the threat of a syringe filled with HIV-infected blood. While incidents of crimes using similar threats have been seen recently in the Los Angeles area, they are not yet frequent enough to merit a column in criminal statistics.

Many data problems are illustrated by cross-national estimates of the prevalence of heroin use. Three basic heroin indicators are available in most nations: the numbers of deaths in which heroin is causally involved, admissions to treatment clinics, and arrests for heroin offenses. In order to make sense of the three indicators, it is important to consider age and other characteristics of those dying, seeking treatment or being arrested. For example, one would like drug-related mortality measured on an age adjusted (or career-length adjusted) basis. A rise in the number of deaths accompanied by increasing age of decedents may mean little more than that the fixed size population of heroin addicts is becoming increasingly frail as it ages. Constant or declining age of decedents may mean that the addict population is increasing, particularly if the numbers of arrests and admissions are also rising and show no increase in age. Unfortunately, all that is available at the moment are gross mortality figures, i.e. the number of persons dying each year from acute consequences of heroin use. Only a few individual studies have measured mortality from all causes (including violence) for a given cohort of drug users.

Design and Analysis Issues

In the best-case scenario of access to complete, reliable, comparable data on drug use and its consequences, an investigator would still face thorny design and analysis problems that would preclude iron-clad inferences about the effects of national drug policies. First and foremost is the problem of inferring cause and effect. As we illustrated in Figure 9.1, drug policies and problems coexist in a complex net of interrelationships with various other policies and social-contextual factors. This raises the familiar risks of confusing the direction of causality – as when a policy change is a reaction to a drug problem – or overlooking a third variable that causally influences both policies and outcomes.

The reader is no doubt familiar with the strengths and limitations of cross-sectional and longitudinal designs in this regard, so we will only briefly summarize some of the key concerns (Cook and Campbell, 1979). The major difficulty with cross-sectional designs is the natural confounding of the independent variable of interest - e.g. penalties for personal possession of cannabis – with a host of other differences between countries. To some extent, this can be corrected statistically, but only to the extent that one has indicator variables for all relevant confounds, which is highly unlikely. Within-nation longitudinal analyses – e.g. before-and-after comparisons of policy changes – control for many of these potential confounds, but are vulnerable to 'history' and 'maturation' artifacts (Cook and Campbell, 1979). For example, the decriminalization of marijuana in many American states during the 1970s coincided with a variety of other broad social, political, and demographic trends that may have influenced patterns of marijuana initiation and consumption.

Of course, the strongest research designs for evaluating public policies is the randomized field experiment or the controlled clinical trial. Authorities have generally resisted such approaches in the drugs arena; a good case study is the 1972 attempt by the Vera Institute of Justice to conduct a limited heroin maintenance experiment in New York City, which was eventually undermined by Congress and the Nixon Administration (Oppenheimer, 1992). It remains to be seen whether a new proposal for a similar experiment in Canberra, Australia will meet a similar political fate (see National Centre for Epidemiology and Population Health, 1991; Chapter 12, this volume). But even when authorities have shown a willingness to 'experiment' with new policies – e.g. needle sharing, decriminalization, the sale of cannabis in coffeeshops – the opportunity to turn such 'experiments' into true, methodological experiments (with random assignment to conditions and systematic data collection) is often overlooked.

In addition to design problems, cross-national comparison poses some serious data-analytic problems. A major problem is selecting the appropriate unit of analysis. Should one compare nations? Or regions? Or cities? Much of drug policy, at least in some countries, is made at the local level. And in all countries, even those with very centralized forms of government, there are inevitably differences between large cities and the rest of the nation. For some countries, we have had difficulty identifying national indicator data for some variables, but have found carefully conducted studies of certain limited locations – cities, neighborhoods, or programs – within those countries. In such cases, can we meaningfully compare data from a neighborhood in one country with national-level indicator data from another?

Where both local and national data exist, the *within-nation* variance sometimes appears to exceed the *between-nation* variance. A good illustration is provided by data on the prevalence of the HIV infection (as measured by seropositivity) among intravenous drug users (IVDUs). There is enormous between-nation variance; in some nations less than five percent of IVDUs are infected; in others, as many as 50 percent are infected (Brenner Hernando-Briongos and Goos, 1991). But there is also tremendous variation across cities within the one nation. For example, Edinburgh has one of the highest rates in Europe, whereas London shows a fairly low rate. The United States also shows enormous variation; in New York the rate is close to 60 percent, whereas in San Francisco it is less than 10 percent. It is difficult to know the extent to which these figures reflect differences in formal policies, in local context, or accidental features of the spatial and temporal diffusion of the virus.

Another unit of analysis problem is the limitations inherent in the use of aggregate data. Aggregated data pose a risk of falling prey to the ecological fallacy – inferring an individual-level association from aggregate-level data (Langbein and Lichtman, 1978). This cuts two ways. We cannot assume that observed aggregate-level associations between policies and outcomes tell us something about how any given individual will respond to policy, nor can we assume that individual-level relationships observed in laboratory or survey research will be replicated at the between-nation level. Aggregate- and individual-level patterns may in fact coincide, but that can only be established empirically through research at both levels.

A final analytic problem is statistical power. When the unit of analysis is the nation, or even the city, it is extremely difficult to obtain an adequate number of observations to support statistical inference. Moreover, the host of variables we are attempting to study in each country guarantees that we will have more parameters than data

points, leaving insufficient degrees of freedom for deriving stable estimates. In principle, one can overcome the power problem by studying
more and more countries, but in practice, the scarcity of appropriate
data, the expense and difficulty of obtaining existing data and making it
usable, and the limited number of culturally and economically similar
nations all place a severe constraint on the number of comparisons that
can be made.

Conclusion: How Can Noisy Data Improve Policy Debates?

At this point, some readers may wonder whether we have backed into a
nihilistic position. Having criticized the overreliance upon casual cross-
national induction in drug policy debates, we have then listed a host of
methodological problems that pose serious difficulties for a more systematic empirical analysis. As historian Virginia Berridge has asked us,
'Are noisy data any better than anecdotes?' (personal commincation,
1992). We take this question sufficiently seriously such that we will conclude this essay by briefly arguing in the affirmative. There are three
major benefits to be derived from systematic cross-national research on
drug policy, even in the absence of more and better data.

The first benefit is new knowledge. Even with all the methodological
problems we have described, we have no doubt that systematic cross-
national research provides valuable new information about the policy-
outcome nexus. Some of this information is not necessarily statistical;
simply describing in more detail the content and implementation of
foreign drug policies is a positive contribution. But even bad outcome
data can tell us more about foreign drug problems than we currently
know. Unlike anecdotes about junkies and broken car windows, for
example, all but the noisiest of indicator data tell us something about
the general range and magnitude of outcomes. Even biased data can be
informative, provided we can identify the direction of the bias. For
example, if a given drug outcome indicator is biased downwards, it
provides a lower-bound estimate; if biased upwards, it gives us an
upper-bound estimate. Thus, even biased data can sometimes tell us
whether 'worst-case scenarios' are actually borne out in practice.

The second benefit is the potential for broadening the US debate
beyond supply-side/demand-side arguments. Comparative studies can
be used to break down the narrowness and ethnocentrism of US policy discourse by forcing a consideration of alternative perpectives and
novel interventions (Oppenheimer, 1992). European concepts like
'normalization' and 'harm reduction' are still not widely recognized in
the USA, but we believe they merit careful consideration, even if they
ultimately fail to garner widespread American support. They will not

receive that consideration unless their operation and consequences are systematically described and analysed.

The final benefit, we hope, is the stimulation and development of improved theory, measurement, and analysis of drug policies and problems. Comparative research makes painfully salient the inadequacy of current problem indicator data systems, particularly in Europe, but also in the USA. In particular, the notion of systematic repeated population surveys regarding drug use has been slow in coming in Europe but – it must be noted – is on the rise, so the future of cross-national comparisons is optimistic. Indeed, recent efforts by several international organizations, such as the newly launched European Drugs Observatory, suggest that investigators five years from now will no longer confront many of the data problems we have encountered in our research. Indeed, we hope that our results, once published, will stimulate new research, providing a target for future investigators who will correct our errors, provide more precise estimates, and detect patterns we failed to uncover. Such critical scrutiny represents scientific progress, so we will welcome it with enthusiasm.

References

Albrecht, H. J. and van Kalmhout, A. (Eds) (1989). *Drug Policies in Western Europe*. Freiburg: Max Planck Institute.

Brenner, H., Hernando-Briongos, P. and Goos, C. (1991). AIDS among drug users in Europe. *Drug and Alcohol Dependence*, **29**, 171–181.

Cook, T. D. and Campbell, D. T. (1979). *Quasi-experimentation: Design and Analysis Issues for Field Settings*. Boston: Houghton-Mifflin.

Grapendaal, M. (1992). Cutting their coat according to their cloth: Economic behavior of Amsterdam opiate users. *International Journal of the Addictions*, **27**, 487–501.

Haaga, J. and Reuter, P. (1991). *Improving Data for Federal Drug Policy Decisions*. Santa Monica, California: The RAND Corporation.

Kahan, J., Setear, J., Bitzinger, M., Coleman, S. and Feinleib, J. (1992). *Developing Games of Local Drug Policy*. Santa Monica, California: The RAND Corporation.

Klein, R. (1991). Risks and benefits of comparative studies: Notes from another shore. *The Millbank Quarterly*, **69**, 275–291.

Langbein, L. I. and Lichtman, A. J. (1978). *Ecological Inference*. Sage University Paper series on Quantitative Applications in the Social Sciences, 07–001. Beverly Hills: Sage Publications.

Laugesen, M. and Meads, C. (1991). Tobacco advertising restrictions, price, income, and tobacco consumption in OECD countries, 1960–1986. *British Journal of Addiction*, **86**, 1343–1354.

Leroy, B. (1992). The European community of twelve and the drug demand: Excerpt of a comparative study of legislations and judicial practice. *Drug and Alcohol Dependence*, **29**, 269–281.

Leuw, E. (1991). Drugs and drug policy in the Netherlands. In M. Tonry (Ed.), *Crime and Justice: A Review of Research*, Vol. 14, pp. 229–276. Chicago: University of Chicago Press.

MacCoun, R. J. (1993). Drugs and the law: A psychological analysis of drug prohibition. *Psychological Bulletin* 113, (in press).

Messner, S. F. (1992). Exploring the consequences of erratic data reporting for cross-national research on homicide. *Journal of Quantitative Criminology*, 8, 155–173.

National Centre for Epidemiology and Population Health (1991). *Feasibility Research into the Controlled Availability of Opioids*. Canberra: Australian National University NCEPH.

Oppenheimer, G. M. (1992). To build a bridge: The use of foreign models by domestic critics of US drug policy. *The Millbank Quarterly*, 69, 495–525.

Pompidou Group (1987). *Multi-city Study of Drug Misuse: Final Report*. Strasbourg, France: Council of Europe

Reuband, K. H. (1990). Research on drug use: A review of problems, needs, and future perspectives. *Drug and Alcohol Dependence*, 25, 149–152.

Reuter, P. (1984). The (continued) vitality of mythical numbers. *Public Interest*, 75, 135–147.

Reuter, P. (1992), Hawks ascendant: The punitive trend of drug policy, *Daedalus*, 121, 15–52.

Sidney, S. (1990). Evidence of discrepant data regarding trends in marijuana use and supply, 1985–1988. *Journal of Psychoactive Drugs*, 22, 319–324.

Smart, R. G. (1989). Is the postwar drinking binge ending? Cross-national trends in per capita alcohol consumption. *British Journal of Addiction*, 84, 743–748.

Chapter 10
Law Enforcement as a Harm-reduction Strategy in Rotterdam and Merseyside

DUNCAN CHAPPELL, TJIBBE REITSMA, DEREK O'CONNELL and HEATHER STRANG

Drug law enforcement policies and practices in the Netherlands and Britain demonstrate vividly the significance of both cultural values and accidents of history in the development and determination of social policies. Because of their colonial histories, both countries have had long experience with drug producing nations and with opium use. Both countries have been obliged to change their drug enforcement strategies since the dramatic upsurge in use and abuse in the 1960s, but have done so in a manner which reflects the predominant values of their societies. Each has also chosen to adopt less punitive policies towards drug dependent people than is the case in many other countries, whilst maintaining strong penalties for the manufacture and trafficking of illicit drugs. In doing so, the Netherlands and Britain have developed interesting models for the use of law enforcement as a harm-reduction strategy. These models are discussed in this chapter and their application is examined in two major metropolitan areas: Rotterdam in the Netherlands and Merseyside in Britain.

Dutch Policy and Practice

Prior to the 1960s, the use of opiates in the Netherlands was largely confined to small numbers of ethnic Chinese, a small group of health professionals and those who had become addicted following the prescription of opiates for medical use (Wijngaart, 1988a). During the 1960s, opium use spread into other social groups, especially middle-class youth, but demand for heroin remained low until 1972 when suddenly it became available at high purity and low price. Wijngaart (1988b) believes that this resulted from the targeting of Western Europe by drug traffickers following the collapse of lucrative drug markets in South-east Asia after the United States of America withdrew from Vietnam.

By 1977 it was estimated that there were 5000 heroin addicts in the Netherlands. That population is currently estimated at 15–20 000, and is believed to be stable, possibly declining and ageing. About 5000 addicts are believed to be in Amsterdam, and a further 3000 in Rotterdam. Currently, the Dutch drug scene is characterised by a stable heroin market, falling cannabis use and increasing use of cocaine and 'designer' drugs (Wardlaw, 1992).

Dutch legislation governing the availability and control of drugs differs little from most other countries, except for the distinction between cannabis and 'drugs presenting unacceptable risks', made in the 1976 amendments to the Opium Act, which is the legislative basis of current policy. It is rather in the application of its laws that the Netherlands has developed its own approach.

Drug abuse in the Netherlands is not seen as primarily a law enforcement problem, but rather as a matter affecting health and social well-being (Korthals Altes, 1987). The underlying principle in Dutch drug policy is the containment of the problem; the goal is not eradication of illicit drug use but rather harm minimisation. This is commonly described as 'normalisation', that is, demand reduction through the social integration of drug users (Van Vliet, 1989). The aim is to ensure that as many users as possible come into contact with welfare/treatment agencies; currently it is estimated that around 70 per cent of users do so (Marshall, Anjewierden and Van Atteveld, 1990). Thus, the policy is to overlook the technical criminality of use in order to make services as accessible as possible and to ensure that drug users are not caused more harm by the criminal justice process than by the use of the drugs themselves.

The Dutch prefer to use the criminal law to the least extent possible in dealing with drug *users* and this is particularly exemplified in the policy of *de facto* decriminalisation of the use and sale of small quantities of cannabis. This has been achieved through prosecutorial guidelines issued in accord with the 'expediency principle' contained in the Dutch Code of Criminal Procedure, which allows the Public Prosecutions Department the discretionary power to refrain from bringing criminal proceedings (Wardlaw, 1992). This principle has been used as well in the development of national guidelines on the intensity of police investigation, the use of police custody, prosecutorial alternatives and penalties for different substances in different circumstances which are set out in the 1976 Opium Act Guidelines. There is widespread recognition that the criminal law is limited in its effectiveness regarding any aspect of the problem other than trafficking and the manufacturing of drugs. This is where enforcement efforts are concentrated, in a manner very much in line with other countries.

The Rotterdam Situation

Rotterdam is the Netherlands's second largest city, with a population of nearly 600 000 in a nation of 15 million people. Within the context of overall Dutch drug policy, individual jurisdictions such as Rotterdam exercise a good deal of autonomy. The Rotterdam Council receives grants for the conduct of its drug programmes from the central government; this is supplemented from the Council's own finances.

Local drug policy is balanced cooperatively between the city's police force and five private foundations which are entirely funded through the Council and which offer medical and welfare assistance to addicts. These foundations are overseen by the Public Health Service, which employs a drug coordinator to advise the City Council. The Service is also responsible for the Rotterdam Drug Information System, which contains anonymous data on all addicts seeking assistance from the foundations.

The City Council is aided in its decision making on drug policy and programming by an advisory committee which consists of the directors of the five foundations, representatives of the police, the Public Prosecutor's office, the Social Service department and the director of the local prison. The Council annually revises its drug policy programme on a detailed basis, including the resourcing and responsibilities of each foundation.

The police role in the administration of drug policy towards drug dependent people in Rotterdam is completely integrated with other agencies. The 'harm reduction' principle in the police context means that trafficking is pursued whilst the drug user is left alone as much as possible. This applies to both 'hard' and 'soft' users and low level dealers. Only if they cause 'unacceptable annoyance' to other citizens, especially in residential areas, do the police take action. The view is that drug addiction is no excuse for socially unacceptable behaviour.

In large cities such as Rotterdam, concentrations of users tend to be quite visible in certain locations, such as the central railway station. In response to this, a special police station has been opened, which offers methadone, needle exchange and other facilities in association with welfare agencies. Thus police are in close and constant communication with users.

Where arrest becomes necessary, methadone is available via the police physician if the user is detained longer than six hours. Considerable emphasis is placed on local knowledge by individual police officers in their day-to-day relations with users, whilst responsibility for dealing with large scale drug trafficking is assigned to special drug enforcement units in the large cities.

Thus police in Rotterdam, as elsewhere in the Netherlands, are part of an integrated, multidisciplinary team, who all share the goal of containing the illicit drug problem and ensuring that addicts are 'normalised' rather than marginalised through their illicit activities. There is, however, an obvious paradox in what is expected of police officers in such a regime; on the one hand, they must adhere to a vigorous policy of combatting drug trafficking and drug-related crime; on the other, they must cooperate with health and welfare agencies in the implementation of a policy where users of these very same drugs are dealt with as rarely as possible by the criminal justice system. This paradox places considerable strain on police who are constantly making difficult judgments about what is tolerable and what is not. Drug enforcement policy at the local level requires a continuous process of decision-making by police as to what measures need to be taken, what their aim should be and what problems they are intended to solve. It is a credit to the pragmatism of the Dutch that although the illicit drug problem has not been solved – it was never expected to be – it is controlled to the extent that, compared with other European countries, it is seen to be at an acceptable level (Visser, 1992). The balancing act continues.

British Policy and Practice

Historically, opiates have been widely used in Britain and for most of the nineteenth century they were freely available over the counter. As the medical profession asserted its authority, however, the disease theory of drug misuse became more influential and underpinned the move towards the control of drugs, but through medical rather than penal provisions (Wardlaw, 1992). The Rolleson Report (1926) legitimised the disease concept of opiate addiction and of maintenance prescribing, which was the basis of the 'British system' until the 1960s, although it should be noted that law enforcement has been used throughout this century against non-dependent opiate users and against users of other drugs.

Maintenance prescribing of heroin continued until the 1960s and worked well while there were only a few hundred addicts. The situation changed dramatically in the course of the 1960s, however, when the prescribing by naive or unscrupulous doctors of large quantities of heroin to a relatively small number of users and dealers effectively destroyed the 'British system' as it then operated (Judson, 1974). The most significant change was the withdrawal of the right to prescribe except by doctors with a special licence, most of whom worked in the National Health Service Drug Dependence Units. With the introduction of methadone programmes in the 1970s, the prescribing of heroin became increasingly uncommon, and for all practical purposes it no longer exists in Britain. Even in the Liverpool Drug Dependency Clinic, whose programme is led by Dr John Marks, a prominent and continuing advocate of maintenance prescribing, only five out of over 1000 patients between 1985 and 1987 were prescribed heroin (Fazey, 1988).

British government drug policy direction in the late 1970s and early 1980s moved towards the American 'war on drugs' model, with associated increases in law enforcement expenditure, tougher legislation and sentencing policies, and a strong anti-heroin media campaign. One consequence of these changes was a shift away from the domination of the medical profession in the drugs discourse (Strang, 1992).

However, through the 1980s, policy direction changed again: the increasing involvement of a diversity of agencies and professions in the drugs area and the emergence of AIDS as a serious health issue have gradually led to the *de facto* development of the 'harm minimisation' principle. Indeed, the Advisory Council on the Misuse of Drugs (1988) declared that 'the spread of HIV is a greater danger to individual and public health than drugs misuse' (p. 17). Thus a hierarchy of concerns developed about the misuse of drugs, and the containment of HIV became the stated priority.

The Merseyside Situation

The county of Merseyside is situated in the north-west of England and has a population of 1.4 million. It is a densely populated region whose major city is Liverpool, the UK's fourth largest port. Liverpool is the headquarters for Merseyside's nearly 5000 police officers.

Although government policy in relation to the misuse of drugs is broadly enunciated, central Government in the UK does not play as crucial a role in controlling strategy as is the case in many other countries. Individual police forces have always had a good deal of autonomy in how they chose to deal with the problem. Strategy on drug issues, and many others, is decided by the individual Chief Constables of each region. In 1986, Merseyside Police introduced a strategy which has been termed 'Responsible Demand Enforcement'. This means rigorous policing at the dealer level, whilst for the user a completely different policy operates.

Merseyside Police, like their Dutch counterparts, recognise that some level of drug misuse is inevitable and cooperate with local health authorities in the operation of a harm reduction policy which permits flexibility in the way in which enforcement is carried out (Wardlaw, 1992). The Mersey Health Authority places great emphasis on their needle exchange programmes, and agreement was reached that police would not carry out any activity near the clinics or prosecute for possession of drug paraphernalia. In addition, the police agreed to provide everyone arrested or detained (not only for drug offences) with literature advising on drug clinics where assistance with drug problems could be sought.

Prior to 1986, crime in the Merseyside region had been increasing.

As a consequence of the introduction of the policy of responsible demand reduction, both the street demand for heroin and drug-related crime began to fall. Importantly, Merseyside became the region with the lowest HIV figures in the United Kingdom, and that remains the case. Merseyside currently has the highest concentration of registered drug users and their average age is over 25 and getting older, clearly illustrating the success of the policy.

Other areas of Britain have now implemented similar initiatives with the same positive results, whilst the police themselves feel more comfortable in the good working relationships they have created with medical and welfare agencies. Overall, heroin demand has continued to fall but other illicit drugs, especially amphetamines, cocaine and MDMA ('Ecstasy') are now emerging as a problem. Merseyside Police are now consulting with the various agencies in preparing an initiative aimed at these particular substances.

Commentary

In many countries, including Australia, the debate about strategies to deal with the problem of illicit drug use has tended to revolve around the question of demand reduction versus supply reduction. Law enforcement programmes and policies have usually been conceptualised purely in terms of their role in supply reduction, and have frequently been subjected to severe criticism for their failure to contain drug abuse (Wardlaw, 1992). It has not generally been recognised that this failure is a consequence of unrealistic expectations on the part of governments and communities concerning what law enforcement can achieve to this end.

As a result of this perceived failure of supply reduction strategies, there have been moves in some countries to direct law enforcement efforts more towards demand reduction. This has involved much closer collaboration between police, education, prevention and treatment agencies. Police in Rotterdam and Merseyside have undertaken a crucial and pioneering role in the implementation of this new enforcement policy direction.

In both the United Kingdom and the Netherlands, local authorities, including police, are able to exercise a great deal of autonomy in the provision of services. Such autonomy does not exist in Australia, for example, though the existence of the federally-funded National Campaign Against Drug Abuse (NCADA) provides a level of consistency in drug policy development between the eight Australian jurisdictions which has proven very successful.

NCADA's stated aim is 'to minimise the harmful effects of drugs on Australian society' through a variety of educational, treatment and law enforcement strategies. It is governed by the Ministerial Council on

Drug Strategy, consisting of law enforcement and health ministers from all Australian jurisdictions. As might be expected, differences do arise from time to time between medical and policing objectives, and the emotional nature of the drug debate and its highly political nature mean that there exists in Australia great difficulty in discussing alternative policies.

An example of the difficulty in achieving such rational debate about strategies differing significantly from the mainstream has been the problems surrounding the proposal to conduct a feasibility study into the provision of opioids to heroin-dependent people in the Australian Capital Territory (ACT) (National Centre for Epidemiology and Population Health, 1991). Issues involved in this proposal are being researched jointly by the Australian National University's National Centre for Epidemiology and Population Health and the Australian Institute of Criminology (see Chapter 12, this volume).

The first stage of this study aimed to determine whether a trial to provide opioids, particularly heroin, in a controlled manner was feasible in principle. After a detailed examination of all the issues, it was decided that, even though many problems would need to be resolved, a trial was feasible and that a proposal should be developed for the structuring of such a trial.

The proposal has been endorsed by police officers expert in both Dutch and Merseyside drug policing strategies (Lofts, 1992; Penrose, 1992; Visser, 1992), but remains controversial as far as Australian police are concerned. Reaction has varied from outright rejection by the former New South Wales Police Minister, Mr Pickering, to strong support by the Tasmanian Police Commissioner, Mr Johnson (Bammer and Gerrard, 1992).

One of the obvious conclusions to be made when examining the range of possible policing strategies is the need for policies regarding illicit drugs – and all other areas of social policy-making – to be congruent with other features of the society for which they are designed. The strategies adopted in Rotterdam exist in the context of a society traditionally tolerant of differences, with lower expectations of law enforcement intervention in illegal activities than is the case in Australia. For example, one of the major concerns regarding the proposed ACT opioid study relates to the consequent likelihood of an increased visibility of a drug problem known to exist but presently able to be largely ignored by the community generally. It is irrelevant to be judgmental towards Australian society's reaction to the possibility of policing practices which now exist in Rotterdam and Merseyside: it is, however, vital to take such reactions into account.

Like the Netherlands, Australia has explicitly stated that its aim is the minimalisation of the harmful effects of drugs on society rather than the eradication of illicit drugs (Wardlaw, 1992). Problems with interpretation of this statement exist, however, and law enforcement and treatment agencies have chosen to define harm minimalisation in different ways. The opportunity exists, nonetheless, for the experiences of Rotterdam and Merseyside to be incorporated into the ongoing development of Australian drug policing policy. Their successes are evident; it remains for their practices to be adopted to the local scene in common sense ways.

References

Advisory Council on the Misuse of Drugs (1988). *AIDS and Drug Misuse*. Part 1. London: HMSO.

Bammer, G. and Gerrard, G. (Eds) (1992). *Heroin treatment: New Alternatives*. Proceedings of a Seminar held 1 November 1991. Canberra: National Centre for Epidemiology and Population Health.

Fazey, C. (1988). *The Evaluation of Liverpool Drug Dependency Clinic: The First Two Years 1985–87*, Research Evaluation and Data Analysis, Liverpool.

Judson, H. F. (1974). *Heroin Addiction in Britain: What Americans can Learn from the English Experience*, New York: Harcourt Brace Jovanovich.

Korthals Altes, F. (Dutch Minister of Justice) (1987). Drug policy in the Netherlands. Paper presented at the International Conference on Drug Abuse and Illicit Trafficking, United Nations, Vienna.

Lofts, M. (1992). Policing the Merseyside drug treatment programme: The Cheshire Experience. In G. Bammer and G. Gerrard (Eds). *Heroin Treatment: New Alternatives*. Proceedings of a Seminar held 1 November, 1991. Canberra: National Centre for Epidemiology and Population Health.

Marshall, I. H., Anjewierden, O. and Van Atteveld, H. (1990). Towards an 'Americanization' of Dutch drug policy? *Justice Quarterly*, 7, 391–420.

National Centre for Epidemiology and Population Health (1991). *Feasibility Research into the Controlled Availability of Opioids*. Canberra: Australian National University.

Penrose, R. (1992). Experiences and developments of the drug misuse strategy within the 'British system. In G. Bammer and G. Gerrard (Eds). *Heroin Treatment: New Alternatives*. Proceedings of a Seminar held 1 November, 1991. *Canberra: National Centre for Epidemiology and Population Health.*

Rolleston Report (1926). *Report of the Departmental Committee on Morphine and Heroin Addiction*. London: HMSO.

Strang, H. (1992). Education. In *Comparative Analysis of Illicit Drug Strategy* (National Campaign Against Drug Abuse Monograph Series No. 18). Canberra: AGPS.

Van Vliet, H. J. (1989). Drug policy as a management strategy: some experiences from the Netherlands. *International Journal on Drug Policy*, 1, 27–29.

Visser, B. (1992). In search of a balance between repression (enforcement) and normalisation. In G. Bammer and G. Gerrard (Eds). *Heroin Treatment: New Alternatives*. Proceedings of a Seminar held 1 November, 1991. Canberra: National Centre for Epidemiology and Population Health.

Wardlaw, G. (1992). Overview of national drug control strategies. In *Comparative Analysis of Illicit Drug Strategy* (National Campaign Against Drug Abuse Monograph Series No. 18). Canberra: AGPS.

Wijngaart, G. F. van de (1988a). A social history of drug use in the Netherlands: Policy outcomes and implications. *Journal of Drug Issues*, 18, 481–495.

Wijngaart, G. F. van de (1988b). Heroin use in the Netherlands. *American Journal of Drug and Alcohol Abuse*, 14, 125–136.

Chapter 11
Prohibition as a Necessary Stage in the Acculturation of Foreign Drugs

ERIK FROMBERG

No human society exists where no psychoactive drug or drugs are taken. Intoxication seems to be a universal human need (Siegel, 1989; Szasz, 1975). Whether Fijians drinking kava, Mongolian shamaans using the fly agaric, khat-chewing Yemenis or Westerners drinking alcohol, members of all human cultures have found ways to alter their minds by the use of pyschoactive substances. No culture exists that denies the right to intoxication altogether.

This does not mean that this right can be exercised under all circumstances; the use of a local psychoactive substance is always surrounded by a number of written and unwritten rules that regulate its use. The kind of drug being locally used is dependent on what nature, albeit occasionally with a little help, has to offer and has to do with its pharmacological properties, assuming that it is psychoactive. The inhabitants of some regions of the world, like South America, are provided by nature with large numbers of plants containing psychoactive drugs, while others, like Europeans, have pitifully few and so have had to resort to the fermentation of grapes or barley (the Mongolians even to the fermenting of mare's milk) to obtain alcohol.

So every culture developed its own ways to handle its drugs, ways that are products of a co-evolution of the society and the naturally available drugs, in the same way that orchids and their pollinators are products of co-evolution.

When societies are suddenly confronted with a new drug, they have no previously developed sociocultural rules to regulate its use. The result is often unchecked use, which can have a highly destructive effect on a large number of members of that society. The introduction of alcohol among Indian tribes in the USA or among Inuit in Canada and Greenland may not be good examples of this, as the role of alcohol-pushing arms peddlers may obscure the true picture, but the sudden availability of large amounts of alcohol in concentrated form due to the industrial application of the distillation process in western Europe and the availability of heroin in South-east Asia are good examples. Although heroin appeared in these countries only after opium became repressed (Westermeyer, 1976), societal regulations that governed the use of opium in these societies did not function with regard to heroin, in the same way that rules applying to beer and wine did not, at least for a time, function for spirits.

Sometimes these effects can be mitigated; when the new drug in question is introduced as part of a complete new and dominant culture, the rules of this new culture can be taken over as well. When, on the other hand, it is just the drug which is introduced, no existing rules apply and the drug can have very negative effects on society, independent of its pharmacological properties.

Socio-immunology

There is an old Dutch saying '*Wat de boer niet kent, lust hij niet*', literally translated as 'What the farmer does not know, he dislikes'. This saying illustrates an inborn fear of new things. New things can be dangerous and the carefulness that results from this fear has an important survival value – so important that it is deeply rooted in all vertebrate brains. It is thus considerably deeper rooted than its surface layer, the cerebral cortex, and as such hardly under rational control. This behavioural pattern is observable not only in individuals, but also at the level of whole societies.

Societies are not simple collections of human individuals, but collections of humans sharing more or less the same values and norms. These norms cement the interdependent individuals into a society. In this sense, a society can also be considered as an organism. Societies reject things that are opposed to societal norms, the reaction being a kind of immunological reaction. Once individuals act contrary to societal norms, this behaviour provokes fear and rejection not because of the intrinsic behaviour, which may be as innocent as the sudden wearing of long hair by males over thirty years ago, but because this behaviour attacks the glue that holds individuals together in a society – the norms and values. Societies defend themselves against behaviour that is considered anti-social. In this way, deviant behaviour provokes a kind of socio-immunological reaction.

One of the norms that seems to govern our Western, predominantly Christian society is that chemical happiness is something to be avoided at all price, unless obtained by the drug that has been used in Europe since times immemorial: alcohol. Other drugs such as coffee and tobacco have, indeed, somehow been integrated in our culture, but only after a period of social disapproval, if not prohibition (Van de Wijngaart, 1991). Thus the use of psychoactive substances other than those 'belonging' to our culture can be thought of as an alien agent provoking socio-immunological defence reactions.

Prohibition as an Allergy

The first stage of defence of the society against any new agent, in this case drugs, is social disapproval, this being the equivalent of a normal immunological defence. The more legalistic a society is, the more this social disapproval tends to prohibitionism. In other words, the more that formal law is considered the ultimate expression of societal values, the more prohibitionist the societal reaction. The social disapproval reaction of society is not different in nature from our body's reaction when a foreign protein enters and can be regarded as a normal socio-immunological reaction.

However, in the human body, useful, protective immunological reactions can become counterproductive in two different ways: as an allergy and as autoimmune disease. Allergies are conditions in which our defence system mobilises and attacks harmless intruders (hay fever being an example, where the sufferer's immune system attacks completely harmless pollen); autoimmune diseases are conditions in which our defence system against foreign proteins does not recognize our own proteins and attacks them as if they were foreign.

Every immunological reaction implies a state of war. In an allergy, the organism fights a harmless enemy; in an autoimmune disease the organism fights a war against itself. In both cases, a lot of energy is spent without reason. In the latter case one harms oneself directly, and in the former case one loses a lot of energy that could be used for better things (better in terms of survival) and harms oneself secondarily too. The present 'war on drugs' combines aspects of both conditions. To explain this, let us first return to society as a organism.

As described above, the reaction to drugs, defined as foreign psychoactive substances, starts as 'normal' social disproval and prohibition, the normal immunological reaction to foreign invaders. In this situation, the prohibition is simply a measure that can be evaluated for its effectiveness in protecting the society against the foreign invader.

However, if the society is very legalistic, this is not sufficient; the foreign agent, even if innocuous, must be attacked, even if this turns out to be ineffective. Users are criminalised because the agent has to be fought. Effectiveness is not a measure; it is the principle that counts. In this sense, the prohibition being enforced is more an allergy than a normal reaction. As in all allergies, more damage is done by the defence reaction than the foreign agent could ever do. The drugs we fight are harmless compared to those we accept, such as alcohol and tobacco. Every physician can easily explain that alcohol is much more toxic than, for example, heroin, but this does not prevent many physicians from being comparatively heavy drinkers and from supporting the war against heroin. They show the over-reaction that is typical of an allergy. This defensive reaction of society provokes secondary reactions, such as secondary deviance and other inflammatory symptoms.

The War on Drugs: An Autoimmune Disease

Now, autoimmune diseases, according to present-day medical knowledge, start by fighting an external invader that becomes connected in some way to one's own proteins, which only then are attacked as a consequence of this connection. In our case, the foreign invader 'drugs' became somehow connected to one's own societal imperatives and the defence, prohibition, starts to attack society itself; the 'war on drugs' is an autoimmune disease.

How has the social rejection of drug use become attached to our society's central values to produce such an autoimmune disease? This attachment originates in other aims being served by the identification of drugs as 'devilish' compounds, not to be compared with the psychoactive compounds that the society is accustomed to. Actually, 'drugs' become the scapegoat for all things that go wrong in our society. The American dream has never been fulfilled, not even when communism ceased to be a threat, so drugs must be the cause and the war rethoric goes on. To a lesser extent the social democratic ideal has not produced the society western Europe believes in; drugs must be the cause. In this way the link is created between the foreign invader and our own society to produce the autoimmune disease. This turns an allergy into an autoimmune disease.

The symptoms of this disease can be observed in the corruption of other central values of our society, as in the conduct of our law system by undercover operations, the criminalizing of our children, the financial corruption created by a black market etc.

However, allergies do not have to be fatal and Europe, which has not as yet fully entered the war on drugs, does not yet show the symptoms of a fully fledged autoimmune disease. We might say it is in a state of allergy. Now, allergies may disappear with time, as though the body learns that the allergy-causing agent is not as threatening as it supposed. The body adapts to the presence of the agent. Anti-allergic treatment can stimulate this process and it is here that our rational capacity can and has to play an important role. Europe still has the possibility of adapting our immune reaction to reasonable proportions, and reducing the inflammation step by step without disrupting the fabric of our society. Let us consider the process from allergy to adaptation.

Treatment: From Prohibition to Acculturation

A new drug enters a society by being used by a small number of people, who will immediately form a subset or subculture. Let us say this is the cradle of infection. Then the immunological reaction starts: prohibition. The result will be marginalisation and criminalisation of this subset on one hand and protection of the majority on the other. As we have seen, when prohibition is an end in itself, the result is allergy and autoimmune disease. However, prohibition may also be considered as a means. In this case, we can treat the condition. In order to do that, we first have to realise that prohibition has never succeeded, so cannot be an end. Secondly, we acknowledge the positive and negative sides of prohibition as a means. In this phase we start 'harm reduction' for the user group. We reduce the inflammation. The perception that prohibition cannot succeed makes us realise that we have to adapt to the situation that drugs exist and will be used, and that finding ways to handle this is the goal of our policy. The drug has to be acculturated; the culture has to find ways to regulate its use in such a way that as little harm is done as possible.

Actually, the only group that can devise ways to handle the drug is the user group itself. Users are members of the dominant culture on the one hand, but are more or less ostracized by the non-using majority. So the government has to protect them. This process is heavily hampered by the fact that the user group often will not be a real elite and from the point of view of the society as a whole could never have been an example for other individuals.

Nevertheless, the user group is the nucleus that has to develop patterns of regulation and sociocultural norms that enable it to regulate use. These norms, however, will be highly subculturally defined, mainly due to the marginalisation of the user group. But as prohibition slowly lessens, this marginalisation is reduced and the norms regulating use will become more and more derived from the cultural values of mainstream society and less and less from subcultural values. The Dutch cannabis policy may demonstrate this process.

The Dutch Cannabis Experience

The use of cannabis is nothing new in the Netherlands or in the Western World. In the nineteenth century, many European and American patent medicines contained cannabis, mostly as the alcoholic extract, cannabis-tincture. Although their use was labelled medical, these potions were freely available; no legal controls existed. This was not abnormal; pharmacists in the Western World produced many potions containing psychoactive drugs, the cocaine-containing *Vin mariani* being just one other well-known example. The use of these potions diminished as stricter controls were imposed on medicines, not primarily to reduce their use, but as protection for the medical and pharmaceutical professions. This made the use of cannabis more or less disappear.

Cannabis reappeared in public in the low countries in the late 1950s, not least through the actions of the Dutch poet, Simon Vinkenoog who became familiar with it in Parisian jazz clubs. Use was at first confined to highly elite circles or young artists and students in Amsterdam and attracted little attention. At first, the Dutch police did not react, probably as a result of their experiences with the use of opium among the Chinese in Amsterdam and Rotterdam which was tolerated. This was possible because the Dutch law system is opportunistic; the public prosecutor is not obliged to prosecute as in legalistic law systems, but only prosecutes as he sees reason to do so. The Dutch apply the penal code not as an end but as a means of social control. As opium smoking within the Chinese community posed no problems, the public prosecutor and the police saw no reason to interfere, however illegal the use might have been.

When smoking marijuana became more common in the early 1960s, it drew attention from the medical profession, and a small group of conservative doctors, started a vehement crusade. This was picked up quickly by the public prosecutors, especially as tabloid papers such as the *Telegraaf* took up the crusade. This resulted in Vinkenoog being sentenced to nine months jail for the possession of two-and-half grams of marijuana. This may be considered normal in countries such as the USA and the UK, but already in the early 1960s this sentence was considered draconian by many Dutch people, not least by many judges who were confronted with accusations against their sons' friends and who quickly realised that the penalties they gave inflicted more harm than the use of the drug itself. So, in the mid-1960s, a public debate raged on the use of drugs, especially cannabis, that went undecided for some years. During that time the number of cannabis users increased. Smoking cannabis became nationally and internationally a passport that showed one belonged to a group of people that would change the world: the hippies. Smoking pot became the equivalent of revolt. The norms regulating cannabis use were derived from this subculture and had nothing to do with mainstream society.

The stalemate between drug 'hawks' and 'doves' was broken when, in around 1970, a Rotterdam hashish dealer was caught in the possession of a couple of hundred kilograms and was subsequently acquitted. The prosecutors' witness, the director of the National Forensic Laboratory, could not prove that the hashish seized answered the description of hashish given by our Narcotic Law that dated from 1928. This was not only true for the seized hashish but for all hashish, so the 'hawks' started to press for a change of legislation as much as the 'doves'.

To solve the problem, the government assembled an advisory committee called, after its presiding member, the Baan Committee, that reported in 1972 (Baan, 1972) and recommended the decriminalization of the possession of drugs for personal use. Comparable committees set up at the same time in Canada (the Le Dain Committee) and the USA (the Shafer Committee) reached the same conclusions. However, while in these countries the reports disappeared into oblivion and were being negated by their governments, the Dutch Ministerial Council discussed the Baan Report and at first voted by majority for the complete legalisation of cannabis (I. Vorrinck, at that time, Minister of Public Health, personal communication). It was because of heavy pressure from the Ministries of Foreign Affairs and Economic Affairs that this was not realized. Their argument against complete legalisation was that the Netherlands already had an isolated position with regard to the Israeli–Arab conflict (it was at the time of the first oil crisis) and could not afford an isolated position in another area.

As a compromise, they decided cannabis should be defined as a drug whose use was considered an acceptable risk (a soft drug) as opposed to all the other drugs whose use was at the time considered an unacceptable risk (hard drugs). According to the new narcotic law, the maximum penalties for trade in hashish were significantly lower than for hard drugs. Moreover the possession of cannabis for personal use became a misdemeanor. The amount to be considered as for personal use was put at 30 grams, not by law but by a directive of the Prosecutor General. This finally became law in 1976, but the government's proposal of the law in 1973 had already ended the first phase of Dutch policy: the phase of criminalisation by prohibition. As far as I know, since 1976 no one has been prosecuted for simple possession for personal use of cannabis.

Cannabis use was recognized as something different from hard drug use in the eyes of the Dutch general public. It was and still is socially rejected by large parts of the population, but a sustained allergic reaction was prevented. Now a phase of desensitization could follow.

The next development was that within certain youth centres where drug use took place, so called 'house dealers' were set up to fight market adulteration and the sale of hard drugs such as the heroin that had entered Europe in 1972 (courtesy of CIA involvement in the 'Golden Triangle'). A cannabis dealer that was trusted by the staff of such a centre was allowed to sell hashish without police interference. Certainly, there were prosecutions when this practice started but these have resulted in a general acceptance of the system. In this way, the retail trade in hashish and marijuana, however illegal, became a tolerated thing, albeit only inside certain establishments such as the Melweg, Paradiso and many other youth centres where the trade was under control of the staff.

This defined the second stage in which use became further regulated and private retail sale became more or less accepted. In this way, use was accepted within limits, in these youth centres, and as a result sub-cultural norms waned and mainstream norms waxed. The general public lost interest because the use disappeared from sight. No more dark dealers at Dam square hissing 'Hash, hash'; retail was cleanly organised in the youth centres out of sight.

The third stage, going public, started when Mellow Yellow, the first 'coffeeshop', opened in Amsterdam. Now retail trade took place in the open. No entrance fee for entering a youth centre is necessary; you simply walk in, choose the cannabis brand you like, buy an amount (generally either for DFl 10 or DFl 25) and walk out. Even drinking coffee is not necessary although most coffeeshops have their regulars for whom the shop is a social centre, like any decent public house.

After some uncertainty this practice was also tolerated. Under a central directive of the Prosecutor General, which is known as the AHOY, direct public retail sale of cannabis was declared tolerable. The limits to tolerance were defined by AHOY which stands for: no Advertising, no Hard drugs, no *Overlast* (Dutch for hindrance to the general public) and no Youth (youth being defined as under 16, this being the same age required for the buying of alcohol). The number of coffeeshops has since grown steadily to a current estimate of 1500, about one fifth of them in Amsterdam (Kuipers, 1991a).

The Future

There are presently three factors that will bring an end to this phase: (1) the increased need for local governments to regulate coffeeshops; (2) the perception by some that the internationally operating wholesale dealers are involved in other criminal behaviour than the cannabis trade; and (3) the European unification as embodied by the Schengen Treaty.

Although the number of Dutch cannabis users has not changed significantly over the last 15 years, life-time incidence fluctuating round 10% of the population as a whole (Kuipers, 1991b), the trade has changed first by an increasing number of foreigners buying cannabis in the Netherlands, and secondly by an increasing transfer to other countries. The latter is not primarily due to the different policy of our country, but is merely the consequence of the fact that the Netherlands (with Rotterdam harbour as the biggest in the world) is the largest single transfer site in Europe for all goods, whether legal or illegal.

Another, more recent development is a continuously increasing production of high quality cannabis in the country, which is now rated by some as the fifth or sixth greatest cash crop. It should however be noted that, up to now, this local production is hardly at all exported but is substituting for the importation of marijuana from the classic producing countries. Thus, the cannabis trade has become an important, however illegal, economic activity which can in no way be regulated, as other trades are, in terms of quality control, price and taxation.

A number of coffeeshops have become involved in the export trade on the kilogram level, while others, especially in the regions near the borders, are also attracting even larger numbers of clients from the neighbouring European countries who buy at the 10 gram level. This market is regarded negatively by the local population and the municipal governments, who feel, however, unable to regulate the situation if only on technical grounds: the AHOY directive turns out to be very difficult to apply. So local governments feel the need for control over coffeeshops, which can only be realised by some sort of formal legalisation. This is reinforced by the opinion of virtually all Dutch police officers involved with narcotics that bringing cannabis under the narcotic laws has been an historical error and that legislation more or less according to the alcohol laws would be much more effective (Fromberg, 1993).

The Dutch Institute for Alcohol and Drugs, NIAD, has recently prepared a proposal for such a law based on the understanding that local production and sale of cannabis under State control could be a way out of the above problems. In this way, we could on the one hand, reduce harm to individual users and, on the other, to society as a whole by continuing to fight international crime (if it turns out to really exist in this area). Recently a high level public servant responsible for our drug and alcohol policy spoke out publicly for the legalisation of cannabis production in the Netherlands. Pressure from other countries to adhere to their policies, embodied in the Single Convention, will probably have an adverse effect, reinforcing the Dutch determination not to enter the 'War on Drugs' in the American manner. Experience has shown that there are more efficient ways to handle these matters. After 30 years of a formal prohibition that was gradually weakened, legalisation of cannabis is possible without risking a significant increase in use or other strong, negative societal reactions. This is due to the gradual desensitisation of our society to the cannabinoid agent.

References

Baan, P. A. H. (1972). *Achtergronden en Risico's van Druggebruik*. Staatsuitgeverij, Den Haag: Staatsuitgeverij.

Fromberg, E. (1993). *Verslag Rechercheconferentie Inzake Koffieshops*. Utrecht: NIAD, in press.

Kuipers, H. (1991a). *Enquete onder Politie naar Koffieshops*. Utrecht: NIAD.

Kuipers, H. (1991b). *De Prevelentie van Cannabisgebruik in Nederland. Voordracht op een Rechercheconferentie*. Utrecht: NIAD.

Siegel, R. K. (1989). *Intoxication: Life in Pursuit of Artificial Paradise*. New York: E.P. Dutton.

Szasz, J. (1975). *Ceremonial Chemistry: The Ritual Persecution of Drug Addicts and Pushers*. London: Routledge and Kegan Paul.

Van de Wijngaart, G. (1991). *Competing Perspectives on Drug Use*. Lisse: Lisse and Zeitlinger.

Westermeyer, J. (1976). The pro-heroin effects of anti-opium laws. *Archives of General Psychiatry*, **33**, 1135–1139.

Chapter 12
A Heroin Trial for the Australian Capital Territory? An Overview of Feasibility Research

GABRIELE BAMMER, BOB DOUGLAS, MICHAEL MOORE and DUNCAN CHAPPELL

Introduction

In 1991 the National Centre for Epidemiology and Population Health (NCEPH), in collaboration with the Australian Institute of Criminology (AIC), conducted the first stage of an investigation into the feasibility of a trial to provide opioids, including heroin, to dependent users in a controlled manner. The research was undertaken at the request of the Select Committee on HIV, Illegal Drugs and Prostitution which was established by the Australian Capital Territory (ACT) Legislative Assembly. It was found that the proposal was feasible in principle and recommended that the research move to a second stage, an investigation of logistic feasibility. Research for Stage 2 began in 1992. The research conducted in Stage 1 and proposed for Stage 2 is outlined here, along with the political background to these considerations and a brief examination of current knowledge about drug use in the ACT.

Political Context

In the last 20 years there has been a series of reports on drugs and drug dependency produced by various Australian government-sponsored committees, Royal Commissions and inquiries. In essence, the reports have shown a good deal of consensus on the nature of the problem and appropriate ways of dealing with it, with recommendations focusing on education, treatment and law enforcement. Since 1977 the reports have argued for harm minimisation rather than the elimination of drug use. Only some of the reports considered heroin maintenance for dependent individuals and they generally argued against it, but one called for research using a limited trial (Committee of Inquiry into the Legal Provision of Heroin, 1981). It should be noted, however, that the context in which most of these deliberations took place was rather different from that existing now, particularly as

HIV/AIDS was not an issue until the most recent report. Every report lamented the lack of empirical information on which to base decisions and called for informed public debate and more research (Hartland, 1991; Hartland et al., 1992).

In 1989, the government of the ACT appointed a select committee to inquire into and report on HIV, illegal drugs and prostitution in the Territory with particular reference to:

> (a) The effectiveness of current legal and social controls enabling action to prevent the spread of HIV; (b) the effectiveness of current legal controls on prostitution and drug-taking; (c) alternative social, medical or legal proposals which may assist in restricting the further spread of HIV; and (d) other such matters relating to the issues of HIV in the ACT which the committee considers should be drawn to the attention of the Assembly.
>
> *(Legislative Assembly for the Australian Capital Territory, Select Committee on HIV, Illegal Drugs and Prostitution, 1991, p. iii)*

This was a tripartite committee, with representatives from both major political parties (the Australian Labor Party and the Liberal Party of Australia) and it was chaired by an independent member, Mr Michael Moore.

The Select Committee was particularly influenced in its deliberations by information provided by practitioners and administrators in the Merseyside area of the United Kingdom that prescription of heroin to people registered as being addicted to that drug had beneficial effects in reducing crime and improving quality of life. This was obtained by the chairman of the committee when he attended the first International Conference on the Reduction of Drug-related Harm held in Liverpool in April 1990. The committee also found advocates among Australian practitioners for a trial 'to assess the impact of a policy shift towards the controlled availability of heroin to people already dependent on that drug' (Legislative Assembly for the Australian Capital Territory, Select Committee on HIV, Illegal Drugs and Prostitution, 1991, p. 2). These practitioners were particularly concerned to find more effective ways to reduce harm associated with injecting drug use and specifically to avert an epidemic of HIV infection among injecting drug users (IDUs) in Australia. They argued that there is impressive evidence that IDUs in treatment have a reduced risk of infection and that the legal provision of substances desired by IDUs, but hitherto unavailable, might attract new populations of IDUs into treatment. One of these practitioners, Alex Wodak, had previously proposed, unsuccessfully, that there should be an evaluation of costs and benefits for providing methadone for injecting.

The Stage 1 feasibility research described below was conducted at the request of the Select Committee and Volume 1 of the resulting report was included in full in the Second Interim Report of that committee. That Interim Report recommended that 'the Government approve a feasibility study of the logistics of conducting a trial to provide opioids, including heroin, in a controlled manner' (p. 7). The Second Interim Report was presented to the ACT Legislative Assembly on 15 August 1991. Debate on a motion that the report be noted was adjourned and was not resumed in the life of that Assembly.

In February 1992 elections were held for the ACT Legislative Assembly. In its 19 January policy statement 'Protecting Canberra's Community', the Labor party (which gained eight of the 17 seats) listed under its objectives for the next three years to 'reject *unilateral* action to use Canberra for experimentation with the supply of free heroin' [our emphasis]. There was no reference to the trial proposal in Liberal party policy statements (they gained six seats). The Michael Moore Independent Group (which gained two seats) included in its policy statement, 'Support the proposed opioid trial in the ACT' and that the Government should 'implement the next stage of the heroin study'.

Illicit Drug Use in the ACT

The ACT is a landlocked territory surrounded by the state of New South Wales (NSW) and houses the national capital, Canberra. In 1989, the ACT achieved self-government; it had previously been governed through the Commonwealth. Canberra has a population of about 285 000 people. On its outskirts is the NSW town of Queanbeyan with a population of some 25 000. In some respects Queanbeyan acts as a suburb of Canberra, but in others it is an integral part of NSW.

In the Stage 1 research it was estimated that there are about 1000 dependent heroin users and about three times as many non-dependent users in Canberra. Amphetamines are also used by a large number of illegal drug users and this population overlaps to some extent with the heroin-using population. Cocaine use is much less common. Cannabis is used by nearly all of those who consume other illegal drugs. Heroin is almost always injected and this is also a common route of administration for amphetamines. The smallest amount of heroin which can be purchased in the ACT is a 'deal' for A$50 which would be sufficient to provide one 'hit' for an inexperienced user or one who is non-dependent. For more experienced or dependent users twice the amount would be needed to give the desired effect (Stevens, Dance and Bammer, 1991; McDonald et al., 1993).

A range of both government and non-government agencies provide either treatment or support for illegal drug users. These include a needle and syringe exchange programme, a range of self-help groups, detoxification centres, an oral methadone programme, a therapeutic community, half-way houses, and counselling, referral and information services. The oral methadone programme which caters for 100 users (85 on maintenance and 15 on withdrawal regimes) requires daily pick-up from a hospital-based drug and alcohol unit. The waiting period for entry into methadone maintenance is about two months (Stevens, Dance and Bammer, 1991). Plans to expand the methadone pro-gramme to include pick-up from pharmacies are currently under review.

The incidence of HIV associated with injecting drug use in the ACT is low, although there may be under-reporting. The best estimates sug-gest that there may be 20 injecting drug users who are HIV positive in the ACT (Stevens, Dance and Bammer, 1991; McDonald et al., 1993).

Stage 1 Research

In April 1991, before NCEPH agreed to undertake the feasibility research, leading practitioners in drug treatment and researchers in drug policy were invited to a workshop to discuss the merits of the pro-posal. There was strong support for the need for such investigations and a four-stage strategy for conducting the research was developed. Each stage was seen as a self-contained activity which might or might not recommend follow-on to the next stage. The focus of the first stage was to be on general theoretical issues, Stage 2 was to consider logistic feasibility, Stage 3 was to be a small pilot study and the fourth stage was to be the trial itself.

The Stage 1 research was conducted between May and July, 1991 and was carried out by a team which involved, for greater or lesser periods of time, 21 people. It resulted in two volumes; a volume enti-tled 'Report and Recommendations' (Bammer, 1991; Bammer and Douglas, 1991; Douglas, 1991) and a volume of background papers. The latter covered: an overview of illegal drug use in Canberra (Stevens, Dance and Bammer, 1991); a review of arguments for and against changing the availability of opioids (Rainforth, 1991); the politi-cal context of the Australian debates about drug policy (Hartland, 1991); interest groups and social controversies (Martin, 1991); legal issues (Norberry, 1991); possible options for a trial (Bammer, Rainforth and Sibthorpe, 1991); ethical issues (Ostini and Bammer, 1991); atti-tudes to a trial (Crawford and Bammer, 1991); evaluation by a ran-domised controlled trial (Bammer, Douglas and Dance, 1991); and models of drug use (Stevens, 1991). Valuable information was provided by a Reference Group of over 60 leaders in the field. A small Advisory Committee had oversight of the whole process and provided expert guidance. However, responsibility for the report and its recommenda-tions rests with Dr Bammer and Professor Douglas.

The Stage 1 research had two essential aims. The first was to determine if a trial to provide opioids, particularly heroin, in a controlled manner was feasible in principle. If it was, the next aim was to develop a proposal for the structuring of such a trial.

The investigations began with a broad approach which allowed for a range of possibilities for a trial and essentially had two prongs. First, the potential benefits and costs of changing the controlled availability of opioids were examined. Second, the barriers and constraints which would determine whether or not a trial should go ahead and which would shape it if it did were studied.

The potential benefits and costs were examined by working through the voluminous literature which has been written on this and associated topics (Rainforth, 1991). Commentators have suggested a range of potential benefits and a somewhat smaller number of potential costs (Table 12.1). However, some important cautions must be attached to this. First, much of what is listed on both sides of Table 12.1 is based on what can best be called 'armchair theorising' and is hotly disputed. Second, those challenging the *status quo* have been much more prolific commentators than those defending it and have put a stronger case. It may be that they in fact have a stronger case, or it may be that those supporting the *status quo* do not feel challenged enough to defend it as strongly.

There is also some empirical evidence which casts light on these issues, notably the research of Hartnoll et al. (1980), evidence from the Mersey region about the availability of controlled substances on prescription and evidence from the Netherlands about their policy of 'normalisation' of 'soft' drug use (Bammer, Rainforth and Sibthorpe, 1991; Rainforth, 1991).

Table 12.1 Potential advantages and disadvantages of a trial of the controlled availability of opioids

Potential advantages	*Potential disadvantages*
↓ Spread of HIV	Wrong message, especially to children
↓ Crime	
	↑ Accidents – work and traffic
↓ Dealing	
	No incentives for users to give up
↓ Corruption	
↓ Use	↑ Number of users
Improve health and well-being	
Improve lifestyle	
Alleviate overloading of courts and prisons	
↓ Cost of policing	

The examination of the constraints on a trial involved consideration of legal, ethical and attitudinal issues.

On the legal side there are three important aspects (Norberry, 1991). One is Australia's international treaty obligations. They are not a barrier to the conduct of a trial but they pose significant constraints on how a trial might be structured. Australia would not be in breach of its international treaty obligations if a trial were conducted for medical or scientific purposes. A second aspect is the Commonwealth which controls the importation and manufacture of narcotic goods and has extensive powers in relation to therapeutic goods. There would need to be a number of licences and permissions granted and the Commonwealth would need to notify estimates of heroin importation to the International Narcotics Control Board. Again, this need not be a significant barrier. Third, there would need to be legislative change in the ACT and probably in other states of Australia. In summary, a range of legal or related changes would need to be made for a trial to go ahead, but these changes are feasible if there is political will.

There are a number of ethical considerations that affect the shape of a trial, but again no significant barriers exist (Ostini and Bammer, 1991; Ostini et al., 1993). Ethical monitoring needs to be on-going through Stage 2 and beyond.

The Stage 1 research included surveys of four key groups (Crawford and Bammer, 1991) and the strong support for the notion of a trial shown by three of them was important in reaching the conclusion that a trial was feasible in principle. The question posed was:

> Some people think there are so many problems caused by illegal drug use that something new urgently needs to be tried. They would say the proposed trial should go ahead. Other people think setting up a trial is just too risky because it might make the problems even worse. They would argue that it should not go ahead. Do you think that a trial should go ahead or that a trial should not go ahead?

The results are shown in Table 12.2.

Table 12.2 Opinions on whether or not a trial should go ahead from the general community, police, service providers, users and ex-users

	% General community (n = 516)	% Police (n = 446)	% Service providers (n = 93)	% Drug users/ ex-users (n = 133)
Should go ahead	66	31	71	76
Should not go ahead	27	63	19	14
Don't know	7	7	9	10

The survey of the ACT general community was conducted by telephone and the response rate was 77%. The other surveys used self-completion questionnaires. Those to the police were mailed through the Australian Federal Police Association (the police union to which all but a handful of police belong) and the response rate was 40%. The questionnaires for service providers and users/ex-users were distributed through service agencies and, for users, also friendship networks, so that an accurate response rate could not be calculated.

A range of questions was also asked about the way a trial should be structured and what the effects of a trial were likely to be, and the results (Crawford and Bammer, 1991) informed the proposal which was developed to guide the Stage 2 feasibility considerations (Bammer, 1991).

After the Stage 1 research was completed we decided that it was also important to know if the ACT community is alone in being supportive of a trial. In October 1991 a telephone survey of a random sample of people in Sydney (the capital of NSW) and Queanbeyan was conducted. The responses are shown in Table 12.3.

Table 12.3 Support for a trial by the Sydney and Queanbeyan communities

	% Sydney community	% Queanbeyan community
Should go ahead	58	43
Should not go ahead	34	46
Don't know	8	10
Number of respondents	521	214
% response rates	61	74

Overall, the conclusion was that a trial is feasible in principle, although a number of constraints on how a trial could be structured were identified. We recommended that a second stage of feasibility investigations, namely to examine logistic issues, should be undertaken.

An Initial Proposal for a Trial

As part of the Stage 1 considerations a specific proposal for how a trial could be conducted was developed (Bammer, 1991; Bammer, Rainforth and Sibthorpe, 1991; Bammer, Douglas and Dance, 1991). It needs to be emphasised that this proposal is a beginning point for the discussions and further research being undertaken in Stage 2. The final proposal for a trial may well look quite different. It also needs to be emphasised that, although the Stage 1 considerations found that a trial is feasible in principle, it is an open question whether or not the Stage 2 considerations will find that a trial is feasible in practice.

The key element of the proposal is a randomised controlled trial. People who meet eligibility criteria would be randomly allocated to one of two groups. One group, the 'expanded availability' group, would have a choice of heroin and/or methadone and three routes of administration – injection, smoking and/or oral. The second group would receive oral methadone only; that is a 'gold standard' for treatment now. This is diagrammatically represented in Figure 12.1 below.

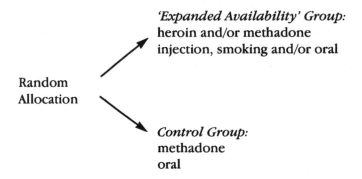

Figure 12.1 Proposal for design of randomised controlled trial

The main questions to be tested with a trial such as this are: can a treatment programme that offers heroin (as well as methadone) and injection and smoking routes of administration (as well as oral) increase the likelihood that participants will be able to: (1) lead a more stable lifestyle in terms of employment, relationships and day-to-day activity; (2) reduce their criminal activity; (3) reduce behaviours which place them at risk of contracting HIV and hepatitis B and C; and (4) increase behaviours important in the maintenance of health and well-being?

We also recommended that methodologies should be developed to address a number of other questions:

1. Can such a treatment program bring into treatment illicit opioid users who have not sought treatment before and can it maintain clients in treatment for a longer time than currently available programs? How satisfied are participants and workers with the program?
2. Can such a treatment program have measurable benefits to society at large, in terms of reducing the level of drug-related problems and the social and economic costs of drug use?

3. Would such a treatment program be cost-effective?
4. Can such a treatment program improve relationships and lifestyle from the point of view of family members and others close to trial participants?
5. Would such a treatment program have a major impact on existing drug treatment services and on law enforcement?

We recommended that a trial should run for two years. Our initial proposal, which we expect to be modified during Stage 2, is that: (1) a trial should be restricted to dependent users; (2) there should be a register and some sort of identification system for trial participants; (3) the drugs should be administered at the distribution points and should not be allowed to be taken away; (4) trial participants should be allowed to have, at a maximum, three doses of heroin per day; (5) there should be a regular review process for people in the trial, where they would be encouraged to move to less harmful practices (meaning that they would be encouraged to use less harmful drugs, and to stop injecting and try using oral or smokable forms of administration); (6) trial participants should be encouraged to use counselling and other forms of treatment; (7) social functioning of trial participants should be regularly assessed and they should be referred to other services like housing and welfare as needed; (8) participants should not be required to pay for trial drugs; (9) there should be sanctions against the diversion of trial drugs; (10) continued use of street drugs should continue to be illegal but it should not be a barrier to participating in the trial; (11) at the end of the trial all participants should have oral methadone available to them.

Each of these suggestions has advantages and disadvantages which are presented in Bammer (1991). They need to be carefully researched and thought through as part of the Stage 2 process.

In November 1991 NCEPH and the AIC organised a day-long seminar (in collaboration with the National Drug and Alcohol Research Centre) to inform key policy makers about the Stage 1 findings and to debate whether or not the research should proceed to Stage 2. There was strong support for proceeding (Bammer and Gerrard, 1992).

Stage 2

There is a significant amount of research which needs to be conducted to determine if a trial is logistically feasible. There are three overarching principles guiding Stage 2:

1. The research should have intrinsic value, so that regardless of whether or not a trial goes ahead, the research should be of value to treatment services or to drug policy generally.
2. Research should be conducted in all relevant disciplines and the

disciplinary findings should be integrated to address the central problem.
3. The Stage 2 process should involve to the greatest extent possible the key interest groups – illicit drug users, service providers, police, policy makers and the community.

An expanded Advisory Committee has been established and a range of reference groups will again be constituted. The information needed for Stage 2 can be divided into five areas: (1) core information (e.g. estimating numbers of users, determining relevant characteristics of ACT-based users, documenting the known information about the psychopharmacological and toxicological effects of opioids); (2) information relevant to trial design and evaluation; (3) information relevant to service provision; (4) information about relevant legal, law enforcement and criminological matters; (5) community and key stakeholder acceptability of a specific trial proposal.

Another way of approaching Stage 2 is to divide the questions and issues to be addressed into the following three groups. The first group are questions directed at feasibility considerations *per se*; the second group are issues which need to be addressed before a Stage 3 pilot study could be undertaken; and the third group are issues which need to be addressed to adequately conduct a Stage 4 trial. There is, of course, overlap between them.

Questions directed at feasibility considerations *per se* are:

1. Is the proposed trial design workable and is it the best possible design?
2. Are the supplementary questions appropriate and can they be adequately answered?
3. Is the service provision as currently designed workable?
4. Why not just improve current treatment services, especially by expanding methadone availability?
5. What are the economic costs of the trial proposal and can they be justified?
6. To what degree is a revised and more detailed proposal acceptable to the community and key stakeholder groups (including users, police, drug service providers and the medical profession generally, and NSW authorities)?

For a pilot study (Stage 3) to be conducted, the following issues would need to be addressed:

1. Legislative change in the ACT, Commonwealth and possibly NSW and Victoria, including information on how to get a licence to import heroin and how best to comply with the Therapeutic Goods Act (1989).
2. Identification of a source of heroin, its conversion into forms usable

in a trial, and provision of secure transport and storage facilities.
3. Provision of secure and appropriate site(s) for service delivery.
4. Tortuous liability regarding trial participants, organisers and staff.
5. Criminal liability.
6. Employment of service providers (training may need to be provided prior to commencement of the pilot).
7. Design of service provision guidelines (e.g. screening, day-to-day operation, methods of determining dosage levels).
8. Identification of a pilot study users group.
9. Design of the pilot study, including its evaluation.
10.Costing of the pilot study.
11.Protection of data collected in the pilot study.
12.Insurance.

Preliminary work for Stage 4 would include the following (many of these issues would also substantially inform the logistic feasibility considerations *per se*).

1. Determination of the best outcome measures.
2. Detailed consideration of trial termination, both if it runs its planned course and if it needs to be terminated early.
3. Determining the philosophy to underlie the service provision.
4. Determination of the details of service provision.
5. Examination of the effects of heroin and other opioids on driving ability, and determination if special consideration needs to be given to the accessibility of distribution sites by public transport and to specially provided transport.
6. Examination of smoking as an acceptable and safe route of administration.
7. Examination of the psychopharmacological effects of heroin and other opioids.
8. Further examination of the economic costs and benefits of a trial.
9. Determination of the eligibility of dependent heroin users who are Queanbeyan residents for a trial.
10.Determination of changes necessary in law enforcement for a trial to proceed (e.g. strengthening of move-on powers).

The more specific question identified in Stage 1 (Bammer, 1991) can be subsumed under these more general areas.

We anticipate being able to reach a conclusion about the logistic feasibility of a trial by mid-1993.

Conclusions

It is clear that a trial such as the one proposed is not without problems. We are attempting to deal even-handedly with both the advantages and disadvantages of the strategy outlined, so that informed decisions can be made about the desirability of proceeding further. The final determination will have to be whether the overall balance between benefits and risks can be improved over the current situation.

Stage 2 has been structured so that it is a stimulus for both research and debate, and so that it has wider applicability in improving services for illegal drug users generally and for informing drug policy considerations. Therefore much can be learnt from the feasibility considerations, regardless of whether or not a trial is eventually conducted.

Postscript

In April 1992, the feasibility research was discussed by the Ministerial Council on Drug Strategy (MCDS). MCDS consists of two Ministers, one each from health and law enforcement, from each jurisdiction (i.e. Australian state and territory) and the Commonwealth. In the resultant resolution it noted 'the progress made by the National Centre for Epidemiology and Population Health (NCEPH) in undertaking a feasibility study, not involving the distribution of any drugs, into heroin treatment options' and recommended that 'the results of the feasibility study be reported to MCDS'.

The ACT Labor government continues to be cautious about the feasibility research which is currently underway. It has, however, agreed to cooperate with some important aspects of the Stage 2 process.

An active programme of formal and informal consultation with key groups is being developed, along with a strategy to keep these groups accurately informed. Part of the information strategy has been the publication of an occasional Newsletter covering research and political developments.

Where possible, research projects are being developed in collaboration with key interest groups. The extent of the research which will be conducted depends largely on external funding, which is being sought through the usual competitive and peer-reviewed channels. The Australian National University awarded A$445 000 over five years from its Strategic Development Fund to employ and support a study coordinator and, to date, two other small grants have been awarded.

The discussion was generated by this proposal at the Third International Conference on the Reduction of Drug-related Harm and subsequently has continued the valuable process of stimulating rational debate. We have also heard that the Stage 1 report is being used to inform guidelines for a heroin trials project being developed in Switzerland.

References

Bammer, G. (1991). Report and recommendations. In *Feasibility Research into the Controlled Availability of Opioids. Vol. 1, Report and Recommendations*, pp. 1–32. Canberra, ACT: National Centre for Epidemiology and Population Health.

Bammer, G. and Douglas, R.M. (1991). Executive summary. In *Feasibility Research into the Controlled Availability of Opioids. Vol. 1, Report and Recommendations*, p. ix. Canberra, ACT: National Centre for Epidemiology and Population Health.

Bammer, G. and Gerrard, G. (Eds) (1992). *Heroin Treatment – New Alternatives. Proceedings of a Seminar Held on 1 November 1991, Canberra*. Canberra, ACT: National Centre for Epidemiology and Population Health.

Bammer, G., Douglas, R. and Dance, P. (1991). Evaluation by a randomised controlled trial. In *Feasibility Research into the Controlled Availability of Opioids Vol. 2, Background papers*, pp. 279–286. Canberra, ACT: National Centre for Epidemiology and Population Health.

Bammer, G., Rainforth, J. and Sibthorpe, B. (1991). Possible options for a trial. In *Feasibility Research into the Controlled Availability of Opioids. Vol. 2, Background Papers*, pp. 117–176. Canberra, ACT: National Centre for Epidemiology and Population Health.

Committee of Inquiry into the Legal Provision of Heroin. (1981). *Report of the NSW Committee of Inquiry into the Legal Provision of Heroin and other Possible Methods of Diminishing Crime Associated with the Supply and Use of Heroin*. Sydney: New South Wales Department of Health.

Crawford, D. and Bammer, G. (1991). Attitudes to a trial. In *Feasibility Research into the Controlled Availability of Opioids. Vol. 2, Background Papers*, pp. 187–278. Canberra, ACT: National Centre for Epidemiology and Population Health.

Douglas, R. M. (1991). Foreword. In *Feasibility Research into the Controlled Availability of Opioids. Vol. 1, Report and Recommendations*, pp. i–iii. Canberra, ACT: National Centre for Epidemiology and Population Health.

Hartland, N. (1991). The political context. In *Feasibility Research into the Controlled Availability of Opioids. Vol. 2, Background Papers*, pp. 53–82. Canberra, ACT: National Centre for Epidemiology and Population Health.

Hartland, N., McDonald, D., Dance, P. and Bammer, G. (1992). Australian reports into drug use and the possibility of heroin maintenance. *Drug and Alcohol Review*, **11**, 175–182.

Hartnoll, R. L., Mitcheson, M. C., Battersby, A., Brown, G., Ellis, M., Fleming, P. and Hedley, N. (1980). Evaluation of heroin maintenance in a controlled trial. *Archives of General Psychiatry*, **37**, 877–884.

Legislative Assembly for the Australian Capital Territory, Select Committee on HIV, Illegal Drugs and Prostitution (1991). *Second Interim Report. A Feasibility Study on the Controlled Availability of Opioids*. Canberra, ACT.

Martin, B. (1991). Interest groups and social controversies. In *Feasibility Research into the Controlled Availability of Opioids Vol. 2, Background Papers*, pp. 83–86. Canberra, ACT: National Centre for Epidemiology and Population Health.

McDonald, D., Stevens, A., Dance, P. and Bammer, G. (1993). Illicit drug use in the Australian Capital Territory. *Australian and New Zealand Journal of Criminology* (in press).

Norberry, J. (1991). Legal issues. In *Feasibility Research into the Controlled Availability of Opioids. Vol. 2, Background Papers*, pp. 87–115. Canberra, ACT: National Centre for Epidemiology and Population Health.

Ostini, R. and Bammer, G. (1991). Ethical issues. In *Feasibility Research into the Controlled Availability of Opioids. Vol. 2, Background Papers*, pp. 177–186. Canberra, ACT: National Centre for Epidemiology and Population Health.

Ostini, R., Bammer, G., Dance, P. R. and Goodin, R. E. (1993). The ethics of experimental heroin maintenance. *Journal of Medical Ethics* (in Press).

Rainforth, J. (1991). Literature review: Arguments for and against changing the availability of opioids. In *Feasibility Research into the Controlled Availability of Opioids. Vol. 2, Background Papers*, pp. 19–52. Canberra, ACT: National Centre for Epidemiology and Population Health.

Stevens, A. (1991). Models and explanations of drug use. In *Feasibility Research into the Controlled Availability of Opioids. Vol. 2, Background Papers*, pp. A4–A10. Canberra, ACT: National Centre for Epidemiology and Population Health.

Stevens, A., Dance, P. and Bammer, G. (1991). Illegal drug use in Canberra. In *Feasibility Research into the Controlled Availability of Opioids. Vol. 2, Background Papers*, pp. 1–18. Canberra, ACT: National Centre for Epidemiology and Population Health.

Part IV
Applications to Specific Substances

Chapter 13
Reduction of Smoking-related Harm: The Scope for Nicotine Replacement*

MICHAEL A. H. RUSSELL

Mr Peter Staples, Commonwealth Minister for Aged, Family and Health Services,has told us that tobacco causes 19 000 deaths per year in Australia – 350 or, as he put it, one Jumbo Jet full of people per week. He also mentioned that this was 72% of all deaths from addictive or abused drugs. In the UK, tobacco kills about 150 000 smokers each year, and some 400 000 die each year in the USA, plus about 1000 UK and 4000 USA non-smokers who die from inhaling other people's smoke. Despite all our efforts to curb and control tobacco over the past 20 years or more, there are still 15 million smokers in the UK, 50 million in the US, and some 25% of children are smokers by the time they leave school at 16. No country has yet achieved a sustained rate of decline in the national prevalence of smoking greater than about 1% per year, and targets for national prevalences below 20% by the year 2000 seem optimistic. Meanwhile, the spread of tobacco use in developing countries proceeds apace. On the basis of current trends, Peto predicts a worldwide death rate from tobacco of 10 million per year by the second decade of the next century (Peto, 1991).

This is indeed a crisis situation – all the more serious because our efforts over the last two decades have been insufficient. Progress has been either too slow or non-existent. One reason for this is that smoking is so addictive. It is now well recognised that cigarette smoking is a form of drug addiction. A landmark in this process was the 1988 report of the US Surgeon General, which concluded that the processes underlying addiction to nicotine are similar to those of other addictive drugs such as alcohol, heroin and cocaine (US Department of Health and Human Services, 1988). What distinguishes nicotine from other widely abused drugs is that its effects are subtle, and it does not cause socially disruptive intoxication, provoke violence or impair performance. The central paradox is that, while people smoke for the nicotine they die

* This chapter is an adapted version of: Internal Paper No. 2, ICRF Health Behaviour Unit, Institute of Psychiatry, London SE5 8AF © ICRF Health Behaviour Unit, 1992.

mainly from the tar and other unwanted components in the smoke. Nicotine itself does not cause cancer or chronic obstructive lung disease, although it probably has a contributory role in causing smoking-related cardiovascular disease.

More rapid progress in our efforts to reduce smoking is held back by smokers' addiction to nicotine. One way to reduce the difficulties of giving up smoking is to provide nicotine from an alternative and less harmful source. Nicotine chewing gum helps people to stop smoking. It is far less harmful than tobacco. It contains no tar or harmful gases, which cause cancer and chronic obstructive lung disease, and the slower rate of nicotine absorption and lower blood levels put less stress on the heart than does nicotine from tobacco smoke.

The *status quo* of the last 5–10 years is about to be shaken by an array of new nicotine replacement products which will soon be available as aids to giving up smoking. These range from nicotine skin patches, which take 6–8 hours to give very flat steady-state peak blood levels (Srivastava et al., 1991), to nicotine vapour inhalers which mimic the transient high-nicotine boli in arterial blood that follow within a few seconds of each inhaled puff of cigarette smoke (Feyerabend and Russell, 1990). Nicotine skin patches from four different pharmaceutical companies are already available in some countries. A nasal nicotine spray, from which rapid absorption gives peak blood levels in about five minutes (Sutherland et al., 1992), is undergoing clinical trials in four countries. A nicotine vapour puffer is at an earlier stage of clinical trial, and nicotine lozenges are being developed as alternatives to the chewing gum.

All kinds of new questions will arise for consideration by policy makers, control agencies and therapists. Which products should be free of medical control and available over the counter? Should the cost of treatment be reimbursed or met by health services? Should long-term use be permitted, or even encouraged, in those who would otherwise relapse to smoking? Should some of these products be promoted on the open market to compete with tobacco?

It is my purpose here to consider how these nicotine replacement products might best be incorporated into ongoing programmes to maximise their potential for reducing tobacco-related harm. The case for nicotine replacement is based largely on evidence of the extent to which progress with educational approaches, restrictive measures and low-tar cigarette programmes has been and will continue to be held back by the addictiveness of tobacco use, and it is within this context that the scope for nicotine replacement is discussed.

Four Main Strategies

There are four main approaches to reduce smoking-related harm: (1) reduce recruitment, (2) increase cessation, (3) reduce the risks of active smoking, and (4) reduce passive exposure to other people's smoke. It is not suggested that focusing on one or two should imply that others be neglected. No single approach is likely to be effective on its own, although theoretically if recruitment could be prevented the other approaches would in time become unnecessary. In some cases progress in one approach may enhance that in another. For example, an increase in cessation among adults is likely to reduce recruitment among their children and to reduce exposure to passive smoking. Restrictions to reduce passive exposure in public places may help to enhance cessation. But positive interactions may not be the rule. Development of less harmful cigarettes, for example, might undermine progress in lowering recruitment and increasing cessation. Striking the right balance may be difficult. It is also obvious that approaches relevant to a developed country with a 'mature' smoking problem may differ from those required to prevent the spread of smoking in a developing country. Issues discussed in this chapter apply mainly to the former.

It is assumed throughout that our main concern is to reduce tobacco-related diseases and that moral objections to recreational and even addictive use of a drug can be discounted provided it is not physically, psychologically or socially harmful to the user or to others.

Motivational Approaches Are Essential but Insufficient

Ever since the hazards of smoking were first widely publicised by the first reports of the UK Royal College of Physicians in 1962 and the US Surgeon General in 1964, campaigns and programmes to control smoking have relied mainly on increasingly intensive health educational approaches in schools, on mass media, and use of posters, warnings on cigarette packets and other forms of publicity about the health risks of smoking. Although successful at motivating people to want to stop and to try stopping, such approaches are relatively ineffective at helping them to succeed (Sutton and Hallet, 1987; 1988). Unfortunately, much of the outcome research in this area has been inadequate. In a review of the effect on smoking cessation of 40 mass media programmes or campaigns, the author concluded that sophisticated meta-analytic techniques were not warranted because 'if we had been restricted to only those studies that satisfied the conditions of minimal scientific validity, there would have been little to review' (Flay, 1987).

More discouraging than the weak effect of motivational approaches on cessation is the lack of any significant effect on preventing recruitment. Intensive intervention in schools with the most sophisticated social learning and health education methods, given over three years, had only a transient effect, with no evidence of any effect at six-year fol-low-up (Flay et al., 1989).

Other less direct motivational approaches include increases in tobacco taxation, restrictions on advertising and promotion of tobacco products, and restrictions on smoking in public places. A number of studies have shown that cigarette sales drop when prices are increased but the response is modest with an elasticity of about –0.5 (Russell, 1973; Godfrey and Maynard, 1988). This means that a price increase of 10% will depress consumption by about 5%. It is not clear how much this is attributable to some smokers quitting or many smokers cutting down consumption. Although few health workers would question that advertising and promotion of cigarettes should be banned, the direct effect of this might be rather small. Addictive drug use spreads only too readily without it. Indeed, as the 1989 US Surgeon General's Report reiterated: 'There is no scientifically rigorous study available to the public that provides a definitive answer to the basic question of whether advertising and promotion increase the level of tobacco con-sumption' (US Department of Health and Human Services, 1989).

Smoking control programmes have tended to focus on the motiva-tional approaches largely because they can be targeted at a national level. They have been successful at motivating smokers and 75% of UK smokers, for example, want to stop. Indeed, the majority have tried more than once (Russell, 1991). However, despite all the campaigns and efforts over many years, fewer than 40% of UK smokers succeed in stopping before the age of 60 (Jarvis and Jackson, 1988), by which time much damage has been done which is at best only partially reversible. It is clear that motivational approaches alone are insufficient for the majority of smokers, and that their paths to successful cessation are blocked by the problem of dependence.

The Addictiveness of Smoking

The importance of help and treatment to complement motivational approaches is well recognised in policies and programmes for alcohol and drug dependence. But this is not the case with smoking. Many people, especially those in the field of health education, have been reluctant to recognise smoking as an addiction that can be helped by treatment. This is difficult to understand in view of how extremely addictive smoking is.

In terms of its intractability, the tendency to relapse after short-term cessation, and the proportion of users who become dependent, ciga-rette smoking is on a par with other addictions. Compulsive smoking is the norm. Smoking is seldom a take-it-or-leave-it intermittent activity practised in moderation on appropriate occasions. Fewer than 10% of smokers are able to smoke occasionally on a non-daily basis. Indeed,

40% of UK smokers light up their first cigarette of the day within 15 minutes of waking, 17% within five minutes (Russell, 1991). Some 50% say that they crave frequently or always in situations when they cannot smoke. A study of drug addicts and alcoholics attending a clinic for treatment found that 57% thought it would be harder to give up smoking than their problem drug, while 72% of alcoholics and 52% of drug users reported that their urges to smoke were as strong or stronger than those to consume alcohol or take drugs (Kozlowski et al., 1989). Without nicotine replacement, stopping smoking can be as difficult to achieve and sustain as is abstinence from heroin or alcohol (Hunt et al., 1971).

As mentioned above, although 75% of smokers want to stop, only 40% at most succeed in stopping permanently before the age of 60. Thus some 60% go on smoking from their teens to their sixties although most of them want to stop and try to stop, often many times over many years. Some carry on smoking despite crippling bronchitis and emphysema, angina or amputations of the feet. Of smokers who have had an operation for lung cancer, some 50% of survivors are smoking again within a year (Davidson and Duffy, 1982). Of smokers who survive a heart attack, 70% take up smoking again within a year, 38% while still in hospital, within five days of transfer from intensive care to another ward (Burt et al., 1974; Bigelow et al., 1986).

More alarming perhaps than the strength of tobacco addiction is the ease with which it develops. Of those children who smoke more than 3–4 cigarettes, some 90% go on to become regular dependent smokers (Russell, 1990). Tolerance is rapidly acquired to the initially unpleasant effects of nicotine, and the nicotine intake from each cigarette is very soon equivalent to that of adults (McNeill et al., 1987). Teenagers also report adult-type withdrawal symptoms when they attempt to quit (McNeill et al., 1986).

Nicotine and Tobacco Dependence

Nicotine is the drug in tobacco that causes addiction (US Department of Health and Human Services, 1988). If tobacco contained no nicotine people would not smoke it, chew it or sniff it. Most tobacco users (at least 90%) absorb sufficient nicotine to obtain pharmacological effects and the venous blood nicotine levels of regular smokers are similar to those of regular oral and nasal snuff users (Russell et al., 1981; Holm et al., 1992). But the comparison ends there.

The modern cigarette is far and away the most effective device for getting nicotine into the brain. The smoke is mild enough to be inhaled deeply into the lungs, from where nicotine is rapidly absorbed to reach the brain within seven seconds. This is more rapid than an intravenous injection, which takes some 14 seconds. The inhaled puff becomes the unit of dosage, so that the average intake of 1 mg nicotine per cigarette (Benowitz and Jacob, 1984; Feyerabend, Ings and Russell, 1985), if taken in say 10 puffs, is taken as a series of 10 intravenous-like shots of 0.1 mg nicotine. Each 'shot' produces a transient high-nicotine bolus in arterial blood to the brain containing nicotine concentrations 3–4 times higher than the levels between puffs and those measured in venous blood after mixing and partial distribution to the tissues (Isaac and Rand, 1969; Rand, 1989).

By altering puff-rate, puff-size and amount of inhalation, smokers unconsciously regulate their nicotine intake to their individually pre-ferred levels and so have finger-tip control over nicotine delivery to their brain. Although blood nicotine levels vary widely between smok-ers, the levels of individual smokers are kept fairly constant from one day to the next.

Nicotine has all the classical hallmarks of an addictive drug. It is psy-choactive and has effects that people find rewarding. Dose-related increases in 'liking' the effects of intravenous nicotine have been demonstrated in humans using standardised procedures (at the US National Addiction Center in Baltimore) used in screening drugs for their abuse potential (Jasinski, Johnson and Henningfield, 1984). In smoking doses, nicotine has stimulant effects on the electrical activity of the brain. It also has calming effects, especially at times of stress, as well as effects on hormonal and other systems throughout the body. Although its subjective effects are pleasurable, they are less dramatic and obvious than those of some other addictive drugs. However, smok-ing doses of nicotine cause activation of 'pleasure centres' in the brain (e.g. mesolimbic dopamine system) which may explain the pleasure and addictiveness of smoking (Grenhoff, Aston-Jones and Svensson, 1986).

Nicotine acts as a primary reinforcer. Animals learn to press a lever to self-inject it at rates comparable to those for cocaine (Spealman and Goldberg, 1982). It induces tolerance, and physical as well as psycho-logical changes occur on withdrawal. Chronic exposure to nicotine induces an increase in the number of nicotinic cholinergic receptors in many parts of the brain, indicating the presence of structural as well as functional changes in the central nervous system of smokers (Schwartz and Kellar, 1983; Benwell, Balfour and Anderson, 1988). Such process-es may play an important part in the development of dependence and the difficulties of giving up smoking. One way to ease these difficulties is to provide nicotine from an alternative and less harmful source.

Nicotine Replacement Treatment

It is clear that some form of help and treatment is necessary to enhance cessation. The term nicotine replacement refers to the use of pure nicotine to replace that which would otherwise be obtained from tobacco use. Nicotine chewing gum was developed in Sweden in the early 1970s as a temporary aid to relieve withdrawal symptoms and so make it easier for people to give up smoking. It has proved a major advance and is now widely used in many countries. Nicotine is absorbed slowly through the lining of the mouth, and blood levels during hourly use average about one third of the peak levels just after a cigarette.

The replacement provided by nicotine gum is only partial, and it provides little of the positive pleasure of smoking. However, it significantly reduces the severity of withdrawal symptoms although it does not always eliminate them. It roughly doubles the success rates achieved by placebo gum or behavioural methods alone. But compliance with adequate gum use is a problem which limits its full therapeutic potential as an adjunct to brief intervention in medical and primary care settings (see Jarvis and Russell (1989) for review).

In general, success rates in smoking cessation depend on the intensity of the intervention. Intensive counselling and support, given individually or in groups, can achieve success rates of around 15–20% abstinence at one year follow-up. With brief advice and support, success rates seldom exceed 5%. A variety of behavioural and other approaches, ranging from hypnosis and acupuncture to aversion therapy and drugs such as tranquillisers and lobeline, have failed to show any specific effect over and above that of attention-placebo controls. There is some suggestive evidence that clonidine, antidepressants or ACTH may have potential value but no reliable data exist to date. Nicotine gum, in contrast, given with intensive support, increases success rates to 30–40% (Jarvis and Russell, 1989). In view of the large number of smokers, intensive treatments with higher success rates are arguably less important than brief interventions that can be widely applied to many more smokers. A success rate of only 10% in a primary care setting may therefore be more useful than 40% success with intensive methods. This view was expressed frankly, if brutally, by a leading activist in the anti-smoking movement who dismissed intensive treatment for smokers as 'trivial interventions with no potential for mass delivery' (Chapman, 1986).

What about the new nicotine replacement products? In more than half a dozen short-term studies, nicotine skin patches have produced significant reduction in craving compared with placebo, as well as higher rates of cessation. So far only two longer term placebo-controlled trials with adequately reliable data have been published. As an adjunct to intensive group therapy, rates of continuous abstinence for six months were 26% and 12% for active and placebo patches respectively (Transdermal Nicotine Study Group, 1991). This is no better than earlier trials with nicotine gum (Jarvis and Russell, 1989).

More encouraging results were obtained from a study in which the skin patches were given with relatively brief support. The rates of sustained abstinence for one year were 17% and 4% in the active and placebo groups respectively (Tonnesen et al., 1991). If a success rate of even 10% is demonstrated in current skin patch trials with brief support in primary care, this would offer real scope for application on a scale sufficient to increase cessation at a national level. The potential advantage of skin patches is the apparent ease of achieving good compliance. Little time is needed for instruction, and therapeutic blood nicotine concentrations can be obtained from Day 1 of cigarette withdrawal. Unlike the gum, there is no evidence of any tendency to become dependent on nicotine patches, and they may also prove useful for weaning people off other more addictive nicotine replacement products.

Some smokers may find it more helpful to receive nicotine more rapidly. The nasal nicotine spray may have a role for the more addicted smokers for whom the gum and skin patch are insufficient. The nicotine vapour puffers and inhalers require further product development before their potential for widespread use can be assessed. Whatever products are used, higher rates of permanent abstinence from smoking could probably be achieved by offering longer term nicotine replacement to smokers who relapse repeatedly after treatment.

The greater the success of treatment approaches to enhance cessation, the less the need will be to consider ways to reduce the risks of active smoking. However, so long as smoking remains widely prevalent, this is one of the more important harm-reduction strategies.

Reducing the Risks of Active Smoking

Strategies to lower the risks of smoking are an important part of the overall programme to reduce smoking-related disease. In the early 1950s, before the harmfulness of smoking was widely known, marked changes in the manufacture of cigarettes were introduced in some countries. These included the introduction of filter-tips and changes in the methods of tobacco processing. As a result, the tar deliveries of cigarettes were reduced substantially and the carcinogenicity of the tar, on a weight-to-weight basis, was also reduced. Epidemiological evidence is now emerging that these changes in cigarettes, introduced in the 1950s, have approximately halved the lung cancer risks among smokers (Peto, 1986). It is too early to assess the additional impact of low-tar cigarettes with ventilated filters introduced in the early 1970s.

Harm reduction principles were considered in detail in the first report of Royal College of Physicians (RCP) in 1962 with recommendations for cigarettes with more efficient filters and the use of modified tobaccos. The report also recommended the adoption of 'safer smoking habits' such as leaving longer butts, and switching to 'safer forms of smoking' such as pipes and cigars (Royal College of Physicians, 1962). The second RCP report in 1971 set out more specific guidelines for those who continue smoking, namely to: smoke fewer cigarettes, inhale less, smoke less of each cigarette, take fewer puffs from each cigarette, take the cigarette out of the mouth between puffs and to smoke brands with low nicotine and tar content (Royal College of Physicians, 1971).

Many countries now have programmes for reducing the tar and nicotine yields of cigarettes, but this and most of the other harm-reduction strategies are undermined by the smoker's need for nicotine. On switching to a pipe or cigars many smokers continue to inhale to maintain their former nicotine intake, so that their health risks are not reduced. The smaller milder cigars now marketed by the Industry are easier to smoke and inhale like a cigarette. It is only non-inhaled pipe and cigar smoking that is less harmful. When smokers cut down the number of cigarettes they smoke, they tend to compensate by puffing harder, inhaling more deeply, and smoking to a shorter butt.

Programmes for low-tar, low-nicotine cigarettes encounter similar problems. Tar and nicotine yields of cigarettes are highly correlated (about 0.9) so that reductions in tar intake are limited by the reluctance of smokers to tolerate similar reductions in nicotine (Wald and Froggatt, 1989; Phillips and Waller, 1991). This gives rise to two problems. One is the progressive loss of satisfaction and acceptability to smokers when nicotine yields get too low. The other problem is the tendency for smokers to undermine the potential health benefits of low yield cigarettes by compensatory increases in puffing and inhalation to enable them to maintain an adequate nicotine intake. Indeed, the logic of expecting smokers who continue smoking because they need nicotine to switch to cigarettes that deliver too little of it is questionable.

Smokers in the past switched very easily from high-tar untipped cigarettes to middle-tar filter-tipped cigarettes, no doubt because the nicotine yields in both cases were well above the 1 mg per cigarette average intake of smokers. However, the acceptability of cigarettes appears to decline sharply as nicotine yields fall below about 0.8 mg. Since their introduction more than 20 years ago, the market share of low-tar brands (<10 mg tar) with nicotine yields around 0.6–0.8 mg has remained below 20%. Brands with ultra-low yields (tar and nicotine yields below 4 mg and 0.3 mg respectively) have also been available but have proved virtually unsaleable. A safer cigarette that no one smokes serves little purpose. It is, therefore, necessary to go back to first principles to develop a more effective strategy.

Tobacco smoke is a mixture of gases and small particles made up of water, tar and nicotine. The tar is a messy mixture of hundreds of toxic chemicals several of which cause cancer (e.g. nitrosamines, benzpyrene). Many of the gases are also harmful. These include carbon monoxide, nitrogen oxides, hydrogen cyanide, ammonia and other toxic irritants such as acrolein and formaldehyde. Due to the high temperatures (over 800 °C) the burning end of a cigarette is like a minature chemical factory. It churns out many more noxious chemicals than are found in unlit tobacco or taken in by use of smokeless tobacco (for example, snuff, which contains no tar or gases). Altogether a total of more than 4000 chemical compounds have been identified in tobacco smoke.

To reduce the risks of smoking, the obvious strategy is to identify those constituents that are harmful and to then eliminate or reduce them as far as possible without seriously impairing acceptability or giving rise to significant compensatory increases in inhalation. The converse of this strategy would be to identify the component that is the major source of satisfaction and then eliminate those that are not crucial to acceptability. Since nicotine is so clearly the single major source of satisfaction, it would be logical either to change the cigarette by maintaining nicotine delivery at an adequate level, while reducing as far as possible all other components that are harmful, or to approach it by the converse route of making nicotine replacement as flavourful and acceptable as possible.

Policies on UK cigarettes are based largely on periodic reports by the Independent Scientific Committee on Smoking and Health (ISCSH). To my knowledge, this is the only influential advisory group to have recognised the importance of maintaining nicotine delivery at a level sufficient to satisfy smokers, while focusing on reduction of other more harmful components less crucial to acceptability and satisfaction. Following earlier suggestions (Russell, 1974; Russell, 1976), the ISCSH cautiously recommended the development of low-tar cigarettes with slightly enhanced nicotine yields (up to about 1 mg) to improve acceptability to smokers and to reduce compensatory increases in the intensity of smoking (Independent Scientific Committee on Smoking and Health, 1983). This Committee has since gone even further down this road by commissioning the monitoring of yields of a variety of noxious smoke components of UK cigarettes (including some of the carcinogenic polycyclic aromatic hydrocarbons and tobacco-specific nitrosamines) with a view to reducing them (Independent Scientific Committee on Smoking and Health, 1988; Phillips and Waller, 1991).

In striking contrast, after an American tobacco company had spent US$300 million to develop a virtually tar-free and far less harmful cigarette (R. J. Reynolds Tobacco Company, 1988), which was a major advance along the lines that the UK Committee is seeking to achieve, its sale in the USA was blocked by bureaucratic technicalities abetted by misguided pressure from health experts. Indeed, the American Medical Association, the Heart and Lung Association, the American Cancer

Society, and others lobbied and spoke against this new cigarette at a special Hearing before a Subcommittee of the House of Representatives (US House of Representatives, 1988). Eventually the product was labelled as a novel nicotine delivery system and attempts to market it as a tobacco product have had to be suspended. Meanwhile the company remains free to actively promote its more lethal conventional cigarettes to the 50 million Americans who still smoke, and the US Government continues to defend the rights of US tobacco companies to export cigarettes to developing countries.

Another example of misapplication or prejudice against harm reduction principles is the recent policy moves to ban the use of smokeless tobacco in EC countries. This would apply to countries like Sweden where oral snuff is used by some 20% of men, many of whom might switch to smoking if snuff is banned. Snuff use is far less harmful than smoking. Besides posing no risk of lung diseases, there is no evidence to date that use of smokeless tobacco increases the risk of cardiovascular disease (US Department of Health and Human Services, 1986). Indeed, the incidence of oral cancer appears to be lower among Swedish snuff users than in smokeless tobacco users in the USA. It is well known that levels of carcinogenic nitrosamines vary between different types of smokeless tobacco, but no data are published to inform users. Moreover, policy makers appear to show little interest in such matters.

Summing Up a Rational Approach

Programmes to control tobacco consumption have become increasingly intensive, comprehensive, and better coordinated over many years. Evidence, since the early 1980s, that passive smoking is harmful to non-smokers has justified more stringent restrictions on smoking in public places. Some countries with well-developed programmes have seen a sustained decline in smoking prevalence, averaging about 1% per year, while in others prevalence is less high than it might otherwise have been. All this is a substantial achievement that has saved many lives, but it is not enough. It provides, however, a sound framework into which new strategies could be integrated.

In addressing the four main approaches to reduce tobacco-related disease it has been argued that use of educational and restrictive measures alone will be insufficient, however much they may be intensified. This is due simply to the addictiveness of tobacco use. It is suggested that national rates of smoking cessation could be increased by widespread use of new nicotine replacement products as adjuncts to treatment for addicted smokers. Consequent reductions in the prevalence of adult smoking might in turn help to reduce uptake of smoking among their children, for which no other effective measures have been demonstrated. Reductions in prevalence will also contribute to reducing passive exposure among non-smokers. This much could and no doubt will be achieved by the most conservative use of nicotine replacement products, i.e. their use as temporary aids to smoking cessation. Acceptance of such use requires little shift in attitude and understanding of policy-makers.

More contentious and difficult for health authorities (although not for smokers) to accept is the notion of long-term and even lifelong nicotine replacement for smokers who would otherwise go back to smoking. This is in fact a logical extension of current low tar programmes to reduce the risks of active smoking. Many lives would be saved if all smokers, rather than a mere 20% of them, could be persuaded to switch to low-tar cigarettes. Most of our health experts and policy-makers would hopefully perceive this as an important step in harm reduction. A much greater step along the same path would be to have smokers switch to pure nicotine products. Although the logic of this step is clear, its novelty and simplicity do not guarantee instant acceptance by those who have not thought along these lines before.

Although it seems self-evident that nicotine alone must be less harmful than nicotine plus tar plus noxious gases, some policy-makers may place undue weight on the potential harmfulness of nicotine itself. They may not be completely reassured by the fact that it has no role in smoking-related cancers or in chronic obstructive lung disease which together account for almost 50% of smoking-related deaths. They may not be reassured that the risk of cardiovascular diseases will be reduced by the elimination of carbon monoxide. Nicotine undoubtedly poses some cardiovascular risk to those who already have heart disease, but this risk is apparent only when it is rapidly absorbed by inhalation, so would apply only to nicotine inhalers and possibly also to the nasal spray. In any case, these risks are countered by adrenergic blockers, which are already given routinely to people with cardiovascular disease. Experts, more competent than I, dismiss the cardiovascular risks as follows. They state: 'That nicotine has a role in the cause of cardiovascular disease has its adherents, but the evidence is not compelling' (Frogatt and Wald, 1989).

Among the commonly used addictive drugs, the safety of nicotine itself would appear to lie somewhere between alcohol and caffeine, probably far closer to caffeine. This would seem a fair exchange for the risks of tobacco. It is very likely that tobacco use could be eliminated more quickly and more completely if replaced by pure nicotine products than it will if no alternative source of nicotine is available. In my view, serious consideration should be given to permit selected nicotine products to be made as palatable and acceptable as possible and actively promoted on the open market. They are unlikely to prove sufficiently pleasant and palatable to compete with tobacco without health authority endorsement and tax advantages to give them a competitive edge. Indeed, taxation and restrictions on tobacco could be applied far more harshly if an alternative product were available.

It is not suggested that nicotine use be presented as something good, but rather as something far less harmful than tobacco. The message of the anti-smoking movement could remain clear and simple. There is only one fight and that is against tobacco and tobacco-related disease. Indeed, the message is more likely to be heeded if those who need it can turn to a substitute source of nicotine. As tobacco is gradually phased out, the battle could shift to avoiding excessive nicotine, if by then it proves to pose an unacceptable burden to health.

Those who fear that such a strategy is too extreme should remind themselves that Peto's forecast of 10 million deaths per year throughout the world by year the 2020 is based on current trends. There is no way that this will be averted by continuing with current strategies. The nicotine replacement strategy suggested is not an alternative strategy, or one that would work on its own. On the contrary, it is argued that its integration into the various components of comprehensive programmes to control tobacco use would be mutually enhancing. So much so that the virtual elimination of tobacco could become a realistic future target.

References

Benowitz, N.L. and Jacob, P. (1984). Daily intake of nicotine from cigarette smoking. *Clinical Pharmacology and Therapeutics*, **35**, 499–504.

Benwell, M.E.M., Balfour, D.J.K. and Anderson, J.M. (1988). Evidence that tobacco smoking increases the density of nicotine binding sites in human brain. *Journal of Neurochemistry*, **50**, 1243–1247.

Bigelow, G.E,. Rand, C.S., Gross, J. Burling, T.A. and Gottlieb, S.H. (1986). Smoking cessation and relapse among cardiac patients. In F.M. Tims and C.E. Leukefeld, (Eds), *Research Monograph 72*, Rockville, Maryland: National Institute on Drug Abuse.

Burt, A., Illingworth, D., Shaw, T.R.D. Thornley, P., White, P. and Turner, R. (1974). Stopping smoking after myocardial infarction. *The Lancet*, **1**, 304–306.

Chapman, S. (1986). *The Natural History of Smoking Cessation: How and Why People Stop Smoking*. London: Health Education Council.

Davidson, G. and Duffy, M. (1982). Smoking habits of long-term survivors of surgery for lung cancer. *Thorax*, **37**, 331–333.

Feyerabend, C. and Russell, M.A.H. (1990). A rapid gas-liquid chromatographic method for the determination of cotinine and nicotine in biological fluids. *Journal of Pharmacy and Pharmacology*, **42**, 450–452.

Feyerabend, C., Ings, R.M.J. and Russell, M.A.H. (1985). Nicotine pharmacokinetics and its application to intake from smoking. *British Journal of Clinical Pharmacology*, **19**, 239–247.

Flay, B.R. (1987). Mass media and smoking cessation: a critical review. *American Journal of Public Health*, **77**, 153–160.

Flay, B.R., Koepke, D., Thomson, S.J., Santi, S., Best, J.A. and Brown, K.S. (1989). Six-year follow-up of the first Waterloo School Smoking Prevention Trial. *American Journal of Public Health*, 79, 1371–1376.

Frogatt, P. and Wald, N. (1989). The role of nicotine in the tar reduction programme. In N. Wald and P. Frogatt (Eds), *Nicotine, Smoking and the Low Tar Programme*, pp. 299–235. Oxford: Oxford University Press.

Godfrey, C. and Maynard, A. (1988). Economic aspects of tobacco use and taxation policy. *British Medical Journal*, 297, 339–343.

Grenhoff, J., Aston-Jones, G. and Svensson, T.H. (1986). Nicotinic effects on the firing pattern of midbrain dopamine neurons. *Acta Physiologica Scandinavica*, 128, 351–358.

Holm, H., Jarvis, M.J., Russell, M.A.H. and Feyerabend, C. (1992). Nicotine intake and dependence in Swedish snuff takers. *Psychopharmacology*, 108, 507–511.

Hunt, W.A., Barnett, L.W. and Branch, L.G. (1971). Relapse rates in addiction programs. *Journal of Clinical Psychology*, 27, 455–456.

Independent Scientific Committee on Smoking and Health (1983). *Third Report.* HMSO: London.

Independent Scientific Committee on Smoking and Health (1988). *Fourth Report.* London: HMSO.

Isaac, P.F. and Rand, M.J. (1969). Blood levels of nicotine and physiological effects after inhalation of tobacco smoke. *European Journal of Pharmacology*, 8, 265–283.

Jarvis, M.J. and Jackson, P. (1988). Cigar and pipe smoking in Britain: implications for smoking prevalence and cessation. *British Journal of Addiction*, 83, 323–330.

Jarvis, M.J. and Russell, M.A.H. (1989). Treatment for the cigarette smoker. *International Review of Psychiatry*, 1, 139–147.

Jasinski, D.R., Johnson, R.E. and Henningfield, J.E. (1984). Abuse liability assessment in human subjects. *Trends in Pharmacological Sciences*, 5, 196–200.

Kozlowski, L.T., Wilkinson, A., Skinner, W., Kent, C., Franklin, T. and Pope, M. (1989). Comparing tobacco cigarette dependence with other drug dependencies. *Journal of the American Medical Association*, 261, 898–901.

McNeill, A.D., Jarvis, M.J., West, R.J., Russell, M.A.H. and Bryant, A. (1987). Saliva cotinine as an indicator of cigarette smoking in adolescents. *British Journal of Addiction*, 82, 1355–1360.

McNeill, A.D., West, R.J., Jarvis, M., Jackson, P. and Bryant, A. (1986). Cigarette withdrawal symptoms in adolescent smokers. *Psychopharmacology*, 90, 533–536.

Peto, R. (1986). Overview of cancer time-trend studies in relation to changes in cigarette manufacture. In D. Zaridze and R. Peto, (Eds), *Tobacco: A Major International Health Hazard*, pp. 211–226. Lyon: IARC Scientific Publications.

Peto, R. (1991). Worldwide mortality from current smoking patterns. In B. Durston and K. Jamrozik, (Eds), *Tobacco and Health 1990: The Global War*, pp.66–68. Perth, Australia: Lamb Printers.

Phillips, G.F. and Waller, R.E. (1991). Yields of tar and other smoke components from UK cigarettes. *Food and Chemical Toxicology*, 29, 469–474.

Rand, M.J. (1989). Neuropharmacological effects of nicotine in relation to cholinergic mechanisms. *Progress in Brain Research*, 79, 3–11.

R. J. Reynolds Tobacco Co. (1988). *Chemical and Biological Studies on New Cigarette Prototypes that Heat Instead of Burn Tobacco*. North Carolina: Winston-Salem.

Royal College of Physicians (1962). *Smoking and Health*. London: Pitman Medical.

Royal College of Physicians (1971). *Smoking and Health Now*. London: Pitman Medical.

Russell, M.A.H. (1973). Changes in cigarette price and consumption by men in Britain, 1946–71: a preliminary analysis. *British Journal of Preventative and Social Medicine*, **27**, 1–7.

Russell, M.A.H. (1974). Realistic goals for smoking and health: a case for safer smoking. *The Lancet*, **1**, 254–257.

Russell, M.A.H. (1976). Low-tar, medium-nicotine cigarettes: a new approach to safer smoking. *British Medical Journal*, **1**, 1430–1433.

Russell, M.A.H. (1990). The nicotine addiction trap: a 40-year sentence for four cigarettes. *British Journal of Addiction*, **85**, 293–300.

Russell, M.A.H. (1991). How to enhance national rates of smoking cessation. pp. In B. Durston and K. Jamrozik, (Eds). *Tobacco and Health 1990: The Global War*, pp. 49–53. Perth, Australia: Lamb Printers.

Russell, M.A.H., Jarvis, M.J., Devitt, G. and Feyerabend, C. (1981). Nicotine intake by snuff users. *British Medical Journal*, **283**, 814–817.

Schwartz, R.D. and Kellar, K.J. (1983). Nicotinic cholinergic receptor binding sites in the brain: regulation in vivo. *Science*, **220**, 214–216.

Spealman, R.D. and Goldberg, S.R. (1982). Maintenance of schedule-controlled behaviour by intravenous injections of nicotine in squirrel monkeys. *Journal of Pharmacology and Experimental Therapeutics*, **223**, 402–408.

Srivastava, E.D., Russell, M.A.H., Feyerabend, C., Masterson, J.G. and Rhodes, J. (1991). Sensitivity and tolerance to nicotine in smokers and nonsmokers. *Psychopharmacology*, **105**, 63–68.

Sutherland, G., Russell, M.A.H., Stapleton, J., Feyerabend, C. and Ferno, O. (1992). Nasal nicotine spray: a rapid nicotine delivery system. *Psychopharmacology*, **108**, 512–518.

Sutton, S.R. and Hallet, R. (1987). Experimental evaluation of the BBC series 'So you want to stop smoking?'. *Addictive Behaviors*, **12**, 363–366.

Sutton, S.R. and Hallet, R. (1988). Smoking intervention in the workplace using videotapes and nicotine chewing gum. *Preventive Medicine*, **17**, 48–59.

Transdermal Nicotine Study Group (1991). Transdermal nicotine for smoking cessation. *Journal of American Medical Association*, **266**, 3133–3138.

Tonnesen, P., Norregaard, J., Simonsen, K. and Sawe, U. (1991). A double-blind trial of a 16-hour transdermal nicotine patch in smoking cessation. *New England Journal of Medicine*, **325**, 311–315.

US Department of Health and Human Services (1986). *The Health Consequences of Smokeless Tobacco: A Report of the Surgeon General*. Maryland: USDHHS, Public Health Service.

US Department of Health and Human Services (1988). *Nicotine Addiction: A Report of the Surgeon General*. Maryland: USDHHS, Public Health Service.

US Department of Health and Human Services (1989). *Reducing the Consequences of Smoking: A Report of the Surgeon General*. p.516 Maryland: USDHHS, Public Health Service.

US House of Representatives. Subcommittee on Health and Environment Hearing (1988). Serial No. 100–68, July 29, 1988. Washington, DC: US Government Printing Office.

Wald, N. and Froggatt, P. (Eds) (1989). *Nicotine, Smoking and the Low Tar Programme*. Oxford: Oxford University Press.

Chapter 14
Application of Harm-reduction Principles to the Treatment of Alcohol Problems

NICK HEATHER

It has been suggested that the concept of harm reduction was invented simultaneously in Merseyside and Amsterdam in 1986. As someone whose career has mainly been devoted to research and treatment in the field of alcohol problems, I find this claim surprising. It may well be true that significant developments in thinking about and responding to problems of illicit drug use and HIV infection took place in Liverpool and Amsterdam at about this time. But to identify this with the origins of harm reduction in relation to drug use in general ignores the much longer history of the concept in the addictions arena and in the alcohol problems field in particular.

A minor aim of this chapter is to demonstrate that, depending on how it is defined, the recognition of harm reduction as an important aspect of the treatment of alcohol problems goes back to the first attempts to evaluate the effects of treatment following the Second World War. The term may not have been explicitly recognised at that time but it is clear that many of the benefits thought to have been derived from treatment coincided with what would now be defined as harm reduction. My recollection is that, from around the late 1970s, the term was formally used to describe some of the objectives and expected benefits of alcohol problems treatment.

More recently, however, there has been an amnesia for past advances in recognising the relevance and importance of harm-reduction principles to alcohol problems treatment, an amnesia that is especially evident in research and practice in the United States of America (and this, as we know, is of considerable influence throughout the world). I shall provide examples of this amnesia and speculate on its origins and functions.

Moreover, meanings of 'harm reduction' in the alcohol problems field have lately become somewhat confused, and the main objective of the chapter is to clarify and distinguish between various uses of the term. I have been able to identify four senses in which harm-reduction principles have been applied to alcohol problems treatment and these will be used to structure this discussion.

'Drinking But Improved'

The first sense of harm reduction is the most obvious. It refers to the status of clients who continue to drink and show alcohol-related problems following treatment but whose levels of consumption and problems are lower than before treatment began.

A category describing such clients can be found in the very first scientific studies of the outcome of treatment directed at total abstinence. In one of the most influential reviews of treatment results, Emrick (1974) examined all outcome studies he could find in the published literature between 1951 and 1971. He noted that the majority of studies reported a rate for 'total improvement', being the sum of clients who were totally abstinent, engaging in harm-free drinking or had shown some degree of improvement in terms of drinking levels or presence of alcohol-related problems. In many cases from direct reporting and in other cases by subtraction, it is possible to calculate from these early papers the proportion of clients who could be said to be 'drinking but improved' compared with pre-treatment status.

So prevalent was this convention for the reporting of treatment results that it led to 'the rule of the thirds', in which one third of treated clients could be expected to achieve abstinence, another third would be drinking but showing improvement, and a remaining third would be unimproved, proportions which Emrick (1974) was able roughly to confirm in his review of the literature. We shall see, however, that the proportion of those who are consistently abstinent following treatment, that is, who achieve the almost universal treatment goal of 'total and lifelong abstinence', is much smaller than one-third.

A second paper by Emrick (1975) as part of the same literature review shocked the alcohol treatment community by its conclusion that alcoholics who had received treatment fared no better than those who had not. This conclusion, combined with Orford and Edwards' (1977) classic comparison of treatment versus simple advice, in which no benefit for the former could be demonstrated at one and two year follow-ups, led to a profound pessimism over the efficacy of treatment for alcohol problems. What is sometimes forgotten, however, is that Emrick's conclusion applied only if the criterion of successful treatment was restricted to abstinence. The summary of Emrick's (1975) paper reads as follows:

> A review of 384 studies of psychologically oriented alcoholism treatment showed that ... mean abstinence rates did not differ between treated and untreated alcoholics, but more treated than untreated alcoholics improved, suggesting that formal treatment at least increases an alcoholic's chances of reducing his drinking problem.
>
> *(Emrick, 1975, p.88)*

An obvious limitation of Emrick's conclusion is that the treated and untreated groups he compared were not randomly assigned and may therefore have differed in respect of unknown variables related to outcome. However, a more recent study by Chick et al. (1988) in Edinburgh did employ random assignment and reached essentially the same conclusion. Chick and his colleagues wished to repeat the Maudsley study (Orford and Edwards, 1977) of treatment versus advice (or brief intervention) while avoiding the drawback of that study that it applied only to married men. They therefore included women and unmarried clients of low social stability in their sample. They randomly allocated 152 attenders at an alcohol problems clinic to one session of advice or to extended in- or outpatient treatment. At the follow-up two years later, 'the group who were offered extended treatment were functioning better, in that, over the year prior to the independently conducted follow-up interview, they had accumulated less harm from their drinking than those only treated briefly' (p.159). But no differences were detected between the groups in abstinence rates or in rates of harm-free drinking.

Another study from which similar conclusions may be reached is the large, multi-centre trial of disulfiram treatment by Fuller et al. (1986), surely one of the most carefully conducted evaluations of alcohol problems treatment ever reported. At the 12 months follow-up, clients given active disulfiram did not show higher rates of abstinence than those in control groups, but there was a group of relatively stable, middle-aged men given disulfiram who drank on fewer days during the follow-up period than control subjects. This difference led Tennant (1986) to dispute the authors' own negative interpretation of their overall findings.

These results from carefully conducted controlled trials, combined with the conclusions from Emrick's (1975) review, suggest that conventional, extended treatment for alcohol problems cannot be justified in terms of rates of total abstinence but only by improvements in the status of those who continue to drink following treatment. From a different starting point, the same conclusion was reached by Gottheil et al. (1982) from their study of clients of a Veterans' Administration hospital treatment programme. These authors also compared their own results from a programme that did not demand total abstinence with those from the abstinence-only programmes studied in the first Rand Report (Armor, Polich and Stambul, 1978) and in Oklahoma by Paredes, Gregory et al. (1979). An outcome category of 'moderate drinking' here included both those who had drunk at low levels during a six month follow-up period and those who had abstained for one month but had drunk heavily on some occasions during the preceding five months. The authors summarize their findings as follows:

If the definition of successful remission is restricted to abstinence, these treatment centers cannot be considered especially effective and would be difficult to justify from cost-benefit analyses. If the remission criteria are relaxed to include the moderate levels of drinking that have been described, success rates increase to a more respectable range of 53% to 67%. When the moderate drinking groups were included in the remission category, remitters did significantly and consistently better than nonremitters at subsequent follow-up assessments.

(Gottheil et al., 1982, p.564)

Other well known follow-ups of treated individuals have reported very low rates of consistent abstinence over the follow-up period. For example, the second Rand Report (Polich, Armor and Braiker, 1980) found that only 7% of clients of NIAAA-funded treatment centres were consistently abstinent throughout a four-year follow-up period. In the Maudsley study (Orford and Edwards, 1977), 4% of those contacted at two years following treatment or advice had not drunk at all since discharge. Rychtarik et al. (1987) found that only 4% of treated individuals had abstained completely throughout a five-year follow-up period. Again, the implication is that alcohol problems treatment cannot be justified by what is almost always its stated goal – complete and permanent abstention from alcohol following treatment.

Given this evidence, it is most curious to note a modern tendency in outcome research to ignore distinctions among those who continue to drink following treatment – a tendency to include all continuing drinkers in a single, poor outcome category. The most outstanding example of this tendency comes from an influential study by Helzer et al. (1985) in which all those who had shown any alcohol-related problem during a three-year period (66.5% of the total sample) were simply grouped together under the heading of 'continued alcoholics'. The degree of problems experienced within this group may have ranged from being late for work because of a hangover on one occasion in three years to almost complete destruction of health, family life and vocational prospects, but no information provided by the authors gives any more details of the drinking or nature and extent of the problems experienced by these clients. This highly uninformative method of reporting treatment outcome seems to reflect a regressive tendency in American research to regard any alcohol consumption of being indicative of a continuing disease process, the existence of which renders variations in drinking behaviour of no interest.

Wider Criteria of Treatment Outcome

The second sense of harm reduction is similar to the first in that it too finds total abstinence from alcohol as the sole criterion of successful treatment to be misleading and unhelpful. Here, however, the emphasis is on the relevance of nondrinking variables reflecting wider aspects of general adjustment in judging the effects of treatment.

The interpretation of harm reduction in this sense begins with the

proposition that the ultimate objective of treatment is not total abstinence or even harm-free drinking but simply an improvement in the
client's overall quality of life. From this point of view, the client's drinking behaviour is not itself the problem to be solved in treatment but
merely a contributing cause of wider problems in living. By the same
token, the modification of drinking behaviour is merely a means to the
higher end of the client's greater well-being and satisfaction in life.

During the late 1960s and the 1970s, considerable progress was
made in explicating this type of harm-reduction approach, particularly
in the work of E. Mansell Pattison. Critiques of alcoholism treatment
concepts with special reference to abstinence were presented by
Pattison (1966; 1968). He reviewed a great deal of evidence available at
that time to show both that total abstinence is by no means necessarily
associated with improvements in other aspects of functioning and that
continued drinking often was associated with such improvements.
Among the conclusions of Pattison (1966) were the following:

1. Improvements in drinking and in social, vocational and psychological adaptation are related but not parallel. Less than total rehabilitation may be the most feasible therapeutic goal in many cases.
2. Abstinence as a criterion for successful treatment is an overstate-
   ment. It is a prescription which should be used judiciously.
3. Abstinence as a criterion of successful treatment is misleading. It may
   be maintained at the expense of total life functioning, as in some
   Alcoholics Anonymous abstainers. Abstinence may also be followed
   by personality deterioration.

The question of the criterion for successful treatment was also
addressed by Belasco (1971). He constructed an index of 'overall
attainment and total life adjustment' among clients discharged from
residential treatment which included 'sobriety' (not necessarily abstinence), occupation and 'ecology' (housing and marital status). He
compared this index with a measure of pathological drinking behaviour
derived from the degree of successful affiliation with Alcoholics
Anonymous and found only a low correlation between these two variables, with discrepancies in both directions. Belasco concluded suc-
cinctly: 'Because of visibility of linkage between pathological (drinking)
behaviour and poor adjustment...many researchers have assumed the
converse of this relationship also to be true. Our evidence casts doubt
on that assumption' (p.42).

Pattison returned to the issues explored in his earlier papers in
three articles published in 1976 (Pattison 1976a,b,c). By this time, he
was more definite and detailed in his recommendations:

Recent advances in alcoholism treatment concepts have been developed that
require clarification and revision of treatment goals. Goals of treatment are

separated into five major areas of Life Health: Drinking Health, Emotional Health, Interpersonal Health, Vocational Health, and Physical Health. The Drinking Health variable is classified further into five possible outcomes: Abstinence, Social Drinking, Attenuated Drinking, Controlled Drinking, and Normal Drinking.

(Pattison, 1976a, p.177)

Pattison (1976a) points out that the importance of the above treatment goals may vary according to the needs of the specific population of problem drinkers in question. For example, the goals relevant to a group of 'Skid Row' alcoholics with very poor general life adjustment will be very different from a group identified through an Employee Assistance Programme, where much higher levels of social, interpersonal and vocational adjustment can be anticipated. Such distinctions are, of course, ignored under a regime of total and lifelong abstinence as the only worthwhile objective of treatment.

Among the different drinking goals identified by Pattison, that of 'attenuated drinking' is most pertinent for present purposes. In contrast to the completely harm-free nature of alcohol consumption suggested by the concept of 'controlled drinking', attenuated drinking implied the tolerance of some continued alcohol-related problems but of less severity than before treatment.

A limited but valuable degree of improvement might well be the deliberate choice of treatment goal if there is reason to believe that an individual will never seriously attempt abstinence, has failed repeatedly to achieve abstinence in previous treatment, or shows life circumstances such that a goal of total abstinence or strictly controlled drinking will be almost certainly unattainable. Part of the reason for the low correlation between drinking status and overall adjustment following treatment is the fact that the 'Skid Row' alcoholic has such major dysfunctions as part of the life-style that there is little potential for major improvements in adjustment even if sober. There is also little incentive for such a person to strive for total abstinence since this would be perceived as making little difference to the overall quality of life. This adds up to a strong case for giving precedence in treatment to relatively modest gains in social, interpersonal, vocational and physical status over radical changes in drinking behaviour. (It might be added here that simple detoxification and medical attention for individuals who do not wish and are most unlikely to reduce a heavy level of drinking, without insistence on alcohol counselling accompanying or following detoxification, is the most straightforward example of harm reduction in practice in the alcohol problems field.)

Despite the reasonableness of Pattison's analysis, there is no evidence that his plea for a broader approach to alcohol problems treatment has been heeded. On the contrary, since he wrote there has been a tendency to narrower, not broader, definitions of treatment outcome.

This may again be illustrated from the article by Helzer et al. (1985) in which dimensions of improvement other than drinking behaviour and alcohol-related problems are not mentioned at all. As for the suggestion that treatment might explicitly be directed towards attenuated drinking, it is as though this suggestion had never been made. To my knowledge, no published research has reported the results of such an initiative and no existing treatment programme has made attenuated drinking a formal part of its objectives. It is likely that, in the current climate of alcohol problems treatment in the United States of America, anyone who proposed the possibility that a goal of treatment might accept some degree of continuing alcohol-related impairment would risk professional ostracism and guarantee exclusion from the band of treatment researchers who receive government support for their work. Again, the reasons for this state of affairs will be discussed below.

Controlled or 'Harm-free' Drinking

This sense of harm reduction might be regarded as a contradiction in terms since the usual meaning of 'controlled drinking' in the field, both as an outcome category following abstinence-oriented treatment and as a goal of treatment itself, has become the complete elimination of alcohol-related harm. More pedantically, it could be argued that this is harm reduction in its most extreme form. The same would apply, of course, to total abstinence.

Nevertheless, the main reason for including this sense of harm reduction here is that it is in fact what many people think of when they apply the idea of harm reduction to the alcohol problems field. This is probably by analogy with other psychoactive drugs, such as opiates, where continuing use or dependence on the substance, but without harm, is a common meaning of harm reduction. However, it could be argued that, in the alcohol field at least, this use of the term is not especially useful since a more radical and innovative meaning of harm reduction implies a countenance of some continuing areas of impairment.

It would be inappropriate here to attempt to summarize the latest evidence on the controlled drinking outcome or the obstacles that have been placed in the way of its greater employment in treatment. The present point, however, is that one unfortunate legacy of the bitter controlled drinking dispute is to have retarded the progress that was being made in recognizing the relevance of harm-reduction concepts to alcohol problems treatment. As a result particularly of the furore that followed the publication of the Rand Reports and of the accusations of fraud directed against the Sobells, treaters and researchers in the field, especially in the United States of America, appear to have become afraid to associate themselves publicly with any nonabstinent goals of treatment (Peele, 1992). Moreover, researchers have become far less willing to examine outcome data to discover whether improvements, either in level of drinking, severity of alcohol-related problems or in more global indices of adjustment, have occurred among those who continue to drink following abstinence-oriented treatment. The point simply is that the retreat from the advocacy of controlled drinking training, even for circumscribed groups of problem drinkers, has also had the effect of jettisoning the conceptual advances that had been made during the 1970s with respect to a broader, more realistic and, indeed, more humane view of treatment.

Behavioural psychologists responsible for developing controlled drinking treatment methods have, in a sense, colluded with these tendencies. Having been forced to go on the defensive in relation to controlled drinking outcomes, they have used their training in quantitative methods to become almost obsessionally concerned with the fine details of drinking behaviour in order to prove a faultless manner of drinking. This has been at the expense of any wider conception of the outcomes or goals of treatment, such as those so articulately described by Pattison (Peele, 1987).

There are undoubtedly other factors that have contributed to this situation. The enormous growth of private, for-profit treatment of alcoholism in the United States of America during the 1980s, which also had its offshoots in other parts of the world, was based largely on the commercialisation of the 12-step principles of Alcoholics Anonymous. This, combined with an increasing fundamentalism in American society and more negative attitudes to alcohol in general (Room, 1987), has resulted in a new hegemony of total abstinence in attitudes and responses to alcohol problems of all degrees of severity.

Harm Reduction from a Societal Perspective

This final sense of harm reduction refers to a reduction by means of community-based interventions in the total number of problems caused by alcohol in a given society. We have seen that the controlled drinking controversy has in some ways been a hindrance to the attempt to develop a harm-reduction approach to alcohol problems. But in this final sense of harm reduction, there is no doubt that the emergence of the controlled drinking goal and its associated methods of behaviour change have contributed to an opportunity to effect a wide-ranging reduction of alcohol problems in society.

In what is already recognised as one of the classic papers of our times, Kreitman (1986) described 'the preventive paradox'. This states that, owing to the distribution of alcohol consumption in the general community, the savings in alcohol-related problems that would be accrued by persuading all heavy drinkers to reduce consumption below medically recommended levels would be less than those achieved by across the board reductions among all drinkers, including moderate and light drinkers.

The logic of this position has a parallel in the field of treatment, which could be called 'the treatment paradox' or, at least, 'the intervention paradox'. This states that, because of their much greater numbers in the community, intervening to reduce the problems of drinkers with only low levels of alcohol dependence would be much more effective in lowering the aggregate of alcohol-related problems in society at large than concentrating on the relatively small numbers of high-dependence 'alcoholics'. In practical terms, it is not being suggested that those showing high levels of dependence and multiple problems should be ignored but only that the focus of interventions should be expanded to include the much larger population of individuals who may have fewer problems each but who contribute to a much greater degree to the total of alcohol-related harm in the general community. Exclusive concentration on 'alcoholics' has left untouched the great bulk of harm caused by alcohol in terms, for example, of health, social welfare, public order and economic efficiency. This is the sense in which workers in the field are now frequently using the term 'harm reduction'.

Interest in this approach has been gathering force for some time now in the United Kingdom and in Australia, but there are recent signs of interest too in the United States of America, as witnessed by a publication of the Institute of Medicine (1990), entitled *Broadening the Base of Treatment for Alcohol Problems*. The interventions in question are typically brief in duration, inexpensive in the use of professional and paraprofessional time, and often use condensed versions of cognitive-behavioural change methods pioneered by psychologists, such as self-control training, relapse prevention and motivational interviewing (Heather, 1989a). Interventions are often 'opportunistic' in that they use the opportunity to screen and intervene for harmful or hazardous alcohol consumption in settings where the prospective client has attended an agency for some other reason than to complain of problems related to alcohol consumption. So far, reports of such methods have been largely confined to medical settings, such as general medical practice and hospital wards, but there is no reason in principle why they should not also be applied in educational, social work, workplace and law enforcement settings.

It must be emphasized that such brief interventions should not be thought of purely in terms of early intervention or 'secondary prevention'. The prevention of more serious problems or more severe levels of dependence from arising may, indeed, be one important benefit of such interventions but they are more properly justified by an appeal to a widening of the scope of alcohol interventions. We know, for example, that many of those excessive drinkers who are the targets of brief interventions will not go on to develop more serious problems (Cahalan, 1970; Cahalan and Room, 1974; Fillmore, 1974; Fillmore et al., 1991). As I have argued elsewhere (Heather, 1989b), the rationale for community-based brief interventions is that they are directed at problems in their own right, not merely at precursors of future problems.

Evidence to date, including the recent results of a WHO cross-cultural trial of brief interventions (Babor and Grant, 1992), encourages the belief that this approach is effective in reducing alcohol-related problems in the general community. But, needless to say, much more work needs to be done, including the development of better screening techniques, improvements in behaviour change methods, explanations of why some individuals fail to respond to brief interventions, the matching of types of change methods with characteristics of individual excessive drinkers, and the discovery of ways to encourage professional workers to become more interested in implementing and maintaining such interventions in their work. Most important, we have no convincing proof as yet that the application of brief interventions on a large scale will lead to long-lasting improvements in public health and welfare.

Implications for Practice

What are the implications of the arguments in this chapter for practice in the field? We have reviewed evidence that treatment for alcohol problems can be justified only if those who continue to drink following treatment are taken into account. Moreover, there is evidence that total abstinence following treatment is not always associated with improvement in non-drinking aspects of life and that continued drinking often is. What then are the consequences of this evidence for the negotiation of treatment goals in clinical settings among those with relatively more serious problems?

I do not wish to be interpreted as arguing that all those attending treatment for alcohol problems should be encouraged to continue drinking or be aimed at a 'controlled drinking' goal. For anyone who prefers not to drink or for whom any drinking is contraindicated on medical grounds, abstinence should clearly be the rule. On the other hand, since it is abundantly clear that the majority of clients will in fact drink at some level following treatment, it seems reasonable to propose that more attention should be paid in treatment to providing skills by which that drinking might be kept under control and not lead to destructive consequences, and to encouraging an increase in confidence among clients that such an outcome is possible. The available evidence would also seem to indicate a much greater use of some form of continued drinking as an explicit goal of treatment and, in cases where abstinence or non-problem drinking is unlikely, the use of the 'attenuated drinking' goal.

Against this, it might be argued that it is only by aiming at the 'perfect' goal of total abstinence that improvements in drinking occur, in the same way that setting high standards in any aspect of life may make it possible for more modest achievements to take place. The lowering of standards in treatment objectives and the tacit granting of permission for drinking, so this argument would go, would inevitably result in poorer outcomes. This is a plausible argument and should be taken seriously.

However, there is no reason why exactly the same logic should not apply to a goal of 'perfect' (i.e. non-problem) drinking. If the goal of treatment is clearly stated to be drinking which does not attract any form of alcohol-related problem, this would serve as a similar kind of ideal target for the less than perfect efforts of problem drinkers to reach that goal. Indeed, one might go further and argue that the goal of total abstinence makes it more likely that uncontrolled and harmful drinking will ensue, for all the reasons suggested by Marlatt and Gordon (1985). If the client has been taught to see drinking in 'black and white' terms, as involving only complete abstinence or totally uncontrolled drinking, he or she will experience a collapse of self-efficacy if any drinking does occur and will not have been provided with any guidance as to how control over drinking can be reinstated. Certainly, there is plenty of evidence that controlled drinking outcomes are negatively correlated with experience of abstinence-oriented treatment and attendance at Alcoholics Anonymous (Peele, 1987). Thus, paradoxically, although the controlled drinking outcome might not usefully be seen as a form of harm reduction in its true sense, the controlled drinking goal could be used realistically to achieve what will be less than optimal but significantly improved outcomes in most cases.

One of the main conclusions that eventually emerged from the Sobell affair is relevant at this point. The study by Sobell and Sobell (1973) remains one of the only controlled trials of treatment directed at total abstinence versus a controlled drinking goal. It will be recalled that Pendery, Maltzman and West (1982), the chief critics of the Sobells, directed their attention almost entirely to the outcome of the group that received controlled drinking training, and ignored the group that received conventional abstinence treatment except to say that this was a group which 'all agree fared badly'. In their reply to their critics, Sobell and Sobell (1984a,b), in common with the independent committee established to investigate the charges against them (Dickens et al., 1982), were able to point out that, while the controlled drinking group did indeed demonstrate a range of continuing alcohol-related problems, the abstinence group showed even more of these problems at follow-up, including more days of drunkenness and a higher number of alcohol-related deaths. Thus, both groups 'fared badly' in the long term but the controlled drinking group showed a greater reduction in alcohol-related harm.

It must be remembered that the context of this discussion is one in which the results of alcohol problems treatment are poor, especially for those with high levels of alcohol dependence and multiple, long-standing alcohol-related problems. At the very least, the situation demands more research into the types of problem drinker who would show greater benefits from some form of continuing drinking as a goal of treatment than from abstinence-oriented treatment. Amid the current research interest in matching problem drinkers to optimal forms of treatment (Miller, 1989), it is disappointing that matching to abstinence versus controlled drinking goals has received so little attention.

With respect to harm-reduction from the societal perspective, the implications of the evidence are clearly that there should be a wide-ranging application of brief, cost-effective interventions aimed at a goal of reduced drinking for low dependence harmful and hazardous drinkers. However, it might again be objected that the same harm-reduction objectives could be achieved more efficiently by total abstinence. The current situation in the United States of America is crucial to this point. During the 1980s, there has been a threefold increase in the number of people in the community who say they have received some kind of treatment for alcohol problems, as well as a large increase in membership of Alcoholics Anonymous (AA) (Room and Greenfield, 1991). This has occurred at the same time as there has been a substantial decrease in per capita consumption in the USA. It would appear then that large numbers of drinkers, who must include many of the low dependence individuals who are the prime targets for brief moderation-oriented interventions, have been urged to pursue a goal of abstinence. The consequences of this massive expansion of abstinence-oriented treatment resources are not yet clear but they could conceivably include a general reduction of alcohol-related harm in the community. Should not total abstinence therefore be the preferred goal of brief interventions in the community?

There are reasons to think that this does not follow. First, data presented by Room (1989) suggest that the majority of those included in this expansion of the abstinence goal continue to drink after treatment and that the main effect of treatment is to reduce the proportion of those who drink at high levels, as might be expected from the evidence reviewed earlier in this chapter. Thus the same logic that applied to the results of treatment for more serious cases also applies here: since clients are going to drink anyway, they should be explicitly helped to keep this drinking as free from harm as possible. Moreover, even if a proportion of low dependence drinkers manage to maintain total abstinence – for example, 'high-bottom' converts to AA – there will clearly be another proportion, of unknown but presumably substantial size, who do not find abstinence the answer to their problems and this group should receive assistance to moderate their drinking. Finally, it is likely that a large expansion of abstinence-oriented treatment could only be envisaged in a country like the USA with a high existing rate of alcohol abstention and cultural support for abstinence from widespread religious affiliation. In more secular cultures with much lower rates of abstinence, like the United Kingdom and Australia, the promotion of a new abstinence ideology in the community at large would be unlikely to succeed.

Summary and Conclusions

This chapter began by pointing out that the concept of harm reduction had a history in the alcohol problems treatment field, either explicit or implicit, dating from about the end of the Second World War and some features of this history were briefly traced. Four senses of harm reduction in this field were identified: (1) harm reduction in the sense of the traditional concept of 'drinking but improved' following treatment; (2) harm reduction in the sense of an appeal to wider criteria of successful treatment outcome in the evaluation and in the planning of treatment; (3) harm reduction in the limited sense of 'controlled' or harm-free drinking following treatment; and (4) harm reduction as referring in the wider sense to brief, community-based interventions aimed at reducing the aggregate harm due to alcohol consumption in society at large. It was also pointed out that older achievements in recognising and applying a harm-reduction perspective to alcohol problems treatment appear to have been forgotten in more recent times, owing largely to a renewed obsession with total abstinence as the only conceivable solution to alcohol-related problems, particularly in the USA.

The implications of the evidence reviewed for intervention are simple and obvious: an expansion in research and practical applications of treatment directed explicitly at some form of continued but less harmful pattern of drinking. Although no responsible student of alcohol problems treatment could seriously suggest that there are never good scientific grounds for the recommendation of total abstinence in treatment, it is equally clear that the denigration of nonabstinent goals and outcomes which has been witnessed over the last decade has not been based on scientific considerations. The amnesia for past achievements in developing a harm-reduction approach to alcohol problems which has been referred to in this chapter is based, not on evidence or logic, but on the politics and economics of treatment provision, and an ideological commitment to abstinence as a way of life. One incidental benefit of a renewed interest in realistically attempting to reduce the harm caused by alcohol to individuals and to society might be that it helps to re-establish the discipline as a genuine scientific discourse.

References

Armor, D.J., Polich, J.M. and Stambul, H.B. (1978). *Alcoholism and Treatment.* New York: John Wiley & Sons.

Babor T.F. and Grant, M. (Eds). (1992). *Project on Identification and Management of Alcohol-related Problems. Report on Phase II: A Randomized Clinical Trial of Brief Interventions in Primary Health Care.* World Health Organization: Geneva.

Belasco, J.A. (1971). The criterion question revisited. *British Journal of Addiction,* 66, 39–44.

Cahalan, D. (1970). *Problem Drinkers: A National Survey.* San Francisco: Josey Bass.

Cahalan, D. and Room R. (1974). *Problem Drinking Among American Men.* New Brunswick: Rutgers Center of Alcohol Studies.

Chick, J., Ritson, B., Connaughton, J., Stewart, A. and Chick, J. (1988). Advice versus treatment for alcoholism: A controlled trial. *British Journal of Addiction,* 83, 159–170.

Dickens, B.M., Doob, A.N., Warwick, O.H. and Winegard, W.C. (1982). *Report of the Committee of Enquiry into Allegations Concerning Drs Linda and Mark Sobell.* Toronto: Addiction Research Foundation.

Emrick, C.D. (1974). A review of psychologically oriented treatment of alcoholism: I. The use and interrelationships of outcome criteria and drinking behavior following treatment. *Quarterly Journal of Studies on Alcohol,* 35, 523–549.

Emrick, C.D. (1975). A review of psychologically oriented treatment of alcoholism: II. The relative effectiveness of different treatment approaches and the effectiveness of treatment vs. no treatment. *Quarterly Journal of Studies on Alcohol,* 36, 88–108.

Fillmore, K.M. (1974). Drinking and problem drinking in early adulthood and middle age. *Quarterly Journal of Studies on Alcohol,* 35, 819–840.

Fillmore, K.M., Hartka, E., Johnstone, B.M., Leino, E.V., Motoyoshi, M. and Temple, M.T. (1991). A meta-analysis of life course variation in drinking. *British Journal of Addiction,* 86, 1221–1268.

Fuller, R.K., Branchey, L., Brightwell, D.R., Derman, R.M., Emrick, C. D., Iber, F. L., James, K. E., Lacoursiere, R. B., Lee, K. K., Lowenstram, I., Maany, I., Niederhiser, D., Nocks, J. J. and Shaw, S. (1986). Disulfiram treatment of alcoholism: A Veterans' Administration cooperative study. *Journal of the American Medical Association,* 256, 1449–1455.

Gottheil, E., Thornton, C.C., Skolada, T.E. and Alterman, A.L. (1982). Follow-up of abstinent and nonabstinent alcoholics. *American Journal of Psychiatry,* 139, 560–565.

Heather, N. (1989a). Brief intervention strategies. In R.K. Hester and W.R. Miller (Eds), *Handbook of Alcoholism Treatment Approaches.* New York: Pergamon Press.

Heather, N. (1989b). Psychology and brief interventions. *British Journal of Addiction,* 84, 357–370.

Helzer, J.E., Robins, L.N., Taylor, J.R., Carey, K., Miller, R.H., Combes-Orme, T. and Farmer, A. (1985). The extent of long-term moderate drinking among alcoholics discharged from medical and psychiatric treatment facilities. *New England Journal of Medicine,* 312, 1678–1682.

Institute of Medicine (1990). *Broadening the Base of Treatment for Alcohol Problems.* Washington DC: National Academy of Sciences Press.

Kreitman, N. (1986). Alcohol consumption and the preventive paradox. *British Journal of Addiction*, **81**, 353–363.

Marlatt, G.A. and Gordon, J.R. (1985). *Relapse Prevention: Maintenance Strategies in the Treatment of Addictive Behaviors*. New York: Guilford.

Miller, W.R. (1989). Matching individuals with interventions. In R.K. Hester and W.R. Miller (Eds), *Handbook of Alcoholism Treatment Approaches*. New York: Pergamon.

Orford, J. and Edwards, G. (1977). *Alcoholism*. Maudsley Monograph No. 26. Oxford: Oxford University Press.

Paredes, A., Gregory, D., Rundell, O.H. and Williams, L. (1979). Drinking behavior, remission and relapse: The Rand Report revisited. *Alcoholism: Clinical and Experimental Research*, **3**, 3–10.

Pattison, E.M. (1966). A critique of alcoholism treatment concepts with special reference to abstinence. *Quarterly Journal of Studies on Alcohol*, **27**, 49–71.

Pattison, E.M. (1968). A critique of abstinence criteria in the treatment of alcoholism. *International Journal of Social Psychiatry*, **14**, 268–276.

Pattison, E.M. (1976a). A conceptual approach to alcoholism treatment goals. *Addictive Behaviors*, **1**, 177–192.

Pattison, E.M. (1976b). Nonabstinent drinking goals in the treatment of alcoholism. *Archives of General Psychiatry*, **33**, 923–930.

Pattison, E.M. (1976c). Nonabstinent drinking goals in the treatment of alcoholics. In R.J. Gibbins, Y. Israel, H. Kalant, R.E. Popham, W. Schmidt and R.E. Smart (Eds), *Research Advances in Alcohol and Drug Problems*, Vol. 3. New York: John Wiley and Sons.

Peele, S. (1987). Why do controlled-drinking outcomes vary by investigator, by country and by era? Cultural conception of relapse and remission in alcoholism. *Drug and Alcohol Dependence*, **20**, 173–201.

Peele, S. (1992). Alcoholism, politics and bureaucracy: The consensus against controlled-drinking therapy in America. *Addictive Behaviors*, **17**, 49–62.

Pendery, M.L., Maltzman, I.M. and West, L.J. (1982). Controlled drinking by alcoholics? New findings and a re-evaluation of a major affirmative study. *Science*, **217**, 169–175.

Polich, J.M., Armor, D.J. and Braiker, H.B. (1980). *The Course of Alcoholism: Four Years after Treatment*. Santa Monica: The Rand Corporation.

Room, R. (1987). Changes in the cultural position of alcohol in the United States: The contribution of alcohol oriented movements. Paper presented at, *Alcohol and Social Science: An International Forum on Drinking Patterns in Relation to Social Change*, Torino, Italy, September/October.

Room R. (1989). Worries, concerns and suggestions: Informal processes in the social control of drinking. Paper presented at Annual Meeting of the Society for the Study of Social Problems. Publication E284, Berkeley: Alcohol Research Group, Medical Research Institute of San Francisco.

Room, R. and Greenfield, T. (1991). *Alcoholics Anonymous, Other 12-Step Movements and Psychotherapy in the U.S. Population, 1990*. Working Paper F281, Berkeley: Alcohol Research Group, Medical Research Institute of San Francisco.

Rychtarik, R.G., Foy, D.W., Scott, T., Lokey, L. and Prue, D.M. (1987). Five–six-year follow-up of broad-spectrum behavioral treatment for alcoholism: Effects of training controlled drinking skills. *Journal of Consulting and Clinical Psychology*, **55**, 106–108.

Sobell, M.B. and Sobell, L.C. (1973). Individualized behaviour therapy for alcoholics. *Behaviour Therapy*, 4, 49–72.

Sobell, M.B. and Sobell, L.C. (1984a). The aftermath of heresy: A response to Pendery et al.'s critique of 'individualized behavior therapy for alcoholics'. *Behaviour Research and Therapy*, 22, 413–440.

Sobell, M.B. and Sobell, L.C. (1984b). Under the microscope yet again: A commentary on Walker and Roach's critique of the Dickens Committee's enquiry into our research. *British Journal of Addiction*, 79, 157–168.

Tennant, F.S.Jr (1986). Disulfiram will reduce medical complications but not cure alcoholism. *Journal of the American Medical Association*, 256, 1489.

Chapter 15
Prospects of Harm Reduction for Psychostimulants

PATRICIA G. ERICKSON

This chapter will examine the evidence that indicates conditions under which the prospects for harm reduction are indeed meaningful and important ones to consider. These are new directions for harm reduction. Very little is known, as yet, about the forms harm reduction may take, and with what impacts, for drugs like cocaine and amphetamine.

Strategies for effective harm reduction will be affected by consequences, patterns of use and control. For a problem to be relevant from a public health perspective, it is necessary that this particular behaviour be both serious and widespread enough to have some bearing on the health of the people in a society. The numbers who have become involved in cocaine and amphetamine use in epidemics that have occurred and recurred globally in this century are such that these drugs warrant consideration. Moreover, amphetamine and cocaine use can result in adverse consequences to users, their families and the community. Problems may include, but are not solely or even predominantly, matters of injection drug use. In fact, not only do problems relate to all major modes of ingestion, but naive or inexperienced users may be at greater risk than the more accomplished ones. Finally, various systems of control – personal, informal and formal – influence patterns of use and consequences. Self-control and restraint practised by the individual are often the focus for harm reduction. Informal controls are rooted in the social group which defines the limits of drug-taking behaviour. Others are structurally determined (e.g. class, employment). Formal controls are the rules set and enforced by the state. These make up the broader social environment of harm reduction (Stimson and Lart, 1991).

The psychostimulants to be considered are cocaine, and to a lesser extent amphetamine. Contemporary users of either or both of these psychostimulants are generally illicit poly drug users (Clayton, 1985); also, they are often heavy alcohol and tobacco consumers. Cocaine and/or amphetamine are hardly ever the first or only drug of choice (Murray, 1984). Thus, it is misleading to identify 'cocaine users' as if

their existence was somehow unique within the drug-taking subculture. Nevertheless, the self-administration of cocaine and amphetamine, their effects and the control issues can be addressed separately
and can provide important insights for harm reduction. What first has
to be considered is what risks are involved, for what users, and what
patterns of use, and what might lessen these risks and promote safer
practices.

Consequences

Cocaine and the amphetamines are CNS stimulants which have similar
pleasurable effects. Users acclaim these drugs' ability to produce alertness, energy, overall feelings of well-being and intense euphoria, and to
combat hunger and fatigue. The principal difference between them
pharmacologically is the much longer half-life of amphetamine;
cocaine's effects peak and dissipate in minutes rather than hours like
that of amphetamine. Both substances carry the risk of serious adverse
consequences, but the likelihood of more frequent administration of
cocaine in combination with its local anaesthetic properties make its
harm potential greater than that of amphetamine. The discussion to follow will deal with the consequences of taking cocaine, and amphetamine where applicable, in relation to mortality, morbidity and
compulsive use.

That cocaine overdose could be lethal was established a century ago
during the first cocaine epidemic, when a number of deaths occurred
as a result of doctor or dentist administered cocaine anaesthesia
(Anglin, 1985) and was re-affirmed during the most recent one as an
increasing number of deaths were attributed to cocaine (Kozel and
Adams, 1985; Jacobs and Fehr, 1987). At high dose levels, the onset of
convulsions and respiratory depression can lead rapidly to coma and
death. The extent to which cocaine's action on the heart may precipitate cardiac arrest or otherwise contribute to heart disease is unclear
(Alexander, 1991). The precise lethal dose of cocaine remains
unknown, moreover, with amounts as small as 20 mg intravenously
(IV) implicated; yet some users may regularly survive taking 10 or more
grams daily (Smart and Anglin, 1987). Not only smoking and IV use,
but also snorting and oral ingestion of large amounts by body packers,
have been associated with cocaine-related deaths (Smart and Anglin,
1987). Autopsy findings are inconclusive in establishing the relationship between blood levels of cocaine, which vary widely, and resulting
fatalities (Ruttenber et al., 1991). Since at postmortem examination
cocaine is frequently detected in conjunction with other substances, its
influence as the cause of death cannot be determined unequivocally
(Ruttenber et al., 1991). Moreover, as Wong and Alexander (1991) have
cautioned, even when cocaine is the sole drug detected, the physically

deteriorated or otherwise compromised health status of the deceased may also cast doubt on cocaine's primary role in the fatality. Thus, reports of 'cocaine-related' deaths, which usually mean 'any level of cocaine detected at autopsy', should be viewed with caution as a valid indicator of deaths caused solely by cocaine ingestion. Nevertheless, this very unpredictability of cocaine, combined with its rare but possible lethal property, urge the consideration of harm reduction to reduce the risk of this most final of outcomes.

In lower doses, cocaine and amphetamine users may experience subjectively unpleasant effects (not unlike those resulting from nicotine and caffeine) such as mild anxiety, tension, nervousness, palpitations, agitation and irritability (Jacobs and Fehr, 1987). Surveys and community studies find that infrequent users rarely have adverse reactions, and do not differ from non-users in mental and physical health status (Newcomb and Bentler, 1986b; Cohen, 1989). Heavier and more frequent users are more likely to experience heightened negative effects and other adverse reactions including insomnia, impotence, weight loss, paranoia and panic attacks (Erickson et al., 1987; Anthony and Petronis, 1991; Waldorf, Reinarman and Murphy, 1991). Treatment or clinical samples provide the highest incidence of serious psychiatric morbidity resulting from large, prolonged ingestion, usually by IV or smoking, of cocaine or amphetamine (Grinspoon and Bakalar, 1985; Kalant, 1987; Hall and Hando, unpublished data, 1991; Rounsaville and Carroll, 1991). The toxic psychosis is the most reproducible feature resulting from heavy cocaine or amphetamine use; its increased incidence marked the numerous epidemics that appeared in various countries since the turn of the century. The symptoms of this serious reaction, featuring hallucinations, extreme paranoia, and sometimes violence, generally disappear quickly when cocaine or amphetamine use ceases for several days. The cause–effect relationship between cocaine use and other forms of psychiatric morbidity is less clear. Even longitudinal studies are inconsistent in indicating whether, for example, depressive symptoms are a risk factor for later cocaine use (Newcomb and Bentler, 1986a) or whether cocaine use leads to depression (Anthony and Petronis, 1991). Nevertheless, although low level social–recreational users express predominantly positive effects of cocaine use, the evidence from surveys, epidemiological, community and clinical studies, shows that heavy cocaine use may be associated with adverse consequences to users' mental health. These findings underline the importance and need for harm-reduction strategies.

Much of the knowledge of cocaine's consequences and the focus of concern is directed at the short-term effects of acute intoxication (Grinspoon and Bakalar, 1985). Although a great deal of research is underway on cocaine, little is known about the long-term effects of chronic use of powder or crack cocaine on major organ systems, bodily functioning and performance (Arif, 1987; Byck, 1987). Direct damage to the nasal passage or lungs related to the frequent repeated mode of ingestion, either by snorting or smoking, has been documented. The life-long practice of coca leaf chewing by indigenous people of South America has been shown to be a remarkably safe form of ingestion. The more potent refined forms present different risks, but do little actual harm to the low dose, occasional user. What is a far less clear is the incidence of serious adverse, long-term reactions among all those who have used cocaine in relation to amount, frequency and duration of use (Foltin and Fischman, 1991; CIBA, 1992). Without unequivocal guidance as to what levels of use are hazardous, approaches to harm reduction must, of necessity, be cautious ones.

One issue of particular relevance to harm reduction that has surfaced during the AIDS epidemic is whether amphetamine, cocaine, and particularly crack use may be linked to risky, repetitive sexual practices and thus increase the probability of HIV transmission. This is a controversial issue and the research is inconclusive (Stimson, 1992). In Australia, daily amphetamine injectors showed slightly lower risk taking practices than opioid injectors (Hall et al., unpublished data, 1991). In the USA, a higher risk of HIV infection among cocaine/crack users was found in New York (Des Jarlais and Friedman, 1988) but in San Francisco, no such relationship was found in a study of daily users (Watters, Cheng and Lorvick, 1991). Since research in several countries indicates wide variability in drug use and sexual practices in different social groups (Feldman and Biernacki, 1988), the influence of social, cultural and economic factors on these practices needs to be understood. It may then be possible to provide a basis for harm-reduction practices that are sensitive to a particular socio-cultural group (Stimson, 1992).

A third type of consequence is the extent to which compulsive, excessive and destructive use is an outcome of exposure to cocaine. Whether called addiction, dependence or uncontrolled use, such a compulsive behaviour pattern was described soon after cocaine hydrochloride became available in the 1880s (Anglin, 1985; Kalant, 1987). It is now part of the conventional wisdom that cocaine is the most addictive substance known to man (or rats) (Akers, 1991). The evidence from animal studies, population surveys, clinical studies and community samples was reviewed by Erickson and Alexander (1989), who concluded that the addictive liability of cocaine has been overstated: between 5% and 10% of those who ever try cocaine will use it weekly or more often; most will not persist or else use infrequently. Of the more frequent users, about one tenth to one quarter develop the compulsive use pattern and get into serious difficulties with cocaine. The more recent studies reviewed later in this chapter (although excluding animal studies; see Brady, 1991) further support these conclusions.

Even crack use, when studied outside of treatment settings, is not necessarily compulsive (Cheung, Erickson and Landau, 1991) and the natural history of the recent crack epidemic in the USA has been described as 'differing little from that of previous epidemics' (Fagin and Chin, 1989, p.606).

The continued emphasis in both popular and scientific literature on cocaine and crack's great or 'instantly addictive' property has serious implications for harm-reduction approaches (Akers, 1991). If the drug dictates the behaviour, and the addict is the victim of pharmacological forces beyond his/her control, then the drug is 'evil' and eradication is the answer. Little trust can be placed in interventions which expect the user to modify or reduce use in less harmful ways. This mechanistic view of the passive user is supported by case studies of the 'worst case scenario' – those who become compulsive users and persist despite extremely destructive consequences to themselves and others. The following quote is typical of many in the literature: 'Crack [cocaine] engenders an almost irrepressible biological drive known as craving and compels many users to search for more crack, heedless of any learned biosocial consequences' (Schwartz, Luxenberg and Hoffman, 1991, p.154). Many more users, however, stop for periods of time, maintain moderate use, stop or regain control over their drug use. Thus the predictive power of the mechanistic view is limited. We are not yet in a position to know why a particular drug's pharmacology acts so devastatingly on some but not others, but it is clearly not the only important factor in explaining compulsive use.

The user's mind set within a larger social setting must also be considered (Zinberg, 1984). In the voluntaristic approach, the user is an active entity capable of making choices, of weighing pleasures against the risks and undesirable effects of drug use (Cheung and Erickson, 1993). Moreover, the individual operates within a web of social, cultural and economic factors that affect decisions about whether, when and how to use a particular drug. From this perspective, the development of strategies for harm reduction is a viable option, with untapped potential to benefit from, and build on, naturalistic assessments of users' own experiences with the drugs.

Indeed, it may be time to stop referring automatically to cocaine and crack as 'highly' or 'extremely' addictive, or even addictive at all (Davies, 1992). Instead, it is preferable to focus on the destructive patterns of use which undeniably sometimes result (Akers, 1991). To redefine the concept of addiction in order to make it fit cocaine (Gawin, 1991) is to ensure that the most extreme pejorative labels can be readily applied. To suggest otherwise is to be 'soft' on cocaine, to be 'on the wrong side' of the issue, or to imply that it is a 'safe' drug (Akers, 1991). This insistence on the tremendous addictive potential of cocaine obfuscates the assessment of its real risks, and by denying users' the ability to control their behaviour, may impede efforts for harm reduction. What is surely one of cocaine's important potential assets for harm reduction, that is, that use can be discontinued without an unpleasant or life-threatening physical withdrawal syndrome, has been neglected.

Patterns of Use

Overview

Epidemics of amphetamine or cocaine use have occurred in several countries during the past century. Although first synthesised in the 1880s, amphetamines were not widely manufactured or prescribed until the 1930s. They were widely used internationally by military and political personnel during the Second World War to counteract fatigue, but details are understandably sketchy (Miller and Kozel, 1991a). The first large-scale, rapid increase in amphetamine use that was recognised as a problem was in postwar Japan. That epidemic had waned by the mid 1950s, but was followed by another in 1970 which escalated and then stabilised at high levels in the 1980s (Suwaki, 1991). Epidemics of mainly injecting amphetamine use also occurred in Sweden in the 1960s, in the USA and Canada in the late 1960s and early 1970s, in the UK in the 1950s and again in the late 1960s, and in Australia in the mid and late 1960s (Hall and Hando, unpublished data, 1991). More currently the lifetime prevalence of amphetamine use in the Australian general population is 6%. Levels of current use have remained low (under 1%) in Canada and in the USA where regional pockets of use are found (Miller and Kozel, 1991a; Single, Erickson and Skirrow, 1991). In most countries which have experienced these epidemics, amphetamine use appears to retain popularity among illicit and especially intravenous drug users. Amphetamine use had been most widespread when militarily and medically prescribed, but became lodged in the illicit drug milieu after legal supplies were drastically curtailed in the 1960s.

The two major cocaine epidemics have been more widely separated than those involving amphetamine. The first wave occurred not long after the extraction of the cocaine alkaloid in 1865. When cocaine became cheaply and widely available in patent medicine in a pure pharmaceutical form, increased consumption occurred in the 1880s and 1890s in Europe (Kalant, 1987; Scheerer, 1991), both in the USA (Musto, 1973; 1991) and in Canada in the early 1900s (Giffen, Endicott and Lambert, 1991) and in Australia in the 1920s and 1930s (Hall and Hando, unpublished data, 1991). The second wave of cocaine use began mainly in the USA and Canada in the 1970s, and rose into the mid-1980s (Erickson et al., 1987; Clayton, 1985). Although declines in the number of users in these two North American countries have occurred during recent years, the use of semi-refined cocaine products has reportedly increased in South America (CIBA, 1992). An influx of cocaine to other parts of the world, especially Europe and Eurasia, has been portrayed as underway or imminent based on increased seizures and reported use among clinical samples (Montagne, 1991; CSIS, 1992; RCMP, 1991). Reliable documentation of a new cocaine epidemic beyond North and South America, however, remains elusive, as what little survey evidence is available shows negligible levels of use in other countries (RAND, 1991).

More detailed knowledge about the extent and patterns of drug use in a country can be derived from a number of sources. The least reliable sources are the indirect indicators found in official statistics such as arrests, convictions, seizures, psychiatric admissions, and coroners' and emergency room reports. Such figures may flag a newly emerging wave of use and problems, but also reflect only fragments of a complex pattern of detection, enforcement and political processes (Clayton, 1985; Goode, 1989; Ben-Yehuda, 1990; Cheung, Erickson and Landau, 1991). Surveys of the general population, based on random probability sampling, provide a broad picture of the proportion of past and current users and the overall frequency of use but find few heavy users. Repeated national surveys allow trends to be examined and generalisations to be made with considerable confidence, but have been done rarely in most countries. Clinical studies conducted in treatment settings reveal the most uncontrolled and destructive patterns of use in those who have sought professional help (Chitwood and Morningstar, 1985; Wallace, 1990). In between these extremes lie community and epidemiological case studies which draw from a wider part of the spectrum of cocaine-use experiences. These studies take a more intensive look at variations in patterns over time, ideally with a longitudinal component or else retrospectively, and consider different precursors and outcomes of use. Each of these approaches has strengths and limitations, but together can help to provide a more comprehensive view than any one single source.

Surveys

The most systematic ongoing studies of drug use in the general adult population and in the student population have been conducted in the USA, and in the province of Ontario, Canada. In Australia and in Canada, national surveys asking about cocaine use have been conducted only once or twice, limiting any conclusions about trends. Nevertheless, all of these studies show broad similarities in patterns of use, despite much higher prevalence of use in the American population. Thus, the proportion reporting ever using cocaine in their lifetime was 11% in the USA (1990), less than 2% in Australia (1989), about 2% in the UK (Ditton et al., 1991), and 3.5% in Canada (1989). A survey in the city of Amsterdam in 1990 found a lifetime prevalence rate of 5.5% for cocaine (Sandwijk, Cohen and Musterd, 1991). In all countries, higher levels of use are found in males, young adults and those with prior illicit drug use. Preferred modes of administration are snorting, with smoking and IV use much less common. Nevertheless, the overall distribution of consumption was this: most of the population never tries cocaine, of those who do, most use it only a few times; most do not continue, but of those who do, frequency of use is low; between 5% and 10% become more frequent users (at least monthly). This general pattern is illustrated by details from Ontario survey research.

In recent adult surveys, Adlaf, Smart and Canale (1991, p. 78) found that of those who had ever used cocaine, about 60% had not used it in the past 12 months. Of those current users, the vast majority reported use of less than once a month, with barely 5% using monthly or more often. Similarly among students, over half reported using cocaine only once or twice in the prior year, and 10% had used 40 or more times (Smart, Adlaf and Walsh, 1991). Moreover, the annual prevalence of cocaine use by Ontario adults has been remarkably stable, between 2% and 3% since 1984. Peak levels of use for students never exceeded 5%, and have shown steady declines since 1985 to about 2% in 1991 (Smart, Adlaf and Walsh, 1991). Crack use has been low and stable, reported by 1% or less of adults and students. These use trends co-exist with increased availability of cocaine, an increase in seizures, greater purity and the lowering of unit price over the past decade in Ontario (RCMP, 1991; Metropolitan Toronto Workgroup, 1991).

Epidemiological case-control studies

James Anthony and colleagues in the USA have probed a unique data source for new findings on initiation and progression of cocaine use (Anthony and Petronis, 1991; Ritter and Anthony, 1991). Between 1980 and 1985, the National Institute of Mental Health Epidemiological Catchment Area (ECA) programme selected large-scale probability samples in five urban sites. The purpose was to investigate the causal associations between the elevation of psychiatric disturbances (using the Diagnostic Interview Schedule) and a wide variety of potential risk factors, including substance abuse. Unlike the national household surveys, the ECA study included an institutional sample. Respondents were interviewed twice, one year apart, enabling the identification of those who progressed in cocaine use during the follow-up interval to the use of cocaine six or more times. Then the new cases of cocaine use were matched in a post-stratification procedure with a non-using sample comparable by age and residential neighbourhood.

The analysis focused on those aged 18–44 years who were candidates for cocaine initiation or progression ($n=4394$). At the follow-up,

78 individuals (1.8%) qualified, and were matched with 131 controls. The final sample was of 73 matched sets (one case and from one to four controls). Their findings revealed a set of personal characteristics – social demographic, prior drug use, role change and psychiatric – that were associated with initiation/progression of cocaine use during the recent epidemic phase (1980–85) in the USA. In the final multivariate model (with the adjusted relative risk shown in brackets) their conclusions were that estimated risk of cocaine initiation/progression was enhanced 'at higher levels of personal income (1.1 with each increment), among persons with recent prior use of marijuana only (10.0), [both marijuana and] other illicit drugs (32.5), among persons who experienced a syndrome of persisting depression (11.6) and among unemployed persons who gained a job (4.7). Risk was lower among married persons and diminished with increasing age' (Ritter and Anthony, 1991, p. 205). This prospective study, therefore, is consistent with the view that fluctuations in cocaine use are embedded in a complex personal and social process. Despite limitations (e.g. no details of frequency, dose or mode of administration were elicited), this research provides a dynamic picture of cocaine use and risk factors.

Community studies

More in-depth information about patterns of cocaine use and actual practices from a wide range of users, but with less generalisability than that obtained in surveys and epidemiological case studies, can be obtained in community studies. As the name suggests, these involve non-institutionalised cocaine users who are at large in their communities, who are recruited through advertising or the snowball sampling method, and who choose to participate in the research. Respondents in such studies tend to under-represent the more affluent, higher socio-economic status cocaine users as well as the more disadvantaged. Although participants are more frequent consumers of cocaine than average, they otherwise share similar characteristics with cocaine users in general (as opposed to the more deviant users in treatment and jailed populations).

A number of such studies have been conducted now in five different countries: Australia (Mugford and Cohen, 1989); the Netherlands (Cohen, 1989); Scotland (Ditton et al., 1991); Canada (Erickson et al., 1987; Cheung et al., 1991; Erickson, Watson and Weber, 1992) and the United States of America (Waldorf, Reinarman and Murphy, 1991). They demonstrate a remarkable degree of consistency in their findings about the possibility of controlled cocaine use, namely that cocaine use is predominantly an infrequent and self-regulating pattern. These results point the way to harm reduction strategies for individual users and their family and friendship networks, whereas epidemiological and population studies direct attention to laws and broader social policies that facilitate harm reduction or augmentation. The findings of two recent community studies will be highlighted before turning to control issues.

In Ontario, the highly variable patterns of cocaine use found in all the community studies were probed through a longitudinal design (Erickson, 1991). One hundred cocaine users who had used at least 10 times in the past year were recruited by advertising, and 54 were rein-terviewed one year later. The majority of respondents (53%) had three years or less experience with cocaine and preferred snorting or smok-ing, although 22 had injected cocaine. Although this study was deliber-ately designed to differ from an earlier one (i.e. Erickson et al., 1987) by recruiting current users who had moved beyond the experimental stage of cocaine use, the number of respondents who also had some experience of crack (79 of the 100) was unexpectedly high. Nevertheless, a pattern of infrequent and de-escalating use was also found in this group of crack users (Cheung et al., 1991). Since crack users did not differ markedly from the cocaine powder only users and indeed all but five were also powder users (Erickson, Watson and Weber, 1992), the combined group of 100 will be discussed below.

As Figure 15.1 shows, mean amount of cocaine used and frequency of use increased after the first year of use, but dropped from maximal

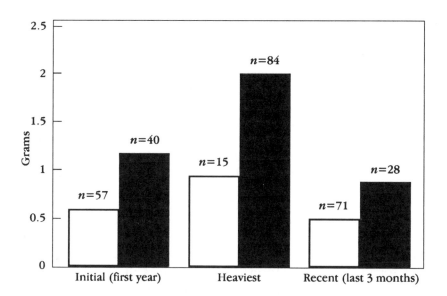

Figure 15.1 Mean amounts of cocaine consumed in three periods of use by fre-quency of use. The number (*n*) does not equal 100 due to some D/K responses. Frequency: (□) once per week or less; (■) more than once per week. (Source: Longitudinal study of cocaine users in the Toronto area – Erickson, 1991)

levels to lower than initial levels in the last three months. During the first year of use, half the respondents were using less than one-half of a gram of cocaine per occasion of use. Initially, respondents were more likely to use once a week or less ($n=57$) than to use more often ($n=40$), but at the heaviest use period, 85% were using more than weekly, consuming a mean amount of about 2g. Less frequent users ($n=15$) were consuming just under 1g on the average. In the last three months prior to the interview, 36 respondents had not used cocaine at all and another 35 were using once a week or less. Those who were still currently using more than once a week ($n=28$) were consuming less than 1g (about 0.75 g) per occasion. The picture presented at the first interview, then, was already one of diminishing frequency and amount of use. This same pattern was observed by Cohen (1989) and Ditton et al. (1991) in their samples of cocaine users.

By the one year follow-up ($n=54$), this pattern was further enhanced (Erickson, 1991). Of the 30% ($n=16$) who had not used either cocaine or crack in the past year, those with and without crack experience were about equally likely to have quit. Of the balance who were still using ($n=38$), the predominant pattern was either a steady decrease, describing 34% of this group, or an erratic start/stop one which characterised 37% of the users. For the remaining one third, use had peaked and declined (10%), fluctuated widely (10%), increased (5%) or been maintained at the same level as one year earlier (3%). In considering the interplay between cocaine and crack use, it is of interest to note that all of the current crack users ($n=16$) also used powder in the past year, and 59% ($n=16$ also) who were former crack users had continued to use powder cocaine in the past year. These results suggest, firstly, that crack is not necessarily a steady diet for users, that complementarity of smoking and intra-nasal routes is possible, and secondly, that some 'de-escalation' of use from crack to powder seems possible. This sample is small and may be unrepresentative of all those who have tried crack, but nevertheless directs us to consider the many alternative patterns to sheer escalation that can occur.

Waldorf, Reinarman and Murphy (1991) interviewed 228 current ($n=122$) and former ($n=106$) heavy users in California, including 45 persons who primarily smoked crack or freebased during their heaviest use period. To qualify for inclusion their respondents had to have used an average of 2g or more of cocaine weekly for at least six months, or have been daily users for at least 12 months. Most, however, had used cocaine for longer times and in greater amounts than the minimum sample criteria. For instance, average weekly intake was 4.69g during period of maximal use (and half had used 2g or more per week for at least one year). Thus, according to the national surveys, these respondents are drawn from the heaviest 5% of the continuum of those who have ever used cocaine.

Their conclusion was that 'no single, uniform career path that all heavy cocaine users ultimately follow' emerged (Waldorf, Reinarman and Murphy, 1991, p. 275). About as many respondents maintained stable use patterns, from periods of 1–10 years, as the number who escalated their use in ways that interfered with their daily roles and responsibilities. Moreover, at different times individuals shifted their patterns of use in ways that involved cutting back as well as escalation. Generally, controlled cocaine users shared these characteristics: 'had a number of meaningful roles which provided a positive identity and a stake in conventional daily life; developed and stuck to routines, rules and rituals that limited cocaine use opportunities; did not abuse alcohol or other drugs, nor did they use cocaine to manage other problems' (p. 153). Since the ways in which respondents quit, regained, or maintained control provide many suggestions for harm reduction strategies, they will be discussed in more detail later.

In summary, these various sources indicate that most cocaine use is experimental, infrequent and short-lived. Most continuous social-recreational users adopt a pattern in which they either maintain a low pattern of use for protracted periods, or else they increase use and then return to even lower levels again. Obviously many possible combinations occur other than simple escalation or termination of use. Although some people get into trouble with cocaine rapidly, the lag time before treatment entry has been found to be 3–5 years for cocaine (Clayton, 1985) and seven months to three years for crack (Wallace, 1990). It is also evident that there is no completely 'safe' period of controlled use. Compulsive, destructive use develops for a minority even after several years of using at stable, moderate levels. Moreover, escalation to problem levels can occur, though less commonly, in the absence of smoking or injecting cocaine; intranasal use can also be uncontrolled use. Risk factors identified for escalation included: being male, younger (adult) age, history of polydrug use, higher income, depressive illness, becoming employed after a period out of work. The next section will examine firstly, the ways in which users themselves control their cocaine use and secondly, the larger issue of control at the community or societal level.

Control

The risks that harm reduction is concerned about are those that threaten the user's or the community's health, safety and well-being (Strang, Chapter 1, this volume). In matters that fall outside the mandate of criminal or regulatory law, individuals have a great deal of leeway. They may choose whether or not to be shot out of a cannon, or to hang-glide, sunbathe, or swim in shark-infested waters. The choice is both personally and culturally determined. Although people like to 'pick their risks', and weigh for themselves whether the pleasure is worth it, they also base their decision on various sources, including culturally pre-digested information (Klaidman, 1991). 'What to favor and what to fear are cultural constructs that enable us to walk right past snarling monsters and run away from little-bitty things. If we want to know why we are fearful about what and whether we should be, this is equivalent to asking the cultural question: How should we live?' (Wildavsky, 1979, p. 36). This section will first look at how users evaluate, confront and mitigate the risks presented by cocaine and what role their social network plays in the informal control process, and then consider the broader context of formal social control.

Informal controls

Numerous studies have documented a high correlation between illicit drug use and use by peers, but rarely examine the process involved or the ways in which peers may restrain harmful use (Dembo et al., 1981; Kandel, 1985). These encompass the constraints operating within the individual's social network (Maloff et al., 1979). Harm reduction practices fall along a continuum of involvement with cocaine, starting with those who are most likely to try cocaine, namely young adults who are already users of other illicit drugs. The cannabis-cocaine connection has been identified as particularly important on the empirical basis that virtually every cocaine user has previously used cannabis, usually frequently (Murray, 1984; Clayton, 1985). Of course, the majority of cannabis users do not become cocaine users. Data are scarce, but a few studies have investigated willingness to try cocaine.

A group of Toronto cannabis offenders interviewed in 1973–1974 indicated quite a favourable attitude to trying cocaine if the opportunity arose and about half had already done so (Erickson, 1982). In the same locale, some 10 years later, a group of mainly recreational cocaine and cannabis users said that they had had no real hesitation in trying cocaine when it was offered (Erickson et al., 1987), but later came to view it as more of a health threat, more subject to social disapproval and shared by fewer friends than cannabis. Many had already quit or intended to stop cocaine use while persisting in cannabis use (Erickson and Murray, 1989). A group of powder cocaine users who had never injected it or smoked crack reported satisfaction with the effects of snorting and fear of the other method (Erickson et al., 1992). In a study of very heavily involved youthful cocaine users in the mid-1980s in Miami, Florida, Inciardi (1991) found a high degree of receptivity to crack, based on friends' and drug dealers' accounts, before youths had tried it. In contrast, a survey by Homel et al. (1990) of young adults in Sydney, Australia, 59% of whom had experience with illicit drugs, reported that only 5% were prepared to try cocaine if offered by a friend. These divergent findings across time and place, in conjunction with the survey findings of low or declining prevalence of cocaine use in most countries (RAND, 1991), suggest that cocaine is not always taken up with great enthusiasm, even among the more predisposed segments of the population.

The historical scenario of the early 1900s painted by Musto (1991) may be apt again: as the populace becomes more aware of the risks posed by cocaine, willingness to experiment declines. The message was somewhat belated in the USA and Canada, but has had time to reach much of Europe and Australia before the upsurge in global availability of cocaine (Homel et al., 1990; Hall and Hando, unpublished data, 1991). Counter to the notion of 'preordained pharmacological progression' is the evidence that social learning and cultural health beliefs can inhibit the uptake of cocaine among non-users (Erickson and Murray, 1989).

The next level of involvement with cocaine is the occasional, leisure or recreational pattern that dominates among the cocaine using population. These users consume small amounts infrequently, may have the occasional day-long 'binge', but maintain low or moderate levels overall. As noted earlier, such users have been studied in Holland, Canada, Australia, the USA and Scotland. Two broad, consistent sets of findings are relevant to harm reduction. The first is that, for a sizeable group of users, control over their cocaine use never becomes an issue, even after several years of exposure. Such users rarely purchase or otherwise seek out cocaine, they use it socially (e.g. parties, special occasions), take part in a number of other non-drug leisure/work activities and have a 'what's all the fuss - take it or leave it' attitude to cocaine.

The other grouping of casual users acknowledge the seductive appeal of cocaine which may take the form of an 'uncontrollable desire' to use it when it's around (Erickson et al., 1987). This recognition leads them to formulate guidelines to restrict its availability and their use. Advice offered to novice cocaine users often was not to try it all, but if they did, limit the amount, stick to snorting and always do it with friends (Erickson, Watson and Weber, 1992). Users developed rules, including these examples: use it only when you can rest the next day; use no more than a certain amount; use no more often than a specified number of times weekly or monthly; don't keep a supply around; never use alone, with certain persons or when depressed; use only in special social situations; never use for work or school (Cohen, 1989; Mugford and Cohen, 1989; Ditton et al., 1991; Waldorf, Reinarman and Murphy, 1991). Users articulate these rules to others in their social network and thus generate informal control (Murphy, Reinarman and Waldorf, 1989). For the majority of cocaine users, self-regulation is the norm, reinforced by the endogenous influence of the social group.

For another group of users, control poses a more serious challenge.

Some users progress to a greater degree of involvement with cocaine, using larger amounts weekly or more often. This does not necessarily imply that total or even partial loss of control must result. Studies that include these heavier users provide numerous examples of those who escalate their use to high levels without becoming compulsive seekers of cocaine and without impeding their daily roles and responsibilities; these users then return to lower levels, usually when their life circumstances change (Erickson et al., 1987). Nevertheless, this heavier pattern is a warning sign, for as Waldorf, Reinarman and Murphy (1991) caution, personal and informal social controls 'are not foolproof' and 'there is nothing necessarily permanent about a pattern of controlled use'. Some of those who get into trouble with cocaine end up in treatment settings. More is known about them (Gawin and Kleber, 1985; Wallace, 1990; Rounsaville and Carroll, 1991). Others, less studied, find ways, on their own and with the support of others, to reverse their disastrous course. Their experiences can help to inform harm-reduction strategies.

The most detailed accounts of heavily involved cocaine users not in treatment have been described in the USA by Waldorf, Reinarman and Murphy (1991) and in Canada by Cheung, Erickson and Landau (1991) and Erickson, Watson and Weber (1992). The most pertinent and consistent observation was that users who developed problems with cocaine found it necessary to impose permanent or temporary abstinence to regain control over the drug and their lives. In the US study of heavy users (45 had regularly smoked crack/freebase) it was striking that many who recognised their use was getting out of hand simply stopped without reporting physical withdrawal symptoms or more than transitory craving (see also Adams and Gfroerer, 1991, for similar survey findings). It was as if the balance tipped, not in one spectacular insight, but as a cumulative process in which the problems finally outweighed the pleasures. For others, the struggle was more protracted. The principal strategy was to 'put distance between themselves and the drug'. This did not usually mean seeking new, non-using friends. In fact, friends were an important resource for offering advice on stopping and for helping to maintain ties to conventional life. They may also have been the first to identify the expansion of cocaine use and the developing problem. There was no one 'magic fix' but rather a variety of strategies that worked for different individuals in different settings.

In the Canadian study of crack users (Cheung, Erickson and Landau, 1991), the major factor affecting the level of crack use was perceived risk of harm. Adverse physical, psychological and financial consequences of crack use cautioned users, and provided a countervailing force to the intense subjective pleasures of the crack high. Since two-thirds had not used crack in the month prior to the first interview and, of those who had, less than half used at least 10 times, it was evident that most were capable of at least temporary abstinence or controlled use; the follow-up a year later showed an increased proportion of non-users (Erickson, 1991). Strategies to control their own use included avoiding people and situations where cocaine would be found, limiting the amount used or the money spent and imposing more self-control (Erickson, Watson and Weber, 1992). Advice offered to daily cocaine users was: get help, quit, use less. None of these results reject the possibility, and indeed reveal such cases, of users who may deny the problems they are having with cocaine and exaggerate their ability to control use. What these recent studies suggest, however, is that friendship networks can be a very potent source of influence on those losing control, and an anchor for those trying to regain it.

An important qualification of these community studies in a variety of countries is that the samples are composed of (in varying degrees) predominantly middle-class, employed, adult, fairly conventional members of Western, developed societies. The relative ease with which most users maintain or regain control ought not to be extrapolated uncritically to, for example, inner-city youth, the unemployed, the disadvantaged, the criminal or other 'underclass' members of either the Western developed nations or the developed countries around the globe. That is not to say that pharmacology is ever destiny, but rather that the interplay between cocaine's pleasurable, reinforcing effects and the informal and cultural controls that reduce harm is likely to vary widely. It is important to know how much accurate knowledge is available about cocaine's risks and what other activities and opportunities are competing with the drug for meaning and focus in a person's life (Waldorf, Reinarman and Murphy, 1991). Nevertheless, the evidence that cocaine users make rational choices, that they weigh pros and cons of drug use, that the possibility exists for sustained controlled use or disentanglement from problematic use, encourage an approach to harm reduction that seeks to mobilize such informal controls.

Formal controls

Formal controls are the rules imposed by the state through criminal or regulatory law. For cocaine, total national prohibition on possession and distribution has been a constant in most western nations since about 1910–1920. Before 1900, cocaine was readily, commercially and legally available to anyone. In the brief, interim transition stage before criminalisation, medical professionals (physicians, dentists, pharmacists, in addition to the patent medicine suppliers) increasingly had the responsibility for distribution at the local/state/provincial levels (Murray, 1987; Musto, 1990). In contrast, amphetamine did not achieve widespread legal availability until the 1930s, a situation that persisted until after the Second World War when a wave of epidemics surfaced in several countries. This led to a much tighter regulation of supply, though amphetamine usually has remained available on medical prescription. Since the 1960s, a large black market in illicitly manufactured amphetamines has persisted in the UK, Australia, Japan, parts of Europe, and also in pockets of countries such as the USA and Canada where cocaine has become much more available (Hall and Hando, unpublished data, 1991; Miller and Kozel, 1991b).

The efforts to control cocaine through both the demand and supply side of prohibition have not prevented a great expansion in global production and trafficking networks since the 1970s (CSIS, 1992). Interdiction efforts have failed to stem the influx of cocaine into the USA and Canada, and measured by lower price and greater purity, the availability of cocaine has dramatically increased in these countries between 1980 and 1990 (Reuter, 1988; Erickson and Cheung, 1993). What I shall consider briefly in this chapter is the matter of how this increased availability appears to relate to user demand and consequences. Consider the most serious consequences, e.g. death, emergency room visits and admissions to treatment, all of which increased in Toronto, Ontario, during the mid to late 1980s, and then appeared to taper off (Single, Erickson and Skirrow, 1991). It is often assumed that harmful consequences increase in linear fashion according to the number of users. In fact, cocaine use was stable or declining, at generally low levels, in the population overall during this period (Adlaf, Smart and Canale, 1991; Smart, Adlaf and Walsh, 1991). This apparent discrepancy may be accounted for by lag effects (i.e. between the time of onset of regular use and the appearance of problems), increased heavy use by a small proportion of the user population, and greater purity of the drug product on the street. The point here is that it is the distribution of consumption that is crucial rather than absolute amount or the total number of users (Skog, 1992). This is germane to harm reduction which aims to influence behaviour at particular points on the consumption curve where the threshold of vulnerability is higher.

A comparison between snowmobile-related and cocaine-related deaths in Ontario will serve to further illustrate this important point (see Figures 15.2 and 15.3). The number of deaths from each cause are of similar magnitude, from about 25 to 35 annually. Between 1986 and 1990, snowmobile use went up, by about 80 000, to 320 000 (indicated by the number of registered vehicles), but the death rate per 100 000 registrations remained nearly constant (Rowe et al., 1992). During the same period, the estimated number of cocaine users in the adult and student population (indicated by any use in the past year) declined, by about 50 000, to 365 000, but the cocaine death rate per 100 000 users increased. The death rate was 5.6 in 1987 and 10.9 in 1989 for cocaine, and 9.9 and 11.0 for snowmobiles in the same years. The implications

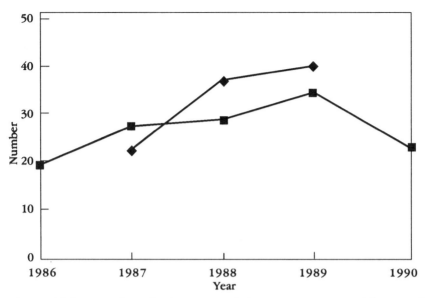

Figure 15.2 Hazardous deaths: snowmobile versus cocaine, 1986–1990. (■) snowmobile; (♦) cocaine. Suicides have been excluded from both data sets. (Sources: Snowmobile-related deaths in Ontario – Rowe et al., 1992; Chief Coroner's Office of Ontario, 1991)

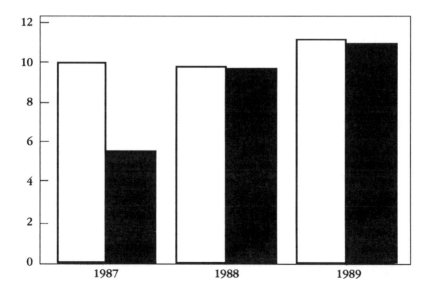

Figure 15.3 Snowmobile-related and cocaine death rates in Ontario, 1987–1989 (per 100 000 registered vehicles and per 100 000 cocaine users. (□) snowmobile; (■) cocaine. (Sources: Snowmobile-related deaths in Ontario – Rowe et al., 1992; Drug use among Ontario adults – Adlaf et al., 1991; Ontario student drug use in survery – Smart et al., 1991; data from the Chief Coroner's Office, 1991)

for preventing snowmobile deaths, in the absence of any other strategy, are quite straightforward: reduce the number of snowmobile users. For cocaine, reducing the number of users is not the simple answer; but reducing harmful practices may be. Thus to direct our formal control policies broadly at suppressing any level of cocaine use is not effective in addressing the harms associated with the heavier and more dangerous patterns.

A second point to be made about formal control is based on the economic argument. While supply side interdiction and enforcement are meant to keep the price high (and of course to pose the risk of arrest as a deterrent), the opposite effect has occurred in both the USA and Canada where prices declined for cocaine in the 1980s. Besides ineffectiveness, Maynard (1992) has also noted that sound data on the effects of enforcement on other related issues such as crime spillover and price-elasticity of cocaine are limited. An interesting historical comparison was made by Musto (1990) who showed that the unit price of cocaine on the street in 1908–1914 and in the early to mid 1980s was, in both periods, about 10 times the average hourly industrial wage (US$3.00 versus US$0.30, and US$50 compared to US$5.00). However, by the end of the 1980s, the cost of cocaine was lower, in buying power, 'than it was on the streets of New York City prior to the Harrison Act [of 1914, the first federal narcotics legislation] and while the legal control of cocaine was vested in the judgement of health professionals' (p. 323). Since the illicit market continued to exist during this health-regulated period, Musto (1990) suggests that the criminal syndicates of those earlier days may have had similar profit margins to the current ones, and that there may be a 'natural market rate' for the street level unit of cocaine. Whether this similarity is coincidence or not, it does provide further evidence that the formal control of cocaine through criminal law is an imprecise way to channel the market behaviour of buyers and sellers.

Implications

Interventions and strategies

This chapter has shown that we need knowledge from the different traditions of research to provide a comprehensive picture of the risks posed by cocaine. There are different kinds of potential risks associated with cocaine use. Some are physical and life-threatening, some compromise mental health and stability, and others are encompassed by compulsive, destructive urges to use cocaine, regardless of the mounting havoc on jobs, finances, loved ones and self-respect. The likelihood that any actual harm will result, however, is far from certain. The highly unpredictable effects of cocaine urge caution. Yet cocaine is not so terrible as it has been portrayed to the public on the wave of near hysteria about its deadly effects. The majority use infrequently, without apparent ill effects and without compulsion.

Based on the convergence of much research that points to a self-regulating pattern of controlled cocaine use, the next step could be to capitalise on this knowledge about informal control to maximise harm reduction among peers. How are we to build a risk-reducing drug subculture? This would require a shift from the prevailing mechanistic to the voluntaristic model, one that appreciates the positive aspects of the subculture in restraining and channelling the drug use of its members, that understands the attractions drug use offers, and that recognises that users weigh pros and cons in making their decisions about consumption. A more voluntaristic approach recognises that it is often inappropriate or futile for non-users to tell experienced drug users how to conduct their lives. Drug users have their own hierarchy of dangerousness that is based on perceived risk and experience (Erickson, 1982).

A barrier to developing such an approach to harm reduction among drug users in any publicly supported community way is that illicit drug users are, by definition, outside the orbit of such mainstream, legitimate support. Interventions that are currently favoured tend to be criminal justice enforcement or abstinence-requiring treatment programmes. Some kind of radical non-intervention – leaving users alone – may be all that most local jurisdictions can offer as an alternative. The drug subcultures themselves already may be building their own harm-reduction practices as knowledge is transmitted covertly. The continued marginalisation of cocaine users undoubtedly slows this process and likely augments harm, especially to new users.

Anti-drug advertising campaigns of the 'just say no' or of the sensationalised scare tactics variety tend to do more harm than good. First, they keep future users ignorant of cocaine's real risks and ways to avoid damaging themselves and second, they lose credibility with drug users for any 'mainstream' source of information about cocaine. Emphasis in the media on the worst-case scenarios of those helpless in the throes of cocaine, or even worse, crack addiction, reinforces the stigma attached to all users. Such perception counters the formation and public acceptance of the notion of a responsible, self-regulating and otherwise conventional group of cocaine users.

And what is the relevance of formal control to harm reduction? The existence of risk and the evidence of some harm resulting from cocaine use may be the basis for some form of state control over availability. It does not presuppose a vigorous criminal prohibition model; moreover, the state does not always stake a claim over the regulation of inherently risky activities. A great deal of choice is allowed the individual in matters not directly harming or disturbing others. One issue is how widespread the activity is, and thus its overall impact on the well-being of the society. Of course, custom and tradition play a crucial role and, for cocaine, that role has been one of efforts at complete state suppression for most of this century. Nevertheless, one can ask what a government might do if it embraced harm-reduction principles. How could government aid and abet this approach if it became an understanding partner? The move from theory to practice requires a pragmatic policy analysis of this question.

What other strategies might be considered to enhance or supplement informal and formal control? Approaches rooted in harm reduction suggest different emphases in education and treatment than those founded in suppression and total abstinence.

Drug education in the schools has not, in and of itself, been shown to have much impact on later behaviour (O'Connor and Saunders, 1992). These authors argue that this is because the value and meaning of being a drug user is not taken into consideration and the benefits of drug use are underestimated. From a harm reduction perspective, education programmes that provide a balanced view of risks and benefits, train those who do use drugs to do so carefully, and avoid reinforcing the values of the nonusers at the expense of stigmatising and marginalising the users, would likely be the most appropriate. Casual or experimental drug users, who have not had the opportunity to absorb safer techniques from a network of regular users, might be particular beneficiaries. Such an approach would be based in assessment of what students know, intended to do, and wanted to change. Even beyond the school setting, active drug users might be recruited to impart knowledge and skills that would minimise risk for those engaged in the activity. A concern with this alternative approach to education is that conveying notions of the acceptability of some forms of drug use might foster a social climate in which increased willingness to use drugs will become normative. Others would argue that as long as cultural reinforcement stops short of active promotion and marketing, social disapproval can still be predominant, without an inevitable accompanying increase in levels of harm.

The community studies reviewed earlier show that users can usually get out of trouble by themselves and 'with a little help from my friends'. Existing programmes for those seeking treatment nearly always focus on abstinence. This emphasis seems appropriate, given the findings that the heaviest but untreated users found abstinence necessary at least for a period (Waldorf, Reinarman and Murphy, 1991). This observation parallels research by alcohol researchers on 'spontaneous (untreated) recovery' from alcohol problems: even if some drinkers returned later to moderate drinking, nearly all imposed a period of abstinence on themselves (Sobell, Sobell and Toneatto, 1991). Greater flexibility in defining abstinence as a short-term, long-term or permanent goal is one implication of harm reduction for treatment interventions. Another implication is to introduce an array of harm-reducing practices into treatment programmes that offer controlled availability. This would attract users who wish to continue use. And the ready access to treatment at an early intervention stage, without stigmatisation (also found to have a positive effect on problem drinkers) could have potential to assist users in avoiding a more harmful escalation of their cocaine problem. Also, the balancing of pros and cons of their cocaine use that led some heavy users in the community studies to cut back or eliminate their cocaine use might be incorporated into a decision-making model for those in treatment. The notion that control is a real possibility could provide an important message to counter the all-powerful image of cocaine that encourages a defeatist or irresponsible attitude in those who might otherwise seek help.

A last comment on interventions relates to the macro or larger environmental conditions that influence drug use. These lie in the purview of the government, not the individual, and are not readily manipulated. Measures to improve the overall health and well-being of the population, and to reduce the poverty and deprivation that contribute to the vulnerability of parts of the population to harmful drug use, are an essential part of harm reduction (Wallack and Holder, 1987). Cocaine use seems more readily controlled when other sources of satisfaction, pleasure and self-esteem are present in the social milieu. Thus, in addition to enhancing individual resources, systemic features must be incorporated as well into an overall public health approach to harm minimisation.

In conclusion, harm reduction is not only possible, but essential, for cocaine and amphetamine. To make this transformation from present approaches requires a new paradigm for illicit drugs. Based on Kuhn (1962, p. 9), the continued existence of anomaly, i.e. that cocaine is shown to be neither as dangerous nor addictive as is popularly believed, will provoke questioning, crisis, and ultimately the adoption of a new approach. As McKenna (1992, p. xviii) says: 'The time has therefore come, in the great natural discourse that is the history of ideas, thoroughly to rethink our fascination with habitual use of psychoactive and physioactive plants. We have to learn from the excesses of the past... [but we cannot] support a view that wishes to divide society into users and nonusers. We need a comprehensive approach...'. We need a new paradigm; we need to recognise the reality and potential of controlled drug use; we need harm reduction.

References

Adams, E.H. and Gfroerer, J. (1991). Risk of cocaine abuse and dependence. In S. Schober and C. Schade (Eds), *The Epidemiology of Cocaine Use and Abuse*, pp. 253–262. Research Monograph No. 110. Rockville, MD: National Institute on Drug Abuse.

Adlaf, E.M., Smart, R.G. and Canale, M.D. (1991). *Drug Use Among Ontario Adults 1977–1991*. Toronto, Ontario: Addiction Research Foundation.

Akers, R.L. (1991). Addiction: The troublesome concept. *Journal of Drug Issues*, **21**, 777–792.

Alexander, B.K. (1991). The impact of research on drug use: Putting cocaine in perspective. Paper presented at the XIV World Conference of Therapeutic Communities, Montréal, Quèbec.

Anglin, L. (1985). *Cocaine: A Selection of Annotated Papers from 1880 to 1984 Concerning Health Effects*. Bibliography Series No. 19. Toronto, Ontario: Addiction Research Foundation.

Anthony, J.C. and Petronis, K.R. (1991). Epidemiologic evidence on suspected associations between cocaine use and psychiatric disturbances. In S. Schober and C. Schade (Eds), *The Epidemiology of Cocaine Use and Abuse*, pp. 71–94. Research Monograph No. 110. Rockville, MD: National Institute on Drug Abuse.

Arif, A. (Ed.) (1987). *Advance Health Consequences of Cocaine Use*. Geneva: World Health Organization.

Ben-Yehuda, N. (1990). *The Politics and Morality of Deviance: Moral Panics, Drug Abuse, Deviant Science and Reversed Stigmatization*. New York, NY: State University of New York Press.

Brady, J.V. (1991). Animal models for assessing drugs of abuse. *Neuroscience and Biobehavioral Reviews*, **15**, 35–43.

Byck, R. (1987). The effects of cocaine in complex performance in humans. *Alcohol, Drugs, and Driving*, **3**, 9–12.

Cheung, Y.W. and Erickson, P.G. (1993). Crack use in Canada: A distant American cousin. In C. Reinarman and H.G. Levine (Eds), *Crack in Context: Myths, Realities and Social Policy*. Berkeley, CA: University of California Press.

Cheung, Y.W., Erickson, P.G. and Landau, T. (1991). Experience of crack use: Findings from a community-based sample in Toronto. *Journal of Drug Issues*, **21**, 121–140.

Chitwood, D.D. and Morningstar, P.C. (1985). Factors which differentiate cocaine users in treatment from nontreatment users. *The International Journal of the Addictions*, **20**, 449–459.

CIBA (1992). *Cocaine: Scientific and Social Dimensions*. Chichester: John Wiley and Sons.

Clayton, R.R. (1985). Cocaine use in the United States: In a blizzard or just being snowed? In N.J. Kozel and E.H. Adams (Eds), *Cocaine Use in America: Epidemiologic and Clinical Perspectives*, pp. 8–34. Research Monograph No. 61. Rockville, MD: National Institute on Drug Abuse.

Cohen, P. (1989). *Cocaine Use in Amsterdam in Non Deviant Subcultures*. Amsterdam: Instituut voor Sociale Geografie, Universiteit van Amsterdam.

CSIS (1992). *Future Trends in Global Drug Consumption*. Seminar held at the Center for Strategic and International Studies, Washington, DC.

Davies, J.B. (1992). *The Myth of Addiction: An Application of the Psychological Theory of Attribution to Illicit Drug Use*. Chur, Switzerland: Harwood Academic.

Dembo, R., Babst, D.V., Burgos, W. and Schmeidler, J. (1981). Survival orientation and the drug use experiences of a sample of inner city junior high school youths. *The International Journal of the Addictions*, **16**, 1031–1047.

Des Jarlais, D.C. and Friedman, S.R. (1988). HIV infection among persons who inject illicit drugs: Problems and prospects. *AIDS*, **1**, 267–273.

Ditton, J., Farrow, K., Forsyth, A., Hammersley, R., Hunter, G., Lavelle, T., Mullen,

K., Smith, I., Davies, J., Henderson, M., Morrison, V., Bain, D., Elliott, L., Fox, A., Geddes, B., Green, R., Taylor, J. Dalgarno, P., Ferguson, I., Phillips, S. and Watt, S. (1991). Scottish cocaine users: Wealthy snorters or delinquent smokers? *Drug and Alcohol Dependence*, **28**, 269–276.

Erickson, P.G. (1982). Illicit drug use, peer attitudes, and perceptions of harmful effects among convicted cannabis offenders. *The International Journal of the Addictions*, **17**, 141–154.

Erickson, P.G. (1991). Some preliminary findings from a follow-up study of cocaine and crack users in Toronto. Paper prepared for 'The Cocaine and Crack Scene' workshop at the International Conference on Drug Policy Reform, Washington, DC.

Erickson, P.G., Adlaf, E.M., Murray, G.F. and Smart, R.G. (1987). The steel drug: Cocaine in perspective. Lexington, MA: DC Heath and Company.

Erickson, P.G. and Cheung, Y.W. (1992). Drug crime and legal control: Lessons from the Canadian experience. *Contemporary Drug Problems*, **19**, 247–277

Erickson, P.G. and Alexander, B.K. (1989). Cocaine and addictive liability. *Social Pharmacology*, **3**, 249–270.

Erickson, P.G. and Murray, G.F. (1989). The undeterred cocaine user: Intention to quit and its relationship to perceived legal and health threats. *Contemporary Drug Problems*, **17**, 141–156.

Erickson, P.G., Watson, V. and Weber, T. (1992). Cocaine users' perceptions of their health status and the risks of drug use. In P. O'Hare, R. Newcombe, A. Matthews, E. C. Buning and E. Drucker (Eds), *The Reduction of Drug-related Harm*, pp. 82–89. London: Routledge.

Fagan, J. and Chin, K-L. (1989). Initiation into crack and cocaine: A tale of two epidemics. *Contemporary Drug Problems*, **17**, 579–616.

Feldman, H.W. and Biernacki, P. (1988). The ethnography of needle sharing among intravenous drug users and implications for public policies and intervention strategies. In R.J. Battjes and R.W. Pickens (Eds), *Needle Sharing Among Intravenous Drug Abusers: National and International Perspectives*, pp. 75–88. Research Monograph No. 80. Rockville, MD: National Institute on Drug Abuse.

Foltin, R.W. and Fischman, M.W. (1991). Methods for the assessment of abuse liability of psychomotor stimulants and anorectic agents in humans. *British Journal of Addiction*, **86**, 1633–1640.

Gawin, F.H. (1991). Cocaine addiction: Psychology and neurophysiology. *Science*, **251**, 1580–1586.

Gawin, F.H. and Kleber, H.D. (1985). Cocaine use in a treatment population: Patterns and diagnostic distinctions. In N.J. Kozel and E.H. Adams (Eds), *Cocaine Use in America: Epidemiologic and Clinical Perspectives*, pp. 182–192. Research Monograph No. 61. Rockville, MD: National Institute on Drug Abuse.

Giffen, P.J., Endicott, S. and Lambert, S. (1991). *Panic and Indifference: The Politics of Canada's Drug Laws*. Toronto, Ontario: Canadian Centre on Substance Abuse.

Goode, E. (1989). The American drug panic of the 1980s: Social construction or objective threat? *Violence, Aggression and Terrorism*, **3**, 327–348.

Grinspoon, L. and Bakalar, J.B. (1985). *Cocaine: A Drug and its Social Evolution*. 2nd edn. New York, NY: Basic Books.

Homel, P., Flaherty, B., Reilly, C., Hall, W. and Carless, J. (1990). The drug market position of cocaine among young adults in Sydney. *British Journal of Addiction*, **85**, 891–897.

Inciardi, J.A. (1991). Crack-cocaine in Miami. In S. Schober and C. Schade (Eds), *The Epidemiology of Cocaine Use and Abuse*, pp. 263–274. Research Monograph No. 110. Rockville, MD: National Institute of Drug Abuse.

Jacobs, M.R. and Fehr, K.O'B. (1987). *Drugs and Drug Abuse:' A Reference Text.* 2nd edn. Toronto, Ontario Addiction Research Foundation.

Kandel, D.B. (1985). On processes of peer influences in adolescent drug use: A developmental perspective. *Advances in Alcohol and Substance Abuse*, 4, 139–163.

Kalant, O.J. (1987). *Maier's Cocaine Addiction*. [Der kokainismus, 1926.] Toronto: Addiction Research Foundation.

Klaidman, S. (1991). *Health in the Headlines: The Stories Behind the Stories.* New York, NY: Oxford University Press.

Kozel, N.J. and Adams, E.H. (1985). Cocaine use in America: Summary of discussion and recommendations. In N.J. Kozel and E.H. Adams (Eds), *Cocaine Use in America: Epidemiologic and Clinical Perspectives*, pp. 221–226. Research Monograph No. 61. Rockville, MD: National Institute on Drug Abuse.

Kuhn, T.S. (1962). *The Structure of Scientific Revolutions*, 2nd edn (Volume 2, No. 2, International encyclopedia of unified science.) Chicago, IL: The University of Chicago Press.

Maloff, D., Becker, H.S., Fonaroff, A. and Rodin, J. (1979). Informal social controls and their influence on substance use. *Journal of Drug Issues*, 9, 161–184.

Maynard, A. (1992). The economics of drug use and abuse. Paper presented at CIBA Foundation Symposium No. 166, *Cocaine: Scientific and Social Dimensions*. Chichester, England: John Wiley and Sons.

McKenna, T. (1992). *Food of the Gods*. New York, NY: Bantam Books.

Metropolitan Toronto Workgroup (1991). *Drug use in Metropolitan Toronto June 1991*. Toronto, Ontario: Metropolitan Toronto Workgroup on Drug Use and Abuse.

Miller, M.A. and Kozel, N.J. (1991a). Introduction and overview. In M.A. Miller and N.J. Kozel (Eds), *Methamphetamine Abuse: Epidemiologic Issues and Implications*, pp. 1–5. Research Monograph No. 115, Rockville, MD: National Institute on Drug Abuse.

Miller, M.A. and Kozel, N.J. (Eds). (1991b). *Methamphetamine Abuse: Epidemiologic Issues and Implications*. Research Monograph No. 115. Rockville, MD: National Institute on Drug Abuse.

Montagne, M. (1991). Descriptive epidemiology of international cocaine trafficking. In S. Schober and C. Schade (Eds), *The Epidemiology of Cocaine Use and Abuse*, pp. 275–296. Research Monograph No. 110. Rockville, MD: National Institute on Drug Abuse.

Mugford, S. and Cohen, P. (1989). *Drug Use, Social Relations and Commodity Consumption: A study of Recreational Users in Sydney, Canberra and Melbourne*. Report to the Research into Drug Abuse Advisory Committee, National Campaign Against Drug Abusers, Canberra, Australia.

Murphy, S.B., Reinarman, C. and Waldorf, D. (1989). An 11-year follow-up of a network of cocaine users. *British Journal of Addiction*, 84, 427–436.

Murray, G.F. (1984). The cannabis-cocaine connection: A comparative study of use and users. *Journal of Drug Issues*, 14, 665–675.

Murray, G.F. (1987). The road to regulation: Patent medicines in Canada in historical perspective. In J.C. Blackwell and P.G. Erickson (Eds). *Illicit Drugs in Canada: A Risky Business*, pp.72–87. Scarborough, On: Nelson Canada.

Musto, D.F. (1973). *The American Disease: Origins of Narcotic Control*. New Haven, CT: Yale University Press.

Musto, D.F. (1990). Illicit price of cocaine in two eras: 1908–14 and 1982–89. Connecticut Medicine, 54, 321–325.

Musto, D.F. (1991). Opium, cocaine and marijuana in American history. *Scientific American*, **265**, 40–47.

Newcomb, M.D. and Bentler, P.M. (1986a). Cocaine use among adolescents: Longitudinal associations with social context, psychopathology, and use of other substances. *Addictive Behaviors*, **11**, 263–273.

Newcomb, M.D. and Bentler, P.M. (1986b). Cocaine use among young adults. *Advances in Alcohol and Substance Abuse*, **6**, 73–96.

O'Connor, J. and Saunders, B. (1992). Drug education: An appraisal of a popular preventive. *The International Journal of the Addictions*, 27, 165–185.

RAND (1991). *American and European Drug Policies: Comparative Perspectives.* Washington, DC: Rand Washington Office.

RCMP (1991). *National Drug Intelligence Estimate 1990*. Ottawa, On: Drug Enforcement Directorate, Royal Canadian Mounted Police.

Reuter, P. (1988). Quantity illusions and paradoxes of drug interdiction: Federal intervention into vice policy. *Law and Contemporary Problems*, **51**, 233–252.

Ritter, C. and Anthony, J.C. (1991). Factors influencing initiation of cocaine use among adults: Findings from the epidemiologic catchment area program. In S. Schober and C. Schade (Eds). *The Epidemiology of Cocaine Use and Abuse*, pp. 190–210. Research Monograph No. 110. Rockville, MD: National Institute on Drug Abuse.

Rounsaville, B. and Carroll, K. (1991). Psychiatric disorders in treatment-entering cocaine abusers. In S. Schober and C. Schade (Eds), *The Epidemiology of Cocaine Use and Abuse*, pp. 227–251. Research Monograph No. 110. Rockville, MD: National Institute on Drug Abuse.

Rowe, B., Milner, R., Johnson, C. and Bota, G. (1992) Snowmobile-related deaths in Ontario: A 5-year review. *Canadian Medical Association Journal*, **146**, 147–152.

Ruttenber, A.J., Sweeney, P.A., Mendleim, J.W. and Wetli, C.V. (1991). Preliminary findings of an epidemiologic study of cocaine-related deaths, Dade County, Florida, 1978–85. In S. Schober and C. Schade (Eds), *The Epidemiology of Cocaine Use and Abuse*, pp. 95–111. Research Monograph No. 110. Rockville, MD: National Institute on Drug Abuse.

Sandwijk, J.P., Cohen, P.D.A. and Musterd, S. (1991). *Licit and Illicit drug use in Amsterdam.* Amsterdam: Instistuut voor Sociale Georgrafie, Universiteit van Amsterdam.

Scheerer, S. (1991). Emergence of an international regime: The case of cocaine. Paper presented at the Conference on *Law and Society*, Amsterdam, The Netherlands.

Schwartz, R.J., Luxenberg, M.G. and Hoffman, N.G. (1991). 'Crack' use by American middle-class adolescent polydrug abusers. *The Journal of Pediatrics*, **118**, 150–155.

Single, E., Erickson, P.G. and Skirrow, J. (1991). Drugs and public policy in Canada. Paper presented at the Conference on *National Drug Policy*, Rand Institute, Drug Policy Research Center, Washington, DC.

Skog, O.-J. (1992). Epidemiological and biostatistical aspects of alcohol use, alcoholism and their complications. In P.G. Erickson and H. Kalant (Eds), *Windows on Science*. Toronto, Ontario: ARF Books.

Smart, R.G. and Anglin, L. (1987). Do we know the lethal dose of cocaine? *Journal of Forensic Sciences*, **32**, 303–312.

Smart, R.G., Adlaf, E.M. and Walsh, G.W. (1991). *The Ontario Student Drug Survey: Trends Between 1977 and 1991*. Toronto, Ontario: Addiction Research Foundation.

Sobell, L.C., Sobell, M.B. and Toneatto, T. (1991). Recovery from alcohol problems without treatment. In N. Heather, W.R. Miller and J. Greeley (Eds), *Self-control and the Addictive Behaviours*. Sydney: Maxwell Macmillan.

Stimson, G.V., (1992). Drug injecting and HIV infection: New directions for social science research. *International Journal of the Addictions*, 27, 147–163.

Stimson, G.V. and Lart, R. (1991). HIV, drugs, and public health in England: New words, old tunes. *International Journal of the Addictions*, 26, 1263–1277.

Suwaki, H. (1991). Methamphetamine abuse in Japan. In M.A. Miller and N.J. Kozel (Eds), *Methamphetamine Abuse: Epidemiologic Issues and Implications*, pp. 84–98. Research Monograph No. 115. Rockville, MD: National Institute on Drug Abuse.

Waldorf, D., Murphy, S.B., Reinarman, C. and Joyce, B. (1977). *Doing Coke: An Ethnography of Cocaine Users and Sellers*. Washington, DC: Drug Abuse Council.

Waldorf, D., Reinarman, C. and Murphy, S. (1991). *Cocaine Changes: The Experience of Using and Quitting*. Philadelphia, PA: Temple University Press.

Wallace, B.C. (1990). Crack addiction: Treatment and recovery issues. *Contemporary Drug Problems*, 17, 79–119.

Wallack, L. and Holder, H. (1987). The prevention of alcohol-related problems: A systems approach. In H. Holder (Ed.), *Control Issues in Alcohol Abuse Prevention: Strategies for States and Communities*. Advances in Substance Abuse: Behavior and Biological Research, Supplement 1.

Watters, J.K., Cheng, Y.-T. and Lorvick, J.J. (1991). Drug use profiles, race, age, and risk of HIV infection among intravenous drug users in San Francisco. *International Journal of the Addictions*, 26, 1247–1260.

Wildavsky, A. (1979). No risk is the highest risk of all. *American Scientist*, 67, p.36. (Cited in Klaidman, S. (1991). *Health in the Headlines: The Stories Behind the Stories*. New York, NY: Oxford University Press).

Wong, L.S. and Alexander, B.K. (1991). 'Cocaine-related' deaths: Media coverage in the war on drugs. *Journal of Drug Issues*, 21, 105–119.

Zinberg, N.E. (1984). *Drug, Set and Setting: The Basis for Controlled Intoxicant Use*. New Haven, CT: Yale University Press.

Chapter 16
Cannabis: Legal Reform, Medicinal Use and Harm Reduction

JOHN P. MORGAN, DIANE RILEY and GREGORY B. CHESHER

Compared to heroin and cocaine, cannabis is seldom prominently discussed in the context of harm reduction. It is however invariably the first drug proposed for reform during any discussion of drug policy; and that discussion often, even unwittingly, involves harm reduction. One could wish to normalize cannabis to reduce at least the real harm of continued criminalization. More than 300 000 people are arrested for cannabis-related offenses in the United States of America annually (Gettman, 1991) and the great majority are charged with simple possession (some may be dealers but the possession offense is more easily proved). Cannabis illegality contributes to the expanded use of workplace and criminal justice urine testing for cannabis metabolite and other drugs in the United States of America. The discovery of small amounts of urinary Δ-9-tetrahydrocannabinol carboxylic acid (Δ-9-THC) by urine surveillance (Morgan, 1988) is a frequent cause of job loss (or non-hiring) and a frequent cause of loss of probation/parole for those supervised by the criminal justice system, whatever their sentencing offense.

Opponents of cannabis reform accept (or actively promote) illegality because they view the normalization of cannabis with great fear. The structure of opposition to altering cannabis prohibition remains unchanged since the late 1970s. Prohibitionists believe: that cannabis is much more dangerous than once thought, and current use causes much clinical and biological harm; that it serves as a 'gateway' drug, introducing users culturally and psychologically to more dangerous drugs; and removal of legal constraint will cause an enormous expansion of consumption, magnifying personal and social costs.

In the past decade, these concerns have been reinforced by the belief that contemporary cannabis is much more potent (higher in Δ-9-THC content by weight) than the American cannabis of the 1960s and 1970s. This 'new' cannabis is believed to be highly dangerous both as an acute intoxicant contributing to accidents and mistakes, and as a chronic toxic agent contributing to impaired immune function, diminished fertility, pulmonary disease and psychopathology.

In the United States of America, cannabis reform is now linked to medical and therapeutic uses of cannabis. Prohibitionists believe that the support of cannabis as medicine is a reformist ruse to legalize the drug. However, the claims of medical utility have gained ground recently with the published preliminary evidence of weight gain caused by Δ-9-THC in a small group of patients with HIV-related wasting (Plasse et al., 1991). The recent discovery of an endogenous ligand for the cannabis receptor reveals the probable existence of a hitherto unknown brain system. A further understanding of this neurological system might have enormous therapeutic potential (Devane et al., 1992).

Therefore, this essay on cannabis and harm reduction shall briefly, and perhaps too broadly, examine the following:

1. What are the claims of cannabis-induced toxicity and what is the proof that such toxicity exists?
2. Does cannabis serve as a gateway drug?
3. Are contemporary cannabis preparations highly potent and what are the potential consequences of such potency?
4. Will drug reform (legalization, normalization or decriminalization) lead to an explosion of use?
5. What are the claims about the therapeutic potential of cannabis?

Cannabis Toxicity

In the early to mid 1970s, there was a prominent movement in the United States of America toward cannabis reform. Individual states had begun to diminish the likelihood of jail time for possession. Preliminary reports of a series of studies of chronic users in Jamaica (Rubin and Comitas, 1975), Costa Rica (Coggins, 1976) and Greece (Fink et al., 1976) indicated a minimum of biological harm. However, at exactly this same time, a counter-reform movement overtly based in toxicology was gathering strength.

In 1974, Gabriel Nahas of Columbia University helped convene a group of clinical scientists who had reported cannabis-induced harm in humans. These men all presented to Senator James Eastland's Internal Security Committee hearings on the harm of cannabis and its implied threat to United States security (US Committee on the Judiciary, 1974). Discussed were claims of immunopathogenicity, pulmonary damage, brain cell damage, amotivational states, and sexual/reproductive damage including decreased testosterone. Nahas in his own book, *Marijuana: Deceptive Weed,* presented these claims as proven fact and mixed in a series of political and conspiratorial ideas as well (Nahas, 1973). He speculated that great Arabic societies had fallen because of cannabis use and that the Communist Chinese planned to promote revolution by amplifying the toxicomania already underway in the West.* Nahas's willingness to accept any anti-cannabis speculation is illustrated by a lengthy discussion on the probable use of cannabis for suicide in Europe, provoked by a single Belgian student who, it was rumored, tried to take his life by smoking a pipebowl full of cannabis. Nahas had presented these ideas earlier in a brief publication discussing 'lethal' cannabis toxication (Nahas, 1971).

In a 1986 article discussing health aspects of cannabis use, Leo Hollister reviewed all of the claims of cannabis toxicity presented to Senator Eastland (Hollister, 1986). He commented on both the large field studies of the 1970s and two prospective 30- and 94-day studies funded by the US government (Cohen, 1976; Jones and Benowitz, 1976): 'If field studies fail to provide evidence of harm from prolonged use of cannabis it is unlikely that experimental studies will do better and such has been the case'. Although he notes that the field studies could miss rare or unusual consequences of great importance: 'Nonetheless, one is forced to conclude that cannabis is a relatively safe drug as social drugs go. To date it compares favorably with tobacco and alcohol, if not with caffeine'.

All interested in drug policy and cannabis owe a considerable debt to Leo Hollister, whose integrity prevented him from joining the chorus of Government-funded scientists claiming to discover cannabis toxicity.[†]

We shall only briefly comment on the important toxicity claims below. Readers are referred to Hollister and other sources for more detail regarding these claims.

Immunity

In some animal and cellular studies exposure to large amounts of cannabinoids alters immune function (Zimmerman et al., 1977). However, studies performed by Nahas presented at the Eastland hearings and later elsewhere claimed that exposure to cannabis impaired *human* cell-mediated immunity (Nahas et al., 1974). These claims and citations of Nahas's early reports were revived by the apparent association in the 1980s between drug use and HIV infection. A variety of

---

*Nahas's style is indicated by the Chinese Communist material. The claim regarding the Chinese plan is actually referenced to a conversation. Someone named M. Heykal was supposedly privy to talk between Chou En Lai and Nasser about these drug plans. We are told nothing more about the eavesdropping Heykal, his credibility nor his conveyance of these plots to Dr Nahas.

†Hollister was very well funded by the Federal government to perform cannabis studies in the 1960s and 1970s. Whether his failure to condemn the drug during the 1980s influenced his support we do not know. We do know from one of the writers of a companion article in the cannabis issue of *Pharmacological Reviews* that the journal was under severe pressure not to publish Hollister's article which was viewed by anti-cannabis forces, particularly Nahas, as a whitewash of the drug.

studies both before and after the emergence of HIV do not confirm any clinical impact of marijuana use on immune function (Lau et al., 1976; Kaslow et al., 1989).

Endocrine and reproductive effects

Decreased levels of testosterone with spermatic morphological abnormalities and impaired sexual functioning associated with cannabis were reported at the Eastland Committee hearings and in a published paper (Kolodny et al., 1974). This triad has never been confirmed. Some studies have repeated the findings of a small decrease in testosterone (although not to abnormal concentrations). However, there has been no confirmation of diminished spermatic production or sexual dysfunction in users. Later studies even call into question the decreased testosterone claims; the original studies may have misrepresented the usual within-day fluctuation in serum testosterone (Mendelson et al., 1974; Abel, 1981).

Reproductive effect

Although marijuana use has been shown to correlate with lower birth weight (Linn et al., 1983), it has been difficult to separate this from other factors, including tobacco and alcohol use. The absence of a definite clinical association between cannabis use and fetal abnormality does not mean that rare serious harm could not occur; however, there is currently no proved association between any dose of maternal cannabis and human fetal harm.

Brain damage and psychopathology

At some time every possible behavioral aberration (panic attacks, amotivational states, acute organic brain syndromes, paranoia, psychosis and the generation of violence) has been attributed to cannabis. The Eastland hearings helped to publicize that cannabis caused an opting-out behaviour labeled the 'amotivational syndrome' (Kolansky and Moore, 1972). There has been little support for any systematic effect on behaviour, including motivation, in any study with any controls. The reports mentioned above link disapproved behavior with antecedent cannabis use; they were accepted and widely publicized because a belief in drug-induced misbehavior characterizes a temperance society. Not so much publicity has attended reported associations between cannabis use and adequate academic performance (Goode, 1971) or the association of moderate cannabis use and positive life adjustment (not true of heavy use or abstinence) (Shedler and Block, 1990). Indeed 'psychopathology', deviant behaviour or adolescent anger may predispose to heavy cannabis use rather than the other way around (Halikas, Goodwin and Guze, 1972).

Acute cannabis effect and its persistence

Cannabis-induced acute effect on perception, psychic changes, mood and cognition are variable, dose-related and affected to some degree by both setting expectation and prior experience (Hollister, Overall and Gerber, 1975). Some individuals experience a euphoric 'high' associated with alterations in time sense, perception and usual thought process; others do not. Psychomotor function such as operating an automobile is impaired if the doses are high enough and the tasks difficult enough. However, low dose studies may not show appreciable impairment in task performance but occasionally improvement. For example, in some closed-course driving experiments, users become exceedingly careful and do not engage in risky behavior which would lower their total scores (Klonoff, 1974).

We believe that the acute use of cannabis may be associated with social and motor impairment and users must be held accountable for the consequences of driving or other hazardous acts. These responsibilities would not diminish under cannabis reform but would appropriately increase.

Most early studies of smoked cannabis noted that a single cigarette or portion thereof produced a 2–3 hour effect. In a large non-crossover study, cannabis effect, as assessed by a computer-based task, was absent three hours after smoking (Dauncy, 1989). This type of between-subject parallel study may be more reliable than usual cannabis studies in which an individual's performance on drug is compared to his own performance on placebo. Experienced users are seldom fooled and the study is not truly controlled. In the Dauncy study, large numbers of individuals were studied once, either after placebo or various cannabis doses. Recently, significant publicity was generated by an uncontrolled study using an airplane-flight simulator indicating a persistence of some aspects of cannabis-induced impairment up to 24 hours after smoking (Yesavage et al., 1985). In attempts to confirm the finding using controls, the authors could not find an effect that persisted beyond four hours (Leirer, Yesavage and Morrow, 1989). However, in a third publication, the same authors renewed their claim of some 24-hour effect (Leirer, Yesavage and Morrow, 1991)*. The second and third publications in the flight simulator series generated little attention. The first study is still frequently cited.

---

*The third airplane stimulator study employed a one-tailed t-test which identified statistically significant effects at 24 hours. We believe that most investigators would not assume that the direction of test changes could move only in a single direction and that this is an inappropriate use of the statistic. A conventional two-tailed test indicates no statistically significant effect 24 hours after use of cannabis.

Pulmonary issues

Since almost all cannabis is consumed in the West by combustion and inhalation, much concern has been directed toward a possible impact on pulmonary function. Forest Tennant presented descriptions of pulmonary damage at the Eastland hearings; he had previously described bronchitis and other problems in young hashish smokers who were also tobacco users (Tennant et al., 1971). Attempts to assess the impact of cannabis smoking have been complicated by the concomitant use of smoked tobacco by most users. Also, customary employment of very deep inhalation and breath holding by cannabis smokers increases the particulate deposit per cigarette, and might increase hazards. However, the difference between the cigarettes smoked daily by the heavy tobacco smoker (40–60) and the heavy cannabis smoker (4–5) probably dimishes the pulmonary risk. Further, only a very few cannabis users are heavy smokers by even this criterion. The character of cannabis effect facilitates its occasional use unlike the character of tobacco which provokes smokers to seek nicotine at frequent intervals. There is general acceptance that neither nicotine nor Δ-9-THC are pulmonary pathogens. The dangers of smoking relate to the concomitant inhalation of combusted hydrocarbon plant material which may cause both pulmonary inflammation and carcinogenesis.

Since 1983, a group of Los Angeles based clinical scientists have followed, monitored and compared pulmonary function in smokers of cannabis only, smokers of tobacco only and a group of smokers of both. The initial evaluation included 144 cannabis smokers who averaged 28 joints per week. The tobacco-only and combined-use groups averaged 28.9 and 18.8 tobacco cigarettes respectively per day. A control group of non-smokers is employed for comparison. A review of the group's work, citing thirteen earlier publications, has recently appeared (Tashkin et al., 1990). Briefly, cannabis-only smokers had functional impairment indicative of damage in larger airways as opposed to the characteristic damage to peripheral airways and alveolar regions in tobacco smokers. Approximately 50 percent of the smoking groups appeared for re-examination in two or three years; the re-examination confirmed these findings. There has been little or no change in the most recent evaluation of the volunteers in 1990 (D.P. Tashkin, personal communication, 1992). Cannabis smokers also demonstrated abnormal histopathologic changes in bronchial biopsies compared to non-smokers. Although of concern, the larger airway changes are not those indicative of progression to chronic obstructive pulmonary disease and emphysema.

These reports indicate that the repeated inhalation of combusted cannabis is damaging to the pulmonary system. There appears to be little reason to fear the chronic obstructive pulmonary crippling lesion of the tobacco smoker but the possibility of carcinomatous change remains. The cannabis smokers studied here are heavy users and unfortunately there are apparently no other ongoing studies. This relatively small group of users is also being followed by the same NIDA-funded group. These studies document to a degree the only biological perturbation associated with chronic cannabis use.

Gateway Drugs

The above subject may not merit a separate heading except in terms of rhetoric. Since cannabis use correlates with the use of more dangerous drugs such as heroin and cocaine, it might be viewed as a 'gateway' drug. Robert DuPont's book, *Getting Tough on Gateway Drugs* (DuPont, 1985) is popular with anti-drug forces. This idea is consistent with policy directed as much toward the symbolic as the substantive. Cannabis is not as toxic as cocaine or heroin; however, young people should resist it because it may lead to hard drug use. It resembles a kind of temptation leading to downfall, like frequenting a pool hall.

The interpretation indicts cannabis as a gateway drug because most users of dangerous drugs have previously used less dangerous drugs. Essentially all users of heroin have previously consumed cannabis, alcohol, caffeine, nicotine and benzodiazepines. All psychoactive drugs use tends to correlate with other psychoactive drug use. This gateway concept, however, seems to resemble identifying driving slowly and safely as a gateway to driving recklessly and unlawfully. The reckless driver has always driven carefully at some point. How often does careful driving proceed to recklessness and does the careful driving cause the recklessness?

Perhaps 60 million Americans have tried marijuana yet slightly more than two thirds have never tried another illegal drug. Cannabis seems more often to be a closed gate than a gateway in that its use signals the terminus of illegal drug experimentation. In describing a group of cocaine users, Erickson and Alexander (1989) noted that all had used cannabis before they had used cocaine; however, the mean time from first cannabis use to first cocaine use was eight years.

Cannabis Potency

For slightly more than a decade, American media have been informed by a group of drug pundits that contemporary cannabis preparations are much more potent than cannabis products of the 1970s. In 1980 and 1986, the *New York Times* carried lengthy, prominent articles discussing the highly potent new cannabis (Brody, 1980; Kerr, 1986). If they exist, what might be the meaning and impact of highly potent cannabis preparations?

Cannabis containing 0.05 percent Δ-9-THC by weight is often judged effective; such a joint weighing one gram would contain 5 mg Δ-9-THC. Even by mouth, a 2.5 mg capsule of Δ-9-THC is both therapeutic in terms of nausea and vomiting and psychoactivity, even distressingly so for some users. A joint containing 10 percent Δ-9-THC would contain 20 times the psychoactive material (100 mg). Ten percent cannabis has been frequently described (Mikuriya and Aldrich, 1988). Anti-reformers believe that such potent material might provoke unwanted effects and surprising toxicity. There is little evidence that such enhanced toxicity exists, probably because smokeable cannabis provides an easy method for autotitration. The onset of cannabis effect is rapid following inhalation and smokers may receive many cues as to dosage. Although the medical literature has conflicting information, a number of recent articles document that smokers inhale lower doses when presented with increasingly potent cannabis (Herning, Hocker and Jones, 1986; Heishman, Stitzer and Yingling, 1989). Therefore, enhanced potency might be a *harm reduction* strategy. The pulmonary pathology described above does not occur because of cannabinoids but because of inhaled particulate material and toxins related to the smoking process. Therefore, presented with potent product, a user engaging in autotitration might inhale less to achieve effect and might therefore reduce the pulmonary hazard. The customary method of smoking cannabis using deep inhalation and breath holding probably does not increase the absorption of cannabinoid (although it has an impact) as much as it increases the deposition of hydrocarbon debris (Taskin et al., 1991).

However, the new highly potent cannabis is a myth. Very potent cannabis preparations, even exceeding 15 percent, occur; but these were present in the early 1970s. The claims of the *New York Times* articles and its informants were based on a NIDA-funded potency monitoring project based at the University of Mississippi. The Mississippi data, however, indicate that since the early 1980s the potency of American domestic cannabis has been very stable (Hawks and Walsh, 1990). These data reflect the current potency of seized domestic cannabis. In the early 1970s, when the monitoring project began, it analyzed only a few DEA-seized *imported* samples. In these seizures low potency Mexican kilobrick material predominated (El Sohley et al., 1984). A comparison of 1980s domestic material exceeding 3 percent Δ-9-THC to fewer than 15 seizures of 1974 Mexican material with less than 0.4 percent Δ-9-THC led to the serious misrepresentation of potency to *NY Times* and wire-service reporters. These improper comparisons may have been made in error but they reflected the desires of media sources, including past and present Federal anti-drug employees Robert DuPont, Sidney Cohen and Richard Hawks, to identify this 'new' cannabis as highly dangerous.

The Impact of Cannabis Reform

There is no consensus on the meaning of 'decriminalization'. In practice it has never meant the total elimination of criminal sanction for the cultivation, possession or sale of cannabis. In the United States of America in the 1970s it was used to denote the reduction of penalties for possession of small amounts of cannabis to punishments other than imprisonment. An examination of decriminalization focuses on the impact of reducing penalties, not eliminating them.

Those who support criminal penalties for cannabis possession believe that such laws act as a deterrent to use. There is minimal evidence that this is so. Substantial increases in cannabis use have occurred in North America despite the enforcement of very punitive measures. Although some non-users of cannabis may cite a fear of punishment, it is unlikely that a significant deterrent effect can exist when the risk of detection and punishment is so low. It requires money and committment for police to have arrested 300 000 Americans annually for cannabis offenses in recent years (Gettman, 1991). However, this probably represents fewer than 1 out of every 100 annual users.

Prior to the 1960s any cannabis use was easily condemned as a menace and was identified with lower social groups and a very small avant-garde set. The evolution of the view that moderate use was not horribly dangerous reflected increased middle-class use. The concept that the drug should not be thought of with harder drugs was enshrined in the 1972 National Commission Report (The Schaffer Commission) (Anonymous, 1972): 'Experimental or intermittent use of this drug carries minimal risk to public health and should not be given over zealous attention' (p.91).

In the 1970s there were many attempts in North America to reform cannabis laws. The movement was fueled not only by the belief that occasional use caused minimal harm but also on an assessment of the costs of increasing enforcement, court use and jailing. By 1978, 11 states populated by one-third of the American population had eliminated jail time as a punishment for cannabis offenses. Thirty other states had provisions for conditional discharge and 12 for clearing of criminal records for first-possession offenders. There are no systematic data on the effects of these American changes but a number of small surveys were done. In Ohio, decriminalization (enacted in 1975) was accompanied by a six percent increase in use from 1974–1978 in those aged 18–24 (Spitzner, 1979). A similar California survey detailed a seven percent increase in 11 months before and after decriminalization. The authors of these documents believed that these modest increases paralleled the increases in states which did not criminalize. Eric Single in evaluating national surveys carried out between 1972 and 1977 noted that use was higher in non-decriminalization states than other states *before and after* changes in the law. States that moderated penalties after 1974 did experience small increases in rates of cannabis use. However, the increase in cannabis use was greatest in non-decriminalization states and the largest proportionate increase occurred in those states with the most severe penalties (Single, 1989).

Self-reported cannabis use was collected in Ann Arbor, Michigan and three neighboring communities during a time when Ann Arbor legally moved through prohibition, reduction of penalty (still with possible imprisonment), misdemeanor (with a maximum of US$5 fine), reinstatement of severe penalty and finally a return to decriminalization. Data collected at four points in time in Ann Arbor indicated no changes in cannabis use as a result of changes in the law (Single, 1989).

Data were also collected by the annual High School Senior Survey. In 1981 this project surveyed use and attitudes in states that decriminalized versus other states. There was no evidence that cannabis use in any state bore a relationship to its legal status. Further, this survey documented that the national decline in cannabis use which began in 1979 and continues to this year occurred alike in states that decriminalized and states that did not (Johnston, O'Mally and Bachman, 1981).

Currently, there is a strong move to recriminalize cannabis in Alaska, which has the most liberal American policy. The state Supreme Court adjudged and reaffirmed that a strong privacy law in the state constitution prevents state intrusion into a private home to search for evidence of consumption (and storage) of cannabis. Although sale and consumption outside the home remain illegal, use inside the home is not. Alaska is not included in the two large NIDA-funded surveys which monitor self-reported drug use, the Household Survey and the High School Senior Survey; therefore, little prior documentation about Alaskan use has been available. Recent studies by Segal document that Alaskans consume more cannabis than their counterparts in mainland states (Segal, 1989). Alaskans for the Recriminalization of Marijuana (ARM) point to this higher prevalance with alarm and used it effectively in a recent referendum vote to recriminalize* (Egan, 1991).

The relatively high prevalence of cannabis use by youthful Alaskans is seen in all psychoactive drug use (legal and illegal). Alaskans outstrip the contiguous states in self-reported consumption of, among others, cannabis, cocaine, LSD and nicotine. It is not clear that the higher prevalence of use in Alaska is related to the law. Segal believes that the high prevalence of all psychoactive drug use in Alaska has to do with a

---

*Despite this vote, cannabis has not been recriminalized in Alaska because of the state constitutional issues outlined. The attitudes and possible actions of the current members of the Alaskan Supreme Court are not clear; the outcome of possible recriminalization also remains unclear.

frontier mentality. Any change in the law may not eliminate Alaskan primacy in youthful psychoactive drug use.

Reform benefits

There may be important state savings in the costs of enforcement and prosecution of cannabis offenses. Most states that decriminalized experienced a 30–40 percent decline in arrests for possession and sharp declines in incarceration rates. For example, the total cost of cannabis enforcement in California declined from US$17 million in the first half of 1975 to under US$4.4 million in the first half of 1976 (Aldrich and Mikuriya, 1988).

In 1990, the Ohio Governor, Richard Celeste publicly discussed a state legislative plan to recriminalize cannabis. Although careful in his language, Celeste pointed out that the costs of restoring cannabis laws were very high. He described the limitation of criminal justice resources and noted that recriminalization would require a shift of those resources away from harder drugs and other crimes. The Ohio legislature did not pass a recriminalization bill.

The Netherlands

Anti-prohibitionists point to the Netherlands in all discussions of the benefits of drug reform. The Dutch have originated a number of pragmatic approaches to drug policy, which do not rely on legislation to effect social control. The Dutch Code of Criminal Procedure contains an expediency principle which empowers the Public Prosecutions Department to refrain from instituting criminal proceedings if there are other public interests to be considered. Although cannabis remains *de jure* illegal, no action is taken by police to detect possession for personal use; selling or possession up to 30 grams of cannabis is *de facto* legal. The sale of cannabis is undisturbed in licensed 'coffee shops' where the sale or use of alcohol is prohibited. These shops are monitored to prevent the sale of other drugs or larger quantities of cannabis, or sale to minors. The Dutch believe that this policy has effectively separated the cannabis market from that for more dangerous drugs. There are more than 300 coffee shops in Amsterdam where cannabis can be sold and comparable shops exist in The Hague, Rotterdam and other cities. These 1976 changes have not been followed by an increase in Dutch use of cannabis. In 1976, 13 percent of those 17–18 had occasionally used hashish or marijuana and in 1985, the prevalence in 17–18 year olds had actually decreased to 6 percent (Ministry of Welfare, Health and Cultural Affairs, 1985).

A survey reported in 1991 (Wijngaart, 1991) indicated that 12 percent of high school seniors in the Netherlands had ever used cannabis.

This compares to more than 59 percent of those surveyed by the HSSS in the USA (Johnston, O'Mally and Bachman, 1991). Current use (monthly prevalence) in Dutch high school students is strikingly lower in the Netherlands than in the USA: 5.4 percent against 29 percent respectively (Wijngaart, 1991). Despite *de facto* cannabis decriminalization in the Netherlands, there has been no expansion of use. Cannabis has been normalized and users are not subject to arrest, nor are they socially marginalized. The decision to use or not use cannabis resembles a decision to use or not use caffeine, and the selling of cannabis has little relationship to the illicit selling of other drugs; there is little retail black market in cannabis in the Netherlands outside the coffee shop market.

South Australia

The Cannabis Expiation Notice System came into effect in South Australia on 30 April 1987. Under this system, adults found to possess small amounts of cannabis (less than 100 grams of marijuana or 20 grams of hashish) are issued an expiation notice (citation). If the prescribed fine is paid within 60 days, the offense is not prosecuted in court and no conviction is recorded.* Rates of marijuana use have not changed in South Australia since the introduction of this system. This conclusion rests upon a series of school children (13–16 year olds) surveyed between 1986 and 1989 who were compared to a control (non-expiation) state's surveys; household surveys of general population drug use were also conducted throughout Australia in 1985 and 1988 by the National Campaign Against Drug Use (NCADA) and compared South Australia to other states. All surveys indicated no change in South Australia's rates of cannabis use related to the introduction of on-the-spot fines and there were no significant differences in rates of use between South Australia and other Australian states which had not changed cannabis legislation (Christie, 1991).

Medical Cannabis in the United States of America

In the United States of America various issues converge in framing the debate about medical cannabis. An ongoing legal challenge to the DEA listing of cannabis as a dangerous drug with no medical utility in Schedule 1 of the Controlled Substance Act has had some success but has not achieved its goal. The availability of a legal Δ-9-THC capsule for the treatment of nausea and vomiting has recently expanded to other uses and a peculiar American program supplying standardized smoke-

---

*An American 'country-rock' band called Barefoot Jerry once recorded a song about an expiation notice. It was called *'Tokin' Ticket'*.

able cannabis, grown on a federally funded farm in Mississippi, has recently been curtailed.

Dronabinol

An American drug company received approval in 1986 to market 2.5, 5.0 and 10 mg capsules of synthetic Δ-9-THC dissolved in sesame oil. This decision emerged from evidence that cannabis and Δ-9-THC were effective in the treatment of nausea and vomiting, particularly that secondary to use of cancer chemotherapeutic agents (Sallan, Zinberg and Frei, 1975). The product has the generic name dronabinol and is marketed under the trade name Marinol®. Until recently, gross sales were adequate for continued marketing (approximately US$8 million per annum). Dronabinol is stringently controlled and listed as a schedule II product highly subject to abuse. Since it entered the market, there has been no evidence of any substantial diversion to illicit sale. The American prescription drug control system does not prevent use of any FDA approved drug for 'non-labeled' indications. When the FDA approves a medicinal for marketing it approves specific labeling of indications for which the manufacturer has submitted acceptable proof of efficacy and may so advertise. Despite such restrictive labeling, physicians often begin to prescribe new medications for other indications. Propranolol was marketed to treat arrhythmias but physicians used it for angina and hypertension. The manufacturer of propranolol ultimately made a new drug application for these indications. Prescribing for non-labeled indications is common and proper because an appropriate clinical use may emerge long before the manufacturer generates proof and makes an application.

Marinol® is labeled only for use in chemotherapy-induced nausea and vomiting. Might physicians use it for other possible indications? Might they prescribe it for glaucoma, migraine headache, spasticity, appetite enhancement, menstrual cramps, nausea and vomiting secondary to other causes? In an unusual fashion, the US Drug Enforcement Agency (DEA) specifically attempted to restrain the use of oral Δ-9-THC outside the single label indication. In a US Federal Register notice, they warned physicians that unlabeled prescribing might be interpreted as a reason to investigate the prescriber (Federal Register, 1986). This threat is very likely without legal foundation but may achieve the DEA's purpose.*

Dronabinol, the legally available Δ-9-THC, has become part of a longer argument regarding cannabis and medication in the United States of America. Robert Randell effectively sued the United States

---

*In response to inquiries, the US Department of Health and Human Services (DHHS) has emphasized that dronabinol may, like other marketed medicinals, be prescribed for unlabeled indications which the prescriber believes to be clinically appropriate (Chow, personal communication).

Government in 1976 over its refusal to permit him access to a needed medication. Randell, with the support of his ophthamalogist, documented that smoking cannabis lowered his intraocular pressure and was therapeutic for his glaucoma. This victory led to the establishment of a compassionate drug program through which by 1992 approximately a dozen patients received standardized cannabis cigarettes legally from a Federal cannabis farm established at the University of Mississippi. These individuals, with help from their physicians, applied for medical cannabis for glaucoma, neurologic illness with spasticity and, just before the termination of the program, HIV-related wasting.

HIV-related wasting and cannabis

The use of smokeable cannabis to treat nausea and vomiting related to AIDS and AZT treatment has become widely discussed in the United States of America. In addition to the anti-nauseant effect, the use of cannabis may independently provoke appetite. The rate of application to the compassionate program was recently increased by AIDS patients. However, in March of 1992, a deputy secretary and physician in the DHHS, James Mason, announced the termination of the smokeable cannabis program, although promising that those previously approved would continue to receive their cannabis. Mason initially cited the potential sexual misconduct of individuals with HIV related to their use of cannabis (Isikoff, 1991). He and others have justified the curtailment of the program on the grounds of the availability of dronabinol, despite the earlier DEA attempt to threaten physicians who might choose to prescribe it more widely.

In December of 1992, Unimed Pharmaceuticals received approval from the FDA for a new label indication for dronabinol, HIV-related wasting. Their experience with the use of this small capsule in patients with HIV has been reported (Plasse et al., 1991). The study involving only a few patients resulted in a modest weight gain in some, but does document what had previously been anecdotal. There is reason to believe that some US officials hope to forestall the use of smokeable medicinal cannabis by encouraging the use of dronabinol capsules; however, the American political movement toward providing smokeable cannabis is stronger than ever. In 1988, a lawsuit requesting rescheduling of marijuana, brought by the Alliance for Cannabis Therapeutics, the Drug Policy Foundation and the National Organization for Reform of Marijuana Laws (NORML) was apparently successful in its challenge of the Controlled Substance Act (Young, 1988). Although the administrative judge agreed completely with the plaintiffs that smokeable cannabis has medical utility, the DEA has the power under the law to ignore such administrative decisions and they have continued to do so (Federal Register, 1989).

Many individuals with nausea and vomiting, and their physicians, might well decide that a swallowed capsule might not be the best choice for treatment, being subject to or even provoking vomiting. In a recent response to a survey mailed to American oncologists, approximately 50 percent stated that they would recommend smokeable illegal cannabis to their chemotherapy patients and more than 40 percent had in fact recommended illegal cannabis for just this purpose (Doblin and Kleiman, 1991). Most cannabis being used by those with HIV-related wasting is illegal smokeable material and such use is commonly discussed in AIDS support groups, by AIDS activists and by physicians in service to AIDS patients. The American FDA (at least some of its staff) has also signaled a willingness to consider a properly done controlled study of smokeable cannabis to effect a new drug application.

Conclusions

A harm-reduction approach to cannabis, painted in broad strokes, would include the following. Cannabis law reform is essential whether that reform is committed legalization, expiation or an enlightened hypocrisy in which existing laws are ignored. Such reform would save the large costs of cannabis law enforcement and could free criminal justice resources for focus on that which is proved harmful to the social community and public order.

Under some systems of reform, the scientific exploration of cannabis as a medicine and as a preferred psychoactive indulgent could take place. The development of cannabis beverages, buccal lozenges, skin patches or other forms could be encouraged to diminish pulmonary hazards. Aerosolized Δ-9-THC has been tried in humans but at the concentrations employed using an alcohol carrier it provoked coughing in most subjects and bronchospasm in a few asthmatic subjects. Recently employing a heated copper filament, scientists have successfully delivered Δ-9-THC as a vapor without the irritation noted above (Tashkin, D. P., personal communication). Such experiments could signal the utility of inhaled Δ-9-THC as a bronchodilator* or the delivery of material in a 'smokeable' form safer for medicinal and recreational purposes.

We strongly recommend public educational attempts to diminish the concurrent use of tobacco and cannabis by combustion. We also strongly recommend that cannabis smokers stop the customary deep inhalation and breath holding which facilitates the deposition of particulate matter without markedly increasing Δ-9-THC delivery. Harm

---

*Because Δ-9-THC is a bronchodilator, some have feared that it may augment the effects of tobacco related irritants. The bronchodilator effect on larger airways may abet the deposition of tobacco particles deeper in the respiratory tree and hasten the deleterious impact of tobacco smoking on small airway and alveolar function.

reduction also includes a commitment to education of youthful users in the character and perils of acute intoxication and acute cannabis effect. Some of the millions of Federal US dollars spent in promoting a futile prohibition and calling it education could be used to teach young people how to manage the effects safely.

The data from several countries indicate that cannabis reform is unlikely to be followed by an explosion of use. Such reform would result in significant cost savings in the criminal justice system and a profound reduction in the harmful criminalization of most users.

References

Abel, E.L. (1981). Marihuana and sex: A critical survey. *Drug and Alcohol Dependence*, **8**, 1–22.

Aldrich, M. and Mikuriya, T. (1988). Savings in California marijuana law enforcement costs attributable to the Moscone Act of 1976: A summary. *Journal of Psychoactive Drugs*, **20**, 75–81.

Anonymous (1972). *Marijuana: A Signal of Misunderstanding (the Official Report of the National Commission on Marijuana and Drug Abuse)*. New York: New American Library Inc.

Brody, J.E. (1980). The evidence builds against marijuana. *New York Times*, **21**, May: C1.

Christie, P. (1991). *The Effects of Marijuana Legislation in South Australia on Levels of Marijuana Use*. Adelaide: Drug and Alcohol Services Council.

Coggins, W.J. (1976). Costa Rica cannabis project: An interim report on the medical aspects. In M.C. Braude and S. Szara (Eds), *Pharmacology of Marijuana*. New York: Raven Press.

Cohen, S. (1976). The 94 day cannabis study. *Annals of the New York Academy of Science*, **292**, 211–220.

Dauncy, H. (1989). *A Psychopharmacological Study of the Interaction between Alcohol and Marijuana*. PhD thesis. Department of Pharmacology, University of Sydney, Australia.

Devane, W.A., Hanus L., Breuer, A., Pertwee, R.G., Stevenson, L.A., Griffin, G., Gibson, D., Mandelbaum, A., Etinger, A. and Mechoulan, R. (1992) Isolation and structure of a brain constituent that binds to the cannabinoid receptor. *Science*, **258**, 1946.

Doblin, R.E. and Kleiman, M.A.R. (1991). Marijuana as antiemetic medicine: A survey of oncologists' experiences and attitudes. *Journal of Clinical Oncology*, **9**, 1314–1319.

DuPont, R.L. Jr (1985). *Getting Tough on Gateway Drugs: A Guide for the Family*. Washington DC: American Psychiatric Press Inc.

Egan, T. (1991) Sitka journal: Life, liberty and maybe marijuana. *New York Times*, May 17.

El Sohley, M.A., Holley, J.H. Lewis, G.S., Russell, M.H. and Turner, C.E. (1984). Constituents of *Cannabis sativa* L. XXIV: The potency of confiscated marijuana, hashish and hash oil over a ten year period. *Journal of Forsenic Science*, **29**, 500–514.

Erickson, P.G. and Alexander, B.K. (1989). Cocaine and addictive liability. *Social Pharmacology*, **3**, 249–270

Federal Register (1986). *DEA Policy Statement on Marinol. 51*, 1746, 13 May.

Federal Register (1989). *Marijuana Scheduling Petition: Denial of Petition. Drug Enforcement Administration (Docket No. 86–22)*. 54, 53767–53785.

Fink, M. Volavka, J. Panayiotopolous, P. and Stafanis, C. (1976). Quantitative EEG studies of marijuana, Δ-9-THC and hashish in man. In M.C. Braude and S. Szara (Eds) *Pharmacology of Marijuana*. New York: Raven Press.

Gettman, J. (1991). Key marijuana indicators. *Marijuana Digest*, 3, 4–5.

Goode, E. (1971). Drug use and grades in college. *Nature*, 234, 225–227.

Halikas, J., Goodwin, D.W. and Guze, S.B. (1972). Marijuana use and psychiatric illness. *Archives of General Psychiatry*, 27, 162–165.

Hawks, R.L. and Walsh, R.L. (1990). *Potency of Marijuana Over the Last Ten Years. Technical Review Brief, Division of Preclinical Research*. Washington DC: National Institute on Drug Abuse.

Heishman, S.J., Stitzer, M.L. and Yingling, J.E. (1989). Effects of tetrahydrocannabinol content on marijuana smoking behavior subjective reports and performance. *Pharmacology, Biochemistry Behavior*, 34, 173–179.

Herning, R.I., Hocher, W.D. and Jones, R.T. (1986). Tetrahydrocannabinol content and differences in marijuana smoking behavior. *Psychopharmacology*, 90, 160–162.

Hollister, L.E. (1986). Health aspects of cannabis. *Pharmacological Review*, 38, 1–20.

Hollister, L.E., Overall, J.E. and Gerber, M.L. (1975). Marihuana and setting, *Archives of General Psychiatry*, 32, 789–801.

Isikoff, M. (1991). Compassionate marijuana use – supplies for medical needs are in jeopardy. *Washington Post* , 12 November.

Johnston, L.D., O'Mally, P.M. and Bachman, J.G. (1981). *Marijuana Decriminalization: The Impact on Youth 1975–1980. Monitoring the Future: Occasional Paper Series, paper 13*. Ann Arbor: Institute for Social Research, University of Michigan.

Johnston, L.D., O'Malley, P.M. and Bachman, J.G. (1991) *Drug Use Among High School Seniors, College Strudents and young Adults, 1975–1990*. National Rockville, Maryland: National Institute on Drug Abuse.

Jones, R.T and Benowitz, N. (1976). The 30 day trip: Clinical studies of cannabis tolerance and dependence. In M.C. Braude and S. Szara.(Eds), *Pharmacology of Marijuana*. New York: Raven Press.

Kaslow, R.A., Blackwelder, W.C., Ostrow, D.G.H., Yerg D., Palenicek, J., Coulson, A.H.G. and Valdisessi, R.O. (1989). No evidence for a role of alcohol or other psychoactive drugs in accelerating immunodeficiency in HIV-1 positive individuals. *Journal of the American Medical Association*, 261, 3424–3429.

Kerr, P. (1986). Increases in potency of marijuana prompt new warnings for youth. *New York Times*, 25 September: A1.

Klonoff, H. (1974). Effects of marijuana on driving in a restricted area on city streets: Driving performance and physiological changes. In L. Miller (Ed.), *Marijuana Effects on Human Behavior*. New York: Academic Press.

Kolansky, H. and Moore, W.T. (1972). Toxic effects of chronic marijuana use. *Journal of the American Medical Association*, 222, 35–40.

Kolodny, R.C., Masters, W.H., Toro, G. and Kolodner, R.M. (1974). Depression of testosterone levels after chronic intensive marijuana use. *New England Journal of Medicine*, 290, 872–74.

Lau, R.J. Tubergen, D.G., Barr, M. Jr., Domino, E.F., Benowitz, N. and Jones, R.T. (1976). Phytohemagglutinin – lymphocyte transformation in humans receiving Δ-9-tetrahydrocannabinol. *Science*, 192, 805–807.

Leirer V.O. Yesavage J.A. and Morrow D.G. (1989). Marijuana, ageing and task difficulty effects on pilot performance. *Aviatiation, Space, and Environmental Medicine*, 60, 1145–1151.

Leirer, V.O., Yesavage, J.A. and Morrow, D.G. (1991). Marijuana carry-over effects on aircraft pilot performance. *Aviatiation, Space, and Environmental Medicine*, 62, 221–227.

Linn, S., Schoenbaum, S.C., Mohson, R.R., Rosner, R., Stublefield P.C. and Ryan K.J. (1983). The association of marijuana use with outcome of pregnancy. *American Public Health*, 83, 1151–1164.

Mendelson, J.H., Kuehnle, J., Ellingboe, J. and Babor, T.F. (1974). Plasma testosterone levels before during and after chronic marihuana smoking. *New England Journal of Medicine*, 291, 1051–1055.

Ministry of Welfare, Health and Cultural Affairs. (1985). *Policy on Drug Use*. The Hague, The Netherlands.

Mikuriya, T.H. and Aldrich, M.R. (1988). Cannabis 1988: Old drug, new dangers – the potency question. *Journal of Psychoactive Drugs*, 20, 47–56.

Morgan, J.P. (1988). Marijuana metabolism in the context of urine testing for cannabinoid metabolite. *Journal of Psychoactive Drugs*, 20, 107–115.

Nahas, G.G. (1971). Lethal cannabis intoxication. *New England Journal of Medicine*, 284, 792.

Hahas, G.G. (1973). *Marihuana – Deceptive Weed*. New York: Raven Press.

Nahas, G.G., Suciv-Foca, N., Armand, J.P. and Morishima, A. (1974). Inhibition of cellular mediated immunity in marihuana smokers. *Science*, 183, 419–420.

Plasse, T.F., Gorter, R.W., Kraskow, S.H., Lane, M., Sjepard, K.V. and Wadleigh, R.G. (1991). Recent clinical experience with dronabinol. *Pharmacology, Biochemistry Behavior*, 40, 695–700.

Rubin, V. and Comitas, L. (1975). *Ganga in Jamaica*. The Hague: Mouton.

Sallan, S.E. Zinberg, N.E. and Frei, E. (1975). Antiemetic effect of Δ-9-tetrahydrocannabinol in patients receiving cancer chemotherapy. *New England Journal of Medicine*, 293, 795–797.

Shedler, J. and Block, J. (1990). Adolescent drug use and psychological health. *American Psychologist* , 45, 612–629.

Segal, B. (1989). Drug taking behavior among school-aged youth: The Alaska experience and comparison with lower 48 states. *Drugs and Society*, 4, 1–144.

Single, E. (1989). The impact of marijuana decriminalization: An update. *Journal of Public Health Policy*, 456–466.

Spitzner, J.H. (1979). *Drug Use in Ohio: 1978*. Columbus: Ohio Bureau of Drug Abuse.

Tashkin, D.P., Fligiel, S., Wu, T.C., Gong, H. Jr, Barbers, R.G., Coulson, A.G., Simmons, M.S. and Beals, T.F., (1990). Effects of habitual use of marijuana and/or cocaine on the lung. In C.N. Chiang and R.L. Hawks (Eds), *Research Findings on Smoking of Abused Substances*. Washington DC: NIDA Res. Monog. 99 USDHHS, US Government Printing Office.

Tashkin, D.P., Gliederer, F., Rose, J., Chang, P., Hui, K.K., Yu, J.L. and Wu, T-C. (1991). Effects of marijuana smoking profile on deposition of tar and absorption of CO and Δ-9-THC. *Pharmacology, Biochemistry Behavior*, 40, 651–656.

Tennant, F.S. Jr, Preble, M., Prendergast, T.J. and Ventry, P. (1971). Medical manifestations associated with hashish. *Journal of the American Medical Association*, 216, 165–69.

US Committee on the Judiciary (1974). *Senate Hearings, 93rd Congress, Marijuana-Hashish Epidemic and its Impact on United States Security*.

Washington DC: US Government Printing Office.

van de Wijngaart, G. (1991) *Competing perspectives on drug use: The Dutch experience*. Amsterdam/Lisse: Swets and Zeitlinger.

Yesavage, J.A., Leirer, V.O., Denari, M. and Hollister, L.E. (1985). Carry-over effects of marijuana intoxication on aircraft pilot performance: A preliminary report. *American Journal of Psychiatry*, 142, 1325–1329.

Young, F.L. (1988). In the matter of marijuana rescheduling petition: Opinion and recommended ruling finding of fact, conclusions of law and decision of administrative law judge. US Department of Justice. Drug Enforcement Administration (Docket No. 86–22) In R.C. Randall (Ed.), *Marijuana Medicine and The Law II*. Washington DC: Galen Press.

Zimmerman, S. Zimmerman, A.M. Cameron, I.L. and Laurence, H.L. (1977). Delta-9-tetrahydrocannabinol, cannabidiol and cannabinol effects on the immune response of mice. *Pharmacology*, 15, 10–23.

Chapter 17
Ecstasy in the United Kingdom: Recreational Drug Use and Subcultural Change

PETER McDERMOTT, ALAN MATTHEWS, PAT O'HARE and
ANDREW BENNETT

Introduction – 'You can be yourself – yeah!'

MDMA is a member of the phenylethylamine family of drugs, related chemically to both mescaline and amphetamine. Consequently, it is often described as a stimulant and/or an hallucinogenic, when in actual fact it is neither. Subjective reports advise us that on an active dose of the drug there is no loss of control or contact with reality. The primary effect is on mood. The structural activity of this drug is so different from others that, it has been argued, the drug deserves a new category (Nicholas, 1986). Terms that have been suggested to describe this category include 'empathogen' (meaning creating a sense of empathy) and 'entactogen' (meaning to touch within).

The first reference to MDMA to reach a broad audience in the UK came in an article in a magazine called *The Face*. This reported on the use of the drug by a small group of people working in the media, pop music and fashion industries who were flying to the United States of America and importing small amounts of the drug for their personal consumption. (Naysmith, 1985).

Over the next two years, the MDMA scene grew slowly but steadily. Two London disc jockeys visited Ibiza in the summer of 1986 and returned with a new style of dance music – created by the DJs themselves – which became known as 'Balearic Beat' (Kaplan et al., 1989). The music consisted of a mixture of late seventies and early eighties disco, and the later mutations of that nightclub oriented sound from Chicago (House), New York (Garage) and Detroit (Techno). Using modern musical technology such as samplers, sequencers and synthesisers, DJs began to create a new musical form that clubgoers found ideally suited the effects of the drug. The Ecstasy/nightclub combination began to spread slowly from the London fashion/music industry elite until 1991, when the rave scene (as the subculture became known) was possibly the biggest youth subculture that Britain had ever seen, a subculture intimately bound up with the use of Ecstasy.

The effects of the drug were to become closely bound up in the artefacts of the newly emerging subculture. For instance, one song that was widely played in the clubs in 1989 was called 'Express Yourself' and gives some insight into the meaning of the experience for young people. The hook lyric proclaims, 'You can be yourself, yeah, yeah'. Although this may seem trite to those who have not shared the experience, most of the people we interviewed felt that this capacity to drop inhibitions and allow yourself to be who you truly were without fear or embarassment was the drug's most rewarding quality. Whereas other drugs like alcohol or LSD produced dramatic changes in the psyche, Ecstasy, in contrast, just allowed people to be themselves, to accept themselves and others. This curious sense of freedom arising from a collective of chemically liberated individuals made the club scene very appealing, not just to teenagers but to people of all ages. When the drug was taken in a club with 2000 other people, it produced a sense of being emotionally synchronised with the crowd, a notion that is amplified by the DJ's use of the music and lighting effects. People would describe how they would make eye contact and, rather than looking away embarassed or being a catalyst for aggression ('Who the fuck d'you think you're looking at?'), strangers would identify a communality, albeit one based on chemistry.

So, from 1987 onwards, nightclubs across the UK witnessed joyous outbursts of mass hugging and kissing. A popular record would be received by 2000 pairs of arms shooting up into the air, as everybody would hold hands, sway blissfully and sing. Given the contrast with our everyday experience, it is not surprising that the experience of the drug and the scene was to become of central importance to the lives of many young people.

'Something is happening here, but you don't know what it is...'

The first two authors became interested in this phenomenon at the end of 1988, when they gained access to a network of young people who were involved with the drug. They spent a great deal of time over the following two years studying this group and the rave scene, research which eventually led to the production of a television documentery ('E is for Ecstasy', *Everyman*, BBC 1).

During the course of this research, we became aware of a growing number of problems that were associated with the drug. Having read most of the published literature available on the drug, we thought it appeared to be fairly safe. However, the set and setting in which the drug was used in the USA, where most of the available research had been conducted, was very different from the way it was now being used in Britain.

In America, the drug had come to the attention of a small group of people who were committed to the continuation of serious research into psychedelic drugs such as Pihkal (Shulgin and Shulgin, 1992) and LSD (Stephens,1987) etc. Because of MDMA's peculiar properties, this group had seen the drug as a useful adjunct to psychotherapy and for a long time it remained a well-kept secret. Although the drug eventually made the transition from the therapist's office to the street, the way it was used in the USA, and the groups that were using it, were very different to this new pattern of use that was emerging in the UK (O'Rourke, 1985; Rosenbaum et al., 1989).

In 1989, the UK saw its first Ecstasy-related death. Although the first was believed to be an idiosyncratic reaction, possibly allergic, as the numbers of people taking the drug grew, the numbers of adverse reactions also grew. This research, combined with the growing number of telephone enquiries to the Mersey Drug Training and Information Centre (MDTIC), pointed to a hunger for information on the effects and the hazards of Ecstasy and the other drugs associated with the dance scene. In September 1991, Mersey Regional Health Authority decided to commission an information campaign aimed at Ecstasy users (McDermott et al., 1992).

At the time the campaign was conceived, there had been virtually no interest in the drug by the medical or drug treatment establishment in the UK, and no research of any substance had been funded or conducted. Apart from the American research, conducted under very different conditions, all the experience of the effects and hazards of this drug lay with the thousands of users who had been carrying out individual and collective experiments. A series of govenment funded television 'drug scare' advertisements had been screened in 1989–1990 and most of the Ecstasy users we spoke to had seen them but did not find them credible representations of the drug, the subculture or the potential risks. Most of those interviewed did not believe that their drug use had caused them any serious problems, though they often felt that the lack of accurate information about the drug, and its illegal status, were problems in themselves.

Furthermore, current drugs services had been preoccupied with their existing clients, opiate users, and most had totally failed to make any attempt to contact this group. In fact, many involved in the drugs field were virtually unaware of the problem. Drug services were for 'addicts', whereas this group was just using drugs recreationally, at weekends. What did a drugs agency have to offer them? The reality was, in fact, not very much (Gilman, 1992).

Everything Starts With an 'E'

It was decided that the form our response would take should be different from other campaigns for a number of reasons. Most importantly, it was felt that the people who were most at risk, and therefore could benefit most from such a campaign, were the many thousands of people who were currently using the drug. There is no evidence that drug prevention campaigns, such as the government's TV adverts, delay or reduce initiation into drug use. However, information may play a role in slowing transitions to heavier or particularly hazardous modes of use (Dorn and Murji, 1992).

The new club-drug scene has a number of characteristics that make it a risk-laden situation. First, many of those involved are young and new to drug taking; therefore they are likely to have little knowledge of the drugs they use. Second, the dominant drug used on this scene, MDMA or Ecstasy, was a relatively new substance that most drugs workers had little knowledge of or experience of dealing with. Our perspective on the problem, and the strategy we adopted in order to deal with it, owed a great deal to the work of Norman Zinberg and Jock Young. From Zinberg, we took the notion that we had to accept that these people were determined to use drugs and, as a consequence, we needed to assist them by facilitating the emergence of a culture of controlled drug use (Zinberg, 1984).

In his book *The Drugtakers*, Young (1972) argues that it is strongly dysfunctional to harass and undermine drug subcultures; instead we should facilitate the emergence of a system of values and norms within that subsulture. Another principle we took from Young was the need for 'positive propaganda'. Drug horror stories fail to mesh with the experience of drug users and so the message is rejected. According to Young, it is only the subculture of drug taking that has the authority to control its members. As he so eloquently explains,

> You cannot control an activity merely by shouting out that it is forbidden; you must base your measures on facts and these facts must come from sources that are valued by the people that you wish to influence... Moreover, information aimed at controlling drug use must be phrased in terms of the values of the subculture, not in terms of the values of the outside world.

The authors decided that the best method of affecting a positive influence upon this group of recreational or non-dependent drug users would be to seek to facilitate the emergence of a set of subcultural rituals and norms aimed at minimising the potential for drug-related harm.

Our field research and literature review had led us to believe that the problems that were associated with Ecstasy could be divided into three categories: drug specific, situational and social. Problems that derive from pharmacological properties of the drug include overdose, allergic or idiosyncratic reactions, anxiety or panic attacks and the possibility of long-term neurotoxicity. Situational problems, those related to set and setting, include dehydration, hyperthermia, exhaustion, panic and problems arising from counterfeit drugs. To date there have been at least 14 deaths in the UK associated with Ecstasy and as many as 50 other severe reactions. One popular hypothesis is that the deaths are caused by heat-stroke due to a combination of Ecstasy, dancing energetically, not drinking enough water and the hot and humid temperature in clubs (Henry et al., 1992).

Finally, use of the drug can also give rise to a number of social problems that encompass relations with family, school or work, the law, and possible personality changes, but the extent to which these should be considered as 'drug problems', rather than normal adolescent rites of passage, is arguable and often depends upon highly subjective criteria.

As an information service, the problem we faced was how to make a positive intervention that would enable us to maximise contact in an appropriate manner and to allocate scarce resources as efficiently as possible. As the Government had recently run an enormous mass media campaign aimed at dissuading young people from using recreational drugs such as Ecstasy, we decided to run an information campaign aimed specifically at those who were determined to continue to use these drugs.

'Reach out and touch somebody's hand...'

Following intense press coverage of the issue after several Ecstasy-related deaths over a short space of time, many drug services began to argue that outreach work should be conducted with this group. We felt that this response was a mistake. Outreach work in the UK emerged in an attempt to contact injecting drug users at risk of HIV. It was an exceptional measure that was necessitated by the need to avert a public health crisis. Ravers are neither hard-to-reach, nor are they such a priority. Grund (1992) argues that outreach should be aimed at those who are most at risk. Ravers do not fall into this category.

Outreach seemed to be unreasonably intrusive in the perceptions of the targeted group, just another form of social policing. If the rationale for such work is reducing drug-related harm or HIV prevention, then such efforts may be more profitably directed to the local pub, where both the extent and the severity of risks and problems will far outweigh those at any rave club. Few would argue that such a response to alcohol was either appropriate or desirable; why should we think it so for other drugs?

One drug agency manager in the Mersey region explained his understanding of this trend towards outreach work among recreational drug users: 'For the first few years, the role of an outreach worker has been to go and sit in a grotty council flat and try to make contact with injectors. Compared to this, going to clubs at the weekend has got to be a high priority. And it's easier, too. In a club, you have access to up to two thousand drug users, all in the same place at the same time'.

If the concept of outreach work is fraught with inconsistencies, the management of such work poses serious logistical problems. Counselling or information-giving in a club where you can't hear yourself think is inappropriate and virtually impossible. Dealing with collapse or overdoses should be the responsibility of club management, who should have staff experienced in first aid and who are just as able to call an ambulance as any outreach worker. When dealing with anxiety or panic attacks (the bad trip syndrome), friends are more likely to be helpful than strangers. Most clubs already sell condoms. As drugs workers, our primary aim is to help prevent problems, not have workers waiting on the sidelines in the hope that one might develop. Our task is to demystify drugs and drug problems, to take power out of the hands of professionals and to empower the drug user, enabling him to make responsible and informed decisions. Outreach work is too often used as a method of perpetuating professional mystique and client dependency on drug workers rather than transferring decision-making skills to drug users who can best understand their own needs.

'Make this world a better place...'

When determining the form and content of the campaign, we set ourselves a number of goals.

1. To provide basic information on the effects of the various drugs commonly used on the club scene.
2. To enable clubgoers to identify potential problems that might arise, and help them to deal with them effectively.
3. To alert them to hazards associated with the set and setting in which the drug may be used.
4. To establish standards for safer, more responsible drug use within the drug subculture.
5. To give drug users a contact point for further information from a source they can trust, should problems arise.

In order to achieve these aims, we felt that the form the information took, and the routes through which it was transmitted, were equally as important as the content. The information should be pertinent to the lives and interests of the intended audience. It must also be accurate and honest, reflecting the positive aspects of drug use as well as the risks and harms that the drug might cause. Finally, the campaign needed to be non-judgmental about the ethical issues inherent in drug use in order to establish a relationship of trust between the information providers and the intended recipients.

As the budget for the campaign was low, we needed to take a creative approach to maximising our audience. Once again, our in-depth knowledge of the subculture gained over the previous two years was invaluable. This was a subculture which was based around holding illegal parties that were not advertised but could attract over 10 000 people by word of mouth. We decided to attempt to utilise the methods and networks that the subculture itself uses to transmit information – flyers, magazine articles and word of mouth.

Flyers are hand-outs that advertise the opening of new clubs or one-off parties. They usually feature a graphic design style that is identifiable with the culture, similar to the graphics associated with the hippie/underground subculture of the 1960s. Flyers are distributed outside clubs, in record shops, clothes shops and other places where ravers congregate. They are often collected by ravers, who pin them on bedroom walls and in scrapboooks as memorabilia and mementos of events or clubs they attended. A local designer, noted for his creative work in this area, was employed to produce a leaflet that would utilise elements of this form.

The leaflet, *Chill Out – A Raver's Guide*, contains basic information about the three main drugs that were used on the club scene – MDMA, LSD and amphetamine. It considers the risks involved in using those drugs, methods to try to minimise the risks, and how to deal with an emergency. Furthermore, the leaflet does not just focus on the drugs but also looks at the other issues involved – the need for sleep and good diet, avoiding dehydration, heat exhaustion etc. Finally, a phone number is available on the leaflet in case further help is required.

As the nature of club culture mitigates against passing out such detailed information in a venue where people have gone to dance and to enjoy themselves, this method of distribution was rejected. If handed out willy-nilly during such an event, we felt that most leaflets would be likely to end up littering the floor, unread. Rather than leaving them behind the desk at drug services, places that are rarely attended by this group, we distributed them initially through specialist record and clothes shops, and through advertisements in fanzines, on radio and in bars, cafés and clubs.

Our resources were limited to an initial print run of 10000 copies of the leaflet, therefore we could only distribute them throughout the region. Yet the need for information on this matter was felt to be increasingly pressing, as the number of deaths and hospitalisations across the country mounted. As yet, no other service was providing the information that was needed. In an attempt to remedy this information shortage and contact a much larger audience, the second component of the campaign was initiated. One of the authors approached the magazine that had carried the original article on MDMA in 1985, *The Face*. This magazine is the most prestigious of the style magazines. Aimed at a readership aged between 18 and 35, continued references to the drug in features on 'stars', in letters and in journalist's asides led us to believe that this was an ideal conduit for a carefully targeted media information campaign.

After protracted negotiations, the magazine published an interview with one of the authors and a visiting Dutch colleague who attempted to summarise the most recent information available on the drug (James, 1991). This may be the first example of utilising the mass media in a harm-reduction information campaign. Confirmation that our choice of this magazine was correct was revealed by the reader response that the piece generated. The following month's issue gave over the whole letters page to the topic and noted that the article attracted the most mail they had had for some time (*The Face*, 1991). Many readers' letters noted the phenomenal rise in the incidence of Ecstasy use in their areas, others identified MDMA-related problems that they or their friends were experiencing, problems that were hitherto not addressed by existing drug service provision. Over the following six months, virtually all the British magazines aimed at this youth audience carried similar articles, often focusing on *Chill Out* and a similar information campaign run by Lifeline based around a cartoon character, Peanut Pete. Given the amount of positive coverage of the issues in the type of magazines that were read by our target audience, we felt that our initiative had been far more successful than we could ever have anticipated.

'... if you can!'

Although the campaign gained an enormous amount of coverage of the various risks and harms associated with MDMA in the youth magazines, we were not expecting the ferocity of the attack that followed from the tabloid press. Over the past four years, British television and the quality newspapers have given a great deal of coverage to the 'new paradigm' in the drugs field. TV programmes such as Granada's *Hooked* series and the BBC's *Open Space* programme, *Taking Drugs Seriously*, are just two examples among many. Serious newspaper columnists and editorials are invariably critical of the 'War on Drugs' mentality and argue for a more pragmatic, harm-reduction approach.

However, this tendency towards realism by the media still only applies to the quality broadsheets and television, and has failed to filter through to the British tabloids, which still cover drug stories in the traditional shock-horror fashion (McDermott, 1992). In an article entitled 'The myth of drug takers in the mass media', Jock Young (1973) has pointed out that the media's portrayal of drug stories is consistently biased. This is not, he argues, a function of random ignorance on the part of journalists, but is grounded in the media's assumption of a consensual ideology that governs the writing of newspaper articles. Most drug stories rely upon a number of myths – myths that were identified and shown to be untrue as early as 1940 by Alfred Lindesmith (1940). These myths are rooted in moral indignation, and are aimed at bulwarking the hypothetical world of the normal citizen and blinkering the audience to deviant realities that exist outside this imaginary consensus. In order to understand why newspaper stories about drugs are systematically skewed, Young argues, one must seek explanation at a structural level. The way in which sections of the media attacked *Chill Out* provides a powerful validation of Young's thesis.

The first author was contacted by a journalist on a local paper, the *Liverpool Echo*, who wanted to know where the information in the leaflet came from. In fact, the information was a summary of all the available literature on the subject, and had been read and appproved by a number of leading experts both on MDMA and on drug education. Locally, it was read and approved by the Director of the Drug Dependency Unit, the Head of Merseyside Police drug squad and other interested professionals. The journalist did not appear to be impressed by this, and intimated that some people in the field were concerned by the content of the leaflet. We later discovered that the concern emanated from her editor who had been outraged by the leaflet and had ordered her to get a critical story.

We were contacted by colleagues in the field who informed us that this journalist had been ringing around in an attempt to find somebody prepared to condemn the leaflet. Apparently, nobody working in the drugs field was prepared to do so but, fortunately for the reporter, there was a general election due in a few months time and Merseyside happens to be a solid Labour stronghold. The newspaper eventually managed to generate a controversy by sending copies of the leaflet to two Conservative MPs, both in marginal seats, asking for their comments.

The item ran as the main story on page one, under the headline, 'Raving mad: MPs' fury over DIY drug brochure for teenagers': 'The Echo today today highlights a glossy drugs leaflet that every Merseyside parent will view with outrage. It is a youngster's guide to taking drugs that looks and reads like part of a sales brochure' (*Liverpool Echo*, 1992a).

Linda Chalker, MP for Wallasey, attacked the leaflet for its message: 'Instead of hammering home the message that drugs are wrong and drugs kill, they are taking the soft option and telling these children how to take them safely'. Her colleague, Ken Hind MP, went even further: 'This is a disgraceful waste of public funds. I shall today send a letter to the Chairman of Mersey Regional Health Authority demanding such funding is immediately withdrawn'.

The following day, the story was picked up by two tabloid newspapers, *The Sun* and the *Daily Star*.* The *Daily Star's* story ran under the headline: 'What a dope: Daft do-gooder tells kids it's OK to use killer drug'. The *Daily Star* also gave its editorial over to the issue, offering advice to Merseyside parents: '... this evil twaddle was written by Centre boss Pat O'Hare and his staff – local parents should find out where these oddballs hang out and then they should storm the place and dump all 20 000 copies of this pernicious pamphlet into the Mersey, followed by Mr. O'Hare' (*Daily Star*, 1992).

The Sun, the paper that introduced the 'page 3 girl' to the British public, retained its usual obsession with sex. Their front page story was headlined: 'Fury at sex guide to E' (*The Sun*, 1992), because of a single reference to sex in the leaflet aimed at raising awareness of HIV in this group. In fact, the leaflet read, 'Sometimes you feel horny as it [Ecstasy] heightens sensations and pleasures of touch – so have condoms with you'.

This national media interest led the *Echo* to devote its front page to the story for the next two evenings. The following night's story was titled, 'Rethink on drug guide' and sought to imply that the regional health authority was about to renounce the leaflet. In fact, a health authority spokesperson said, 'We have no immediate plans to withdraw the leaflet'. Meanwhile, other sections of the media were expressing their support for *Chill Out*. Mick Middles, a columnist on Manchester's counterpart to the *Echo*, the *Manchester Evening News*, wrote:

> The media has universally feigned outrage and plucked a few provocative lines from the leaflet ...It is all too easy for the media to take a line out of context and make the whole project seem like a celebration of this appalling drug. It isn't. It merely accepts the sad fact that many ordinary, intelligent teenagers are caught

---

* Neither paper sells very well on Merseyside, in part because of their continued support for the locally despised Conservative government, but primarily because of their coverage of the Hillsborough football disaster. In 1986, at a Liverpool football match held at Hillsborough stadium in Sheffield, 96 fans died and many more were injured as a consequence of poor crowd control. The game was being broadcast live on TV at the time, and many Liverpool people watched as their friends and relatives had the life crushed out of them.

Widespread popular anger at the tabloids built over the next few days. First, some papers published ghoulish pictures of dead and dying football supporters, in full colour, without any thought for the impact on the friends of the victims. Then, *The Sun* and the *Daily Star* published unattributed police claims that the tragedy had been caused by unruly Liverpool supporters, who had been aggressive, had robbed bodies lying injured or dead, and had urinated on police officers who were attempting to help the victims.

In fact, a public enquiry found that the tragedy was a consequence of police mismanagement of the crowd and poor facilities at the ground, and that the allegations had been made by a senior police officer who resigned over the incident and had been attempting to divert blame from his force. The people of Merseyside began a mass boycott of *The Sun* and the *Daily Star*. Newsagents refused to stock the papers and the few who did found themselves abused by their customers. The circulation of these papers has never recovered in the region, so both papers are continuously seeking stories that will help them to rebuild their circulation in the Merseyside area. The *Echo's* 'Raving Mad' story seemed ideal, appealing to ignorant but concerned parents, and so both papers carried it as their front page story the following day.

up in this Ecstasy subculture and takes it from there. The authority should be commended for attempting to reach the kids via this method.

(Middles, 1992)

This support was also echoed in the *Liverpool Echo*'s sister newspaper, the *Daily Post*, where columnist David Charters (1992) wrote:

Admittedly, it is a defeatist tract, taking the line: the problem is here to stay. How do we cope with it? ... Most of the information is reasoned. The passage saying, 'Ecstasy can make you feel relaxed but energetic, happy, calm, exhilarated, warm and loving' is too glowing, though it is balanced with references to sweating, nausea and vomiting. ...Until the authorities control the spread of drugs, the MDTIC's leaflet has a role'.

On the third evening, the *Echo* gave its front page over to the story once again, this time to report that the Home Secretary, Kenneth Baker, had withdrawn a £15 000 grant to MDTIC from the seized asset fund that was intended to finance an Ecstasy information campaign (*Liverpool Echo*, 1992b). The grant was frozen until after the general election.

By this time, staff on the *Liverpool Echo* had begun to sense that their stance was not only out of step with professional opinion, but also with public opinion. In local radio phone-ins and on television news vox-pop interviews, support for *Chill Out* was overwhelming, particularly among the young whom the leaflet was aimed at. The following week, the *Echo* gave the centre's director, Pat O'Hare, and the leaflet's author, Alan Matthews, space to defend themselves.

It also gave its letters page over to the issue (*Liverpool Echo*, 1992c). Again, public support was overwhelming. Of 16 letters, only three did not support the leaflet. The letters gave some insight into the public's awareness of the harm-reduction philosophy:

As the Echo pointed out, the drug trade in the North West reaps profits of £25 million. This will not be halted overnight. Obviously there must be a demand.

I am writing as the concerned parent of a 19 year-old son to comment on your front page report, 'Raving Mad'. The most accurate part of the story is the headline – but only if applied to yourselves.

I have in my counselling sessions been using the *Chill Out* guide and I have been astounded at the success of this publication, which in my experience has given the drugs agencies credibility with the young drug users.

I am 27 years of age and have been using Ecstasy for the last three years. Like most users I was ignorant of the side-effects attached to its use. Having read the leaflet, I have sat back and actually thought about my drug use.

I was reminded of the outrage expressed when MDTIC introduced a free needle policy for drug users, and how that policy, now copied by others, has helped circumvent the spread of AIDS.

The objectors to this leaflet – the Liverpool Echo, Lynda Chalker and Ken Hind – are in no position whatsoever to comment on a situation they know very little about ...It is about time the whole drugs issue was tackled with some realism, instead of pretending that by making it illegal, the whole problem will disappear.

I think your articles on Ecstasy are on par with the Government warnings – a load of rubbish ...You are meant to be an independent local paper for the good of the community. Tell us the truth and tell it straight.

Like the politicians, the newspapers were attempting to appeal to an imaginary consensus – the worried parent, concerned about their children being 'on drugs'. Furthermore, the newspapers were relying upon common sense notions of how we should deal with drug problems, believing that the public will reject anything other than a 'just say no' approach. The response of the public to the controversy indicates that no such consensus exists. In Liverpool at least, it appears that the public is well aware of the failure of drug prevention campaigns. The evidence of failure is visible all around us – to any parent of teenage children, to anybody who drinks in their local pub, indeed, to anybody between the ages of 13 and 45. Illicit drug use is now a well-integrated part of the social fabric in this area.

These letters also indicate a high level of understanding and acceptance of the harm-reduction policies that were introduced in Mersey Region in order to deal with HIV and AIDS. Rather than opposing a more realistic/pragmatic approach to drug problems, the public appears to be calling for the extension of such policies. Politicians and the tabloid press have not yet managed to catch up with public opinion.

Conclusion: Who Wants Yesterday's Papers?

This controversy arose primarily because of serious contradictions that once underpinned the ideology that governed how we think about illegal drug use. Unless these contradictions are resolved, our attempts to develop a rational and effective response to the problem of ever-increasing illegal drug use are likely to continue to fail.

A major problem lies in our inability to think hard about the issues of pleasure and consciousness change. One of the principles that appears to underpin the government and media ideology is the notion that it is inherently wrong to seek to alter one's consciousness through artificial means. This assumption seems to have its roots in Protestantism and in the modern requirement for the time and work disciplines that were necessary to industrial capitalism.

Though many of the early prohibition laws were a product of the struggle for economic and political dominance by certain sectional interests over others (Berridge and Edwards, 1987; Duster, 1970; Szasz, 1975), more recent laws introduced to regulate the synthetic psychedelics appear to be a direct consequence of the perceived challenge that such drugs posed to the existing ideological order. Drugs such as LSD and mescaline had a perceived revolutionary potential as American hippies began to vocally reject the ideology of the 'American dream' and the Protestant 'work ethic'.

Following the reaction to early advocates of psychedelic drugs such as Timothy Leary, and the subsequent consequences for research into the uses and properties of these drugs, more recent advocates of drug law reform have strenuously avoided any discussion of the pleasurable aspects of such drugs. These new psychedelic advocates talk about the value of drugs such as MDMA as a 'research tool' or as an 'adjunct to psychotherapy'. It is important to ask ourselves whether a group of middle-aged Californian academics sitting around on MDMA listening to Mozart and calling it 'research' can genuinely be prioritised over the behaviour of an 18-year-old kid from the north-west of England who takes MDMA to get out of his face and dance to hard-core Techno music? We think not.

A central issue that is rarely addressed is whether intoxication should be considered an inherently immoral act. If society decides that it is, then we must apply the same sort of sanctions to the use of alcohol and caffeine that we do to heroin. Yet an ever-growing body of informed opinion today believes that decisions about intoxication and drug use are a matter for individual choice, best dealt with as a health issue, rather than being a matter for moral judgment or legal sanctions. Most young people who use drugs are aware of these contradictions and will not listen to grown-ups telling them that it is 'wrong' to take Ecstasy. They point to legally sanctioned drugs – tobacco and alcohol use far outweigh deaths from MDMA use. They will also ask why nobody has taken the trouble to make those risks known in an accessible manner and give information on how to avoid them.

If the argument against using illegal drugs is couched in terms of support for a corrupt and illegal enterprise, young people see this as another point in favour of the legalisation of drugs. Without wishing to get into the legalisation debate here, we suggest only that the widespread use of MDMA in the UK must lend more weight to arguments in favour of interventions aimed at separating the different illegal drug markets. Some measure of liberalisation of cannabis and MDMA markets offers more control over and easier intervention into those markets, while preventing a crossover into the markets for harder drugs such as cocaine and heroin. It is our belief, based upon our experience in Liverpool, that the general public is able to understand such sophisticated concepts and is likely to enbrace them, given the failure of traditional methods of drug control. Unfortunately, interventions of this type remain unlikely to be implemented while politicians and the mass media continue to approach questions of drug control from within an ideology rooted in moral absolutism, rather than taking a pragmatic approach based upon interventions that work as opposed to outdated ideology that does not.

References

Berridge, V. and Edwards, G. (1987). *Opium and the People*. New Haven: Yale University Press.

Charters, D. (1992). Agonising over Ecstasy while the rave goes on. *Daily Post*, 3 February.

Daily Star (1992). What a Dope. 29 January.

Dorn, N. and Murji, K. (1992). *Drug Prevention: A Review of the English Language and Literature*. London: Institute for the Study of Drug Dependence.

Duster, T. (1970). *The Legislation of Morality*. New York: Free Press.

Gilman, M. (1992). Beyond opiates. *Druglink*, 6, 16–17.

Henry, J.A. (1992). Ecstasy and the dance of death. *The Lancet*, 341, 5–6.

James, M. (1991). Ecstasy. *The Face*, November.

Kaplan, C.D., Grund, J-P. and Dzoljic, M.R. (1989). *Ecstasy in Europe: Reflections on the Epidemiology of MDMA*. Rotterdam: Instituut voor Verslavingsonderzoek.

Lindesmith, A. (1940). Dope fiend mythology. *Journal of Criminology and Police Science*.

Liverpool Echo (1992a). Raving mad. 28 January.

Liverpool Echo (1992b). Drugs agency to lose funding. 30 January.

Liverpool Echo (1992c). Letters. 4 February.

Middles, M. (1992). Ecstasy is not Horlicks. *Manchester Evening News*, 4 February.

McDermott, P., Matthews, A. and Bennett, A. (1992). Dealing with recreational drug use. *Druglink*, 7, 12–13.

McDermott, P. (1992). Representations of drug users: Facts, myths and their role in harm reduction. In P. O'Hare, R. Newcombe, A. Matthews, E.C. Buning and E. Drucker (Eds), *The Reduction of Drug-related Harm*. London: Routledge.

Naysmith, P. (1985). Ecstasy (MDMA). *The Face*, 66.

Nicholas, D. (1986). Differences between the mechanism of action of MDMA, MBDB and the classic hallucinogens. Identification of a new therapeutic class: entactogens. *Journal of Psychedelic Drugs*, 18, 305–313

O'Rourke, P.J. (1985). Turn on, tune in, go to the office late on Monday. In *Republican Party Reptile*. London: Paladin.

Rosenbaum, M., Morgan, P. and Beck, J.E. (1989). Ethnographic notes on Ecstasy use among professionals. *International Journal on Drug Policy*, 1, 16–19.

Shulgin, A.T. and Shulgin, A. (1992). *Pihkal*. California: Transform Press.

Stephens, J. (1987). *LSD and the American Dream*. London: Heinemann.

Szasz, T. (1975). *Ceremonial Chemistry*. London: Routlege and Paul.

The Face (1991). Letters. December 1991.

The Sun (1992). Fury at sex guide to E. 29 January.

Young, J. (1972). *The Drugtakers*. London: Paladin.

Young, J. (1973). The myth of the drug taker in the mass medic. In S. Cohen and J. Young (Eds), *The Manufacture of News*. London: Constable.

Zinberg, N. (1984). *Drug, Set and Setting*. New Haven: Yale University Press.

Futher Reading

Beck, J. (1990). The public health implications of MDMA use. In S.D. Peroutka
(Ed.), *Ecstasy: The Clinical, Pharmacological and Neurotoxicological Effects of
the Drug MDMA*. Boston: Kluwer.

Part V
Harm Reduction and Developing Countries

Chapter 18
Harm Reduction or Harm Aggravation? The Impact of the Developed Countries' Drug Policies in the Developing World

ANTHONY HENMAN

The purpose of this chapter is to illustrate the implications of the emerging debate on harm reduction and drug legalization for those countries which are both large producers and traditional consumers of illicit drug plants. The three major illicit drug crops are each analysed in a specific geographical setting: cannabis in Brazil, coca in the Andean countries, and opium in the Golden Triangle.

In Defence of Extremism

There can be little doubt that the policies fostered on developing countries as the result of drug prohibition in the developed industrial states have been almost uniformly negative in their effects. To ignore the accumulating cost of such policies, although expedient for certain governments, international organizations and non-governmental organizations, only lends credibility to the latent authoritarianism of drug prohibition. More importantly, it also fails to address the real social and economic problems facing the developing world which include indebtedness, resource depletion and inequitable world trading patterns. In this context, drug use and production appear much more as a symptom than as a cause.

Indeed, it would be no exaggeration to describe most current official policies in the developing countries as a conscious or unconscious process of harm aggravation. Though proposals for reform may appear 'extremist' in their opposition to the current orthodoxy of the War on Drugs, a clear demand for policy change towards harm-reduction, and ultimately full drug legalization, therefore offers the principal means for developing countries to transcend their present powerlessness. By recognising the proven effectiveness of 'traditional', informal controls over the use of drugs – controls that depend on a wide social consensus rather than on the use of force – developing countries can both encourage respect for their own indigenous cultural practices and contribute positive examples to the wider international community.

Cannabis in Brazil

Though it has become commonplace to lament the growth of social marginality and violent crime in Brazil's major cities, it is seldom pointed out that much of the underlying racism and class discrimination has historically found its symbolic expression in the denigration of cannabis smoking. Brought over from Angola by the eighteenth century, *diamba* was already sufficiently common in Rio de Janeiro in the 1830s to warrant a formal interdiction, probably the first in the New World, directed specifically at the public use of the cannabis water pipes introduced from Africa (Henman and Pessoa, 1986).

By 1916, scientific accounts of cannabis smoking in Brazil began to reproduce the opium-based demonology of the period with only the most cursory attention to local social realities. Since the majority of cannabis users in this period consisted of the descendants of black slaves, campaigns against the killer-weed had a useful function in disciplining an unruly and increasingly urbanized population. Through the insistent broadcasting of negative stereotypes, attitudes among the consumers themselves gradually shifted focus from enthusiastic advocacy to ambiguity and ambivalence, and finally to an identification of cannabis smoking with a life of *malandragem* – hustling, pimping, living off one's wits and petty crime.

Continuing police repression, undertaken with uncontrolled ferocity during the military regime of 1964–1985, led even to remote tribes of Amazonian Indians being subjected to torture for their cultivation of cannabis (Henman, 1980). Though middle-class youths and intellectuals also suffered beatings, electric shocks and extortion as a regular feature of any drugs arrest, the rhetoric of the local War on Drugs found its principal vocation in justifying the physical elimination of gangs of small-scale drug dealers. Death-squad victims – often numbering over fifty in a single week in the slums of Rio de Janeiro – are still, in the new democratic era, predominantly young, black and poor, even if routinely described by the authorities as 'major drug traffickers' (America's Watch, 1987).

Increasingly, however, campaigns against cannabis have created a notable scarcity of this once-common substance in Brazil, thus shifting consumption towards more dangerous forms of drug taking. The intravenous use of amphetamines and cocaine, in particular, has recently been implicated in the rapid spread of HIV. Public health surveys describe the huge increase in the number of cases presenting to medical authorities with problems resulting from the use of solvents, pharmaceutical drugs, alcohol and cigarettes. In short, the offensive against cannabis in Brazil – after decades of consistent harm aggravation – has finally succeeded in producing a thoroughly 'modern' drug problem.

Coca in the Andes

It is important to remember that the early and mid twentieth century campaigns against coca were only very remotely justified by the dangers represented by cocaine. Indeed, the major manifestation of this approach in Peru – the 1950 UN Commission of Inquiry into the Problem of Coca-Leaf Chewing (summarized in Comisión de Estudio de las Hojas de Coca, 1978) – coincided with a period in which cocaine was virtually absent on the world illicit market. It is hard, therefore, to avoid the conclusion that the roots of the West's unhealthy obsession with coca lie in a particularly arrogant form of technocratic intolerance, a modern inquisition governed by the horror of foreign drug plants (Antonil, 1978).

The essentially religious – that is to say, anti-rational – nature of this obsession is amply documented by the total indifference shown towards the considerable scientific output which has sought to situate the use of coca in a more realistic pharmacological, social and cultural context. This has been true even of studies commissioned directly by the United States Government, such as Carter et al. (1980), which were ignored when they reported back favourably on coca. Governed by a peculiar ideal of abstinence, and constrained by the idea that the only way to control the use of a drug is to 'cut it off at source', successive US administrations and international bureaucracies have spent enormous sums on attempts to eliminate coca in the producing areas.

Whether through the 'softly, softly' approach of crop-substitution and alternative development, or by means of more aggressive military operations of forcible eradication, the net result has been predictable: a temporary disruption of the peasant economy, an eventual rise in coca prices brought about by the resulting shortages, and a subsequent incentive to plant coca on new sites (Henman, 1985). This economic logic, as unmysterious and unrelenting as the corresponding falls in coca prices occasioned through cycles of over-production, has nevertheless had a series of deleterious knock-on effects. In the social field, the disarticulation of peasant leadership – split between 'good' farmers who cooperate with crop-substitution and 'bad' farmers who do not – as well as the growing discredit of national institutions, seen as willing servants of outside intervention, have provided legitimacy and fresh recruits for both organized crime and armed political insurgency (Henman, 1990). In the environmental context, coca eradication in one area has only favoured the clearing of new land elsewhere, and thus a growing depletion of primary rainforest in the sensitive sub-montane fringes of the Amazon basin.

Additional problems have been associated with the different specific attempts to find a technical 'fix' that could interrupt the flow of cocaine into the United States. In the late 1980s, trials with the chemical herbicide Spike, a tebuthiuron manufactured by Eli Lilly Co., had to be halted in the face of vocal and effective opposition from the environmental lobby in Peru and the United States of America. Subsequent experiments with the malumbia butterfly, *Eloria noyesi*, were fraught with technical difficulties. Though in its caterpillar stage this pest will strip a coca bush of leaves, it does not actually kill the bush. Given that the caterpillar has many natural predators, it was found that effective crop eradication required repeated reinfestation of a single locality. This in turn necessitated the propagation and dissemination of malumbia butterflies on a truly industrial scale, and spiralling costs which could not be justified in view of the programme's uncertain outcome.

It is in this context that must be situated the 1991 outbreak of a new strain of the root-mould, *Fusarium oxysporum*, first reported in the district surrounding the town of Uchiza in the centre of the Upper Huallaga valley, reputed source of 60% of the world's cocaine. Agronomists at Peru's school of tropical agriculture in Tingo Maria describe this fungus as endemic in coca plantations where it has traditionally occasioned small losses, mainly among old bushes growing on poor or marginal soils. The appearance of a far more virulent strain of the mould, however, is unanimously ascribed by local sources to the spreading of a 'white powder' by UMOPAR and CORAH, the Peruvian anti-narcotic and crop-eradication forces financed by the United States of America.

Ironically, United Nations' personnel at sites of the local crop-substitution projects claim that the new strain of *Fusarium* is decimating food crops and their experimental plots of avocado and citrus fruit, while encouraging the development of new coca plantations in the virgin forests to the north and south. Sceptics point out that extensive coca monoculture in the Upper Huallaga offered ideal conditions for the development of such a pest as *Fusarium*, which may have mutated spontaneously. However, the previous record of the US Drug Enforcement Administration in the area – their experiments with Spike and the malumbia butterfly – together with the undeniable existence of a large item in the US Department of Agriculture budget clearly earmarked for the development of 'coca-specific pathogens' suggests caution in assigning the fungus outbreak entirely to natural causes.

Furthermore, biological warfare against coca makes a degree of opportunistic sense in any strictly military assessment of the threat of armed insurgency in Peru. Depriving the local guerrilla movements of their economic base would seem a desirable move from this narrow perspective, at least in the short term. This should, of course, be weighed against the probability of increased guerrilla recruitment among destitute peasants and the likely spread of guerrilla influence into new coca-growing areas north and south of the main production centres in the Upper Huallaga. As a technique of political and environmental harm-aggravation, then, the ill-considered attempts to wipe out coca will continue to bear their recurrent harvest of poisoned fruit.

Opium in the Golden Triangle

If the Brazilian and Peruvian cases provide illustrations of the impact of vigorous anti-drug policies on drug consumption and production in the developing countries, it is nevertheless in the Golden Triangle, and principally in the West's 'good example' client state, Thailand, that the full implications of such policies are most glaringly apparent. Thailand is repeatedly cited as the only known case of 'successful' crop substitution, and indeed the opium harvest in that country has diminished considerably from the high point reached in the late 1960s. Concurrent prevention and education programmes, lavishly funded by the United States of America, the UN drug bureaucracies, the European powers and Japan, have poured anti-opium propaganda into even the most remote hill-tribe villages. Actively encouraging the young to mock and ridicule their opium-smoking elders, such campaigns have clearly undermined native social structures and with them the mutual respect between sexes and generations which acted in the past as a constraint on problematic opium consumption.

The most visible effect of such policies, other than the hundreds of opium users languishing in Thai gaols, has been to encourage the diffusion of heroin use among young people, and with it the spread of the practice of injecting drugs – resulting in subsequent dissemination of the HIV virus due to sharing of needles and syringes. The switch from opium to heroin was documented as an unintended effect of anti-opium campaigns as early as the 1930s in China (Bensussan, 1946), and formed the substance of a major study carried out on opium by the American psychiatrist, Joseph Westermeyer (1982), in Laos during the Vietnam War. Indeed, one positive advantage of the relative isolation and economic backwardness of Laos in the subsequent period of Communist government (1975–1990) has been the virtual disappearance of the earlier heroin epidemic in that country, arguably as the result of a renewed tolerance of opium-smoking. At present, the advent of heroin injecting and AIDS looks set to accompany the opening up of Laos to external influences; ironically it will be from the 'model' anti-drug state, Thailand, that the threat will come.

Many other, less obvious negative effects of the campaigns against opium become apparent if one scratches below the surface, and numerous studies have attempted to bring these to light (for example, Tapp (1989) and various articles in McKinnon and Vierre (1989)). The destruction of peasant livelihoods which has resulted from the whole-sale disruption of the opium economy is apparent in a widespread drift into prostitution, casual labour and tourism-related service jobs by many members of Thailand's hill-tribe minorities. The Yunnanese traders who traditionally provided credit and retail goods in exchange for a share of the opium harvest have largely abandoned the country-side, causing real hardship and distress, for their role was vital as inter-mediaries and informal bankers in the regional economy.

Nor is this the only form of economic dislocation. The opium-for-rice exchanges between highlands and lowlands have also been dis-rupted, with the result that hill-tribe villages, never self-sufficient in basic foodstuffs, are now facing acute shortages and actual famine. Even the widely-trumpeted introduction of 'alternative crops' has proved a mixed blessing; most of them require more land, more water and greater capital inputs, and in the medium term have exacerbated social conflicts over access to local natural resources. In the final analy-sis, debt-bondage to international aid agencies must seem a distinctly worse arrangement than having to deal with supposedly sanguinary opium warlords.

More subtle social changes are apparent to the careful eye of the ethnographer. In Lisu society, where women traditionally had a major say in both the production and commercialisation of opium, the intro-duction of alternative crops, negotiated directly with the male leader-ship, has resulted in a distinct deterioration of female status. Exchanges of silver jewellery, of great symbolic importance in the negotiation of marriage vows, have been rendered financially unviable by the absence of opium sales. In such a context, it is hardly surprising if the status of wives has deteriorated markedly (Hutheesing, 1990).

Finally, one should also consider the close parallels between the South-east Asian and the Latin American experiences in terms of the use of the drugs pretext as a cover for human rights abuses. Successive military governements in Thailand have received generous funding from the USA, supposedly to stem the flow of heroin, but in fact to prop up the country's overall security apparatus. Even after the Bangkok massacres of May 1992, anti-narcotics assistance continued to flow from Washington to the Thai Armed Forces with total impunity, repeating a pattern which was widely denounced in the US Congress in Washington in the case of the Argentine military regime of the mid 1970s.

More alarming still is the involvement of United Nations agencies in providing legitimacy for the corrupt, repressive and genocidal regime in Myanmar (Burma). In early 1992, the United Nations Drug Control Programme announced with considerable fanfare that it was support-ing moves to set up a trilateral anti-narcotics agreement between Thailand, Laos and Myanmar, and the ministers of these countries met in Bangkok to discuss technical arrangements even while the Myanmarese Army was attempting to exterminate the country's democratic opposition and its Muslim, Shan and Karen minorities. No doubt the UNDCP was little concerned that a renewed anti-opium drive in the Golden Triangle could ultimately result in a refugee crisis of truly Cambodian proportions, and thus to further strains on the UN's already overstretched resources in the region. Taking a totally cynical view, one might even suspect that 'harm aggravation' in the drug field finds its strategic complement in a process of deliberate problem creation in areas of potential military conflict.

Empower the Powerless: A Modest Solution to the Drug Question

The characteristic response to the barrage of malign disinformation designed to discourage the consumption of three of the world's oldest, most useful and most interesting drug plants – cannabis, coca and opium – has been what one could describe as ironic inversion. The Brazilian *malandro* of the 1920s and the Jamaican *rude boy* of the 1950s, whether inserting sly references to cannabis-smoking in the lyrics of a samba, or actively championing the use of ganja during the gin-soaked sunset of the British Empire, provided models of the type of social non-conformism which have subsequently become almost normative among minority illicit drug users. Both in the developing world and in the ghettos of the world's major industrial states, a process has occurred which can only be described as 'ruding up' – a positive identification with negative societal images.

The logic underlying such a development – 'if you think we're fucked up now, wait 'till you see *this*' – has two characteristic effects on drug consumption: a potentially positive one, in which considerable symbolic investment is made in ensuring a respectful and enthusiastic relationship with drugs, and an almost certainly negative one, in which the maladjusted are encouraged to signal their unhappiness through ever more problematic patterns of drug misuse. Ironic inversion of the prevailing anti-drugs discourse thus encompasses not only an affirmative defence of the more benign forms of drug use – such as cannabis legalization campaigns, and the strident pro-coca campaigning of Andean indigenous groups – but also the type of ambivalence and ambiguity, indeed the veritable honesty, which characterises many long-term opium smokers, who are often explicitly aware of both the benefits and the drawbacks of their habit.

In a sense, the various forms of ironic discourse tend to offer extremely accurate messages of prevention and education to potential drug users in their own society: almost unrestricted enthusiasm for the beneficial qualities of the coca leaf, a more qualified enthusiasm for the mildly stupefying effects of cannabis, and enthusiasm tempered by some caution for the potentially addictive enchantment of opium. Nor are these attitudes restricted to the herbal forms of the major drugs; similar approaches, such as warnings to inexperienced users as to the dangers of refined cocaine and opiates, are very much a part of the sub-culture of these drugs, in the developing world as elsewhere. On occasion, such a posture flies in the face of economic rationality; Andrade's (1989) study of small-scale cocaine base dealers in Ecuador, for example, demonstrated that the individuals who stayed in business were very reluctant to expand their regular clientele, and positively avoided selling their product (*basuco*) to novices and problematic users.

In every way these positions, based as they are on a healthy instinct of survival and on considerable collective experience of the drugs in question, are markedly preferable to the hypocrisy and obscurantism of most official authorities in the developing countries. In the corridors of power, the slavish reproduction of internationally approved anti-drug rhetoric combines, not infrequently, with direct or incidental profiteering from the illicit market. Where double standards are all, the morality play of 'going after the drug traffickers' is not just an inquisition and a class war; it is also the Great Lie raised to the level of national policy. In the long term, such mendacity will undoubtably corrode the legitimacy of the state and usher in new forms of political instability, as the Andean and Golden Triangle states have so graphically illustrated in recent decades.

The only positive alternative to a never-ending drug war, then, must be to begin with the process of what I have called ironic inversion itself, and recognise in it a response of attempted re-legitimation by the powerless, the marginalised and the disinherited. Such voices – those of drug users and, indeed, drug producers and traffickers as well – express the need for a grass-roots form of drugs education which respects the opinions of the direct participants. It is possible, for instance, to think of the manager of an opium den not only as a drug trafficker, but also as an outreach worker in the field of AIDS and opiate-dependency prevention. To do so, however, requires a rather radical reversal of the perspectives adopted by the authorities hitherto. And above all, it demands a formal and unqualified recognition of the human rights of drug users, and of drug dealers and drug producers as well.

Such an extension of the human rights logic to groups normally excluded by virtue of their criminal status has important implications in recognising drug users, producers and dealers as persons able to control their own destiny, and therefore as citizens both responsible for their actions and, in the absence of any direct or active prejudice to third parties, worthy of social recognition and respect before the law.

Prisons worldwide are begging to be freed of the enormous overcrowding caused by the 'prisoners of war' locked up by current anti-drug offensives, a large proportion of whom are not even drug users themselves but 'mules' and other small-scale intermediaries enticed into the drug trade by the lack of any other economic options.

The producers of drug crops, too, have long been due recognition as legitimate farmers and it is high time the crop substitution programmes imposed on them in the name of progress be clearly denounced for what they are: crude and colonial attempts at political manipulation. For, even more than a war targeted on groups of particular populations, the current campaigns are felt in the developing countries as a form of strictly economic warfare. Shorn of its rhetorical justification, its self-appointed Divine Right in the banishment of Evil, the War on Drugs is perceived quite simply, and correctly, as the symbolic denial of markets for the products of certain defenceless and impoverished countries. This is all the more galling in that the prohibition of their exports is being enforced by the representatives of those very same countries whose drugs (tobacco, alcohol, pharmaceuticals) are provided with subsidies and incentives, and actively 'pushed' by a system of world-wide marketing.

The time is ripe for challenging this institutionalised double standard. The current President of Bolivia wants to free up coca leaf exports, and in 1992 he has made representations along these lines to the UN, the WHO, and the Organisation of American States. One can confidently predict that he will be followed and emulated by other nations. Once freed of the need to reproduce the prevailing international orthodoxy, developing countries will come to recognise that they possess considerable, unsuspected skills in dealing with their own genuine drug problems. A society is not exposed to the use of coca, opium or cannabis for hundreds of years without developing some collective understanding of the risks and benefits of different forms and contexts of drug consumption.

Perhaps the single, most succint message of 'traditional' drug use lies here: in its recognition of the need for societies to provide positive orientation in the use of drugs, to domesticate drugs by offering a supportive social context for their consumption and to promote a symbolic system which matches the expectations of their eventual users. To this extent, it would be no exaggeration to say that harm reduction may eventually have more to learn from the developing world than it has to teach.

References

America's Watch (1987). *Police Abuse in Brazil*. New York: The America's Watch Committee.
Andrade, X. (1989). *Pequeños Traficantes*. Quito: Fundación Nuestros Jóvenes.

Antonil (1978). *Mama Coca*. London: Hassle Free Press.

Bensussan, I.J. (1946). *L'opium*. Paris: Vigot.

Carter, W.E., Mauricio, M.P., Morales, J.V. and Parkerson, P. (1980). *Coca in Bolivia*. La Paz: US National Institute of Drug Abuse.

Comisión de Estudio de las Hojas de Coca: Naciones Unidas (1978). Conclusiones y recomendaciones. *América Indígena*, 38, 1008–1021.

Henman, A.R. (1980). The war on drugs is a war on people. *The Ecologist*, 8/9, 282–289.

Henman, A.R. (1985). Cocaine futures. In A. Henman, R. Lewis and T. Malyon (Eds), *Big Deal: The Politics of the Illicit Drugs Business*. London and Sydney: Pluto.

Henman, A.R. (1990). Coca and cocaine: Their role in 'traditional' cultures in South America. *Journal of Drug Issues*, 20, 577–588.

Henman, A. and Pessoa, O. (1986). *Diamba Sarabamba: Coletanea de Textos Brasileiros Sobre a Maconha*. São Paulo, Ground/Global.

Hutheesing, O.K. (1990). *Emerging Sexual Inequality Among the Lisu of Northern Thailand*. Leiden: E.J. Brill.

McKinnon, J. and Vienne, B. (Eds) (1989). *Hill Tribes Today: Problems in Change*. Paris and Bangkok: ORSTOM/White Lotus.

Tapp, N. (1989). *Sovereignty and Rebellion: The White Hmong of Northern Thailand*. Singapore: Oxford University Press.

Westermeyer, J. (1982). *Poppies, Pipes, and People: Opium and its Use in Laos*. Berkeley and Los Angeles: University of California Press.

Chapter 19
Harm-reduction Policies and Programmes in Developing Countries

NAOTAKA SHINFUKU

Health, WHO and Consumption of Alcohol and Other Drugs

Health is defined in the WHO Constitution (1946) as a state of physical, mental and social well-being and not merely the lack of disease and infirmity. Based on this definition, WHO has a mandate to develop programmes on mental health, including prevention of alcohol and drug abuse. The traditional focus of WHO has been on collaboration with member states in the prevention of communicable diseases and the strengthening of basic health care. However, diseases related to lifestyles and behaviours have become increasingly important public health and social concerns. This trend has also become evident recently in developing countries. Injuries associated with acute alcohol intoxication and the spread of HIV infection through sharing of injection equipment among injecting drug users are now recognised as major health threats in many developing countries, including some with very scarce health resources. Consequently, WHO has been requested to increase its collaboration with member states to reduce the harm resulting from consumption of alcohol and other drugs.

Special Programme on Substance Abuse

In September 1990, WHO established a new Programme on Substance Abuse (PSA) in response to the increasing problems resulting from alcohol and drugs which have been experienced by a growing number of countries world-wide in recent years. The overall goal of this special programme is, first, to reduce the impact that currently used psychoactive substances have on the health and welfare of populations everywhere and, second, to prevent the emergence of new forms of substance abuse. The specific objectives are: (1) to reduce the demand for addictive substances; (2) to reduce the impact of substance abuse

257

on the health and welfare of individuals and families; (3) to develop effective approaches to the treatment of substance dependence and associated diseases; (4) to collaborate in controlling the supply and use of illicit psychoactive substances; and (5) to integrate relevant health components into all development programmes designed to reduce the supply of illicit narcotic drugs.

Analysis of the Present Situation

Every year the UN Commission on Narcotic Drugs is required to report on the situation and trends in drug abuse and illicit traffic to the Economic and Social Council of the United Nations. According to the report of the Commission which met in Vienna in January–February 1992, the world drug abuse situation is generally stable or even improving, with Africa and South America being the main exceptions to these trends.

The report noted however that the situation is deteriorating in many developing countries in the world with increasing problems associated with cannabis, cocaine, heroin and other psychotropic substances. In North America, consumption of cocaine and cannabis has been decreasing. However, this trend was counterbalanced by increasing abuse of coca-type drugs in South America and of cocaine and cannabis in some Caribbean islands. The situation was reported to be generally stable in Europe, Oceania, Asia and the Far East.

Opioid abuse was reported as a serious problem in all areas except South America. In Europe, Oceania, Asia and the Far East, opioids were the main problem drug. Consumption of heroin showed a decreasing trend in Europe and North America. To some extent this trend was also present in Asia and the Far East where traditional opium use, in particular, was on the decrease. In Africa and the Near and Middle East, however, abuse of opioids, including especially heroin, was increasing. Alcohol consumption and problems associated with amphetamines and other stimulants had increased slightly in Africa and in some countries in Asia and the Far East, in the Near and Middle East and in Oceania.

In summary, the global epidemic of addictive drugs is increasing in developing countries and probably levelling off in many developed countries.

Alcohol

In the past, problems associated with alcohol were unique to developed countries. However, a variety of alcohol-related problems, including accidents and impaired productivity in the work place, road traffic accidents, violence and crime, have become very common in developing countries in recent years. In addition, these countries have difficulty in developing effective programmes for prevention of alcohol-related problems.

The country profiles presented at the Inter-regional Meeting on Alcohol-related Problems held in Tokyo in April 1991 showed interesting contrasts between the complications experienced in developing and developed countries (Programme on Substance Abuse, 1991). Between 1978 and 1988, there has been marked decrease in *per capita* alcohol consumption in most of the developed countries. Australia, Canada, France and West Germany recorded reductions in consumption of more than 10%; Sweden and the United States of America also reported decreases of 7% and 9% respectively. Countries with heavy drinking traditions, such as Ireland, Italy and Spain, reported decreases of 23%, 33% and 22% respectively. Only in the case of Japan and Finland, where *per capita* consumption was relatively low, was alcohol consumption greater in 1988 than in 1978.

Also, in a number of developed countries, declining alcohol consumption was accompanied by a reduction in alcohol-related problems (e.g. alcohol-induced liver cirrhosis, admission to psychiatric hospitals with a primary diagnosis of alcoholism, alcohol-impaired driving and violence associated with alcohol). In contrast to this generally optimistic note from several developed countries, presentations made from some developing countries were alarming. Whereas in many developed countries alcohol consumption peaked in the mid 1970s and has been declining since, alcohol consumption is rising rapidly in many developing countries, particularly in Africa, the Caribbean, the South Pacific and parts of Central and South America.

This situation requires that special attention be paid to the reduction of alcohol and drug-related harm in developing countries, with greater international efforts to alleviate these problems.

WHO Programmes and Strategies on Alcohol and Drugs

WHO's strategies on harm reduction are governed by member states. The policies of WHO on alcohol and drug-related problems are determined by resolutions adopted by the World Health Assembly and Regional Committees.

In the field of drugs, the Single Convention on Narcotic Drugs (1961) and the Convention on Psychotropic Substances (1971) are the basis of WHO activities. These two conventions set the policy guidelines for member states to control production, transportation and the use of narcotic and psychotropic substances.

The main strategy of WHO has been to collaborate with member states to formulate and strengthen comprehensive national policies and programmes for the prevention and control of alcohol and drug abuse. In the past, the Western Pacific Regional Office of WHO has collaborated with member states in the following activities: (1) raising the level of awareness of the public health impact of problems related to alcohol and drug abuse; (2) supporting the establishment and strengthening multi-sectoral inter-disciplinary national programmes; and (3) supporting training and research in the field of alcohol and drug abuse.

National Alcohol and Drug Policy

Encouraging the development of comprehensive national policies on alcohol and drugs has been the key concept in the collaboration of WHO with member states. The concept was new to most member states initially but it has been gradually accepted by member states as a most effective component of national responses to alcohol and drug problems. For government officials from developing countries with very limited resources, programmes to develop treatments for alcohol and drug-dependent persons were neither socio-culturally relevant nor cost-effective. Comprehensive national alcohol and drug policies and programmes include a range of measures designed to limit drug supplies, reduce drug demand and reduce alcohol- and drug-related harm. Supply reduction measures include regulation of production, distribution and taxation. Production is regulated by controlling commercial and domestic outputs, including illegal drugs, and control of imports including agriculture supplies. Distribution is regulated by such measures as controlling the number and location of retail outlets and defining the conditions of permitted sales. Demand reduction involves a range of measures including the regulation of advertising, international agreements to restrict cross-national advertising and promotion, regulation of consumption through pricing policy, encouraging the provision of non-alcoholic beverages, and health education addressed to the general public, specific high risk groups, professional workers and opinion leaders.

Measures Designed to Reduce Alcohol- and Drug-related Harm

Harm reduction covers a variety of activities. Problems associated with intoxication can be reduced by measures intended to prevent traffic accidents, violence, family problems and public drunkenness. The distribution of sterile needles and syringes can reduce the spread of HIV infection among injecting drug users. Chronic problems are prevented by early diagnosis and intervention, improved treatment at primary health care level, improved specialist treatment and improvement of referral procedures. Methadone maintenance programmes for drug users who inject heroin have been introduced in several countries as a practical means of reducing drug-related harm.

This is not an exhaustive list of harm-reduction measures. However, it indicates the main areas that need to be covered in a comprehensive national alcohol and drug policy. This list shows that harm reduction has been an essential part of WHO collaboration with member states. HIV infection and AIDS among injecting drug users has emphasised the importance of harm reduction as part of WHO programmes of cooperation with member states in response to the problems resulting from substance use.

Policy Options and Culture

The Western Pacific regional office of WHO covers 36 countries. The member states differ in size of population, stage of socio-economic development, cultural and religious background. Culture and religion have the strongest impact on the choice of public policies including those related to alcohol and drugs. Brunei and Malaysia have adopted Islam as their nation's official religion. China, Japan and the Republic of Korea are strongly influenced by the traditional Asian values associated with Buddhism and Confucianism. Australia, New Zealand, Papua New Guinea and the island countries in the South Pacific come under Christian influence which places a higher value on individual freedoms over conformity to community values. Different cultures define different policy options on the responses to injecting drug use. Traditionally, no Asian or Islamic country in the Western Pacific Region regards methadone maintenance programmes or the provision of free needles and syringes as an acceptable harm reduction measure for injecting drug users. Also, the fact that methadone and needle and syringe exchange programmes are expensive for developing countries with scarce resources must be considered. However, the introduction in the 1970s and subsequent acceptance of methadone maintenance in Hong Kong, the more recent considerable extension of the methadone withdrawal programme in Thailand in reponse to HIV and the commencement of a needle and syringe exchange programmes in Nepal suggest that more latitude might be available for policy makers than is often claimed.

In some Muslim countries, alcohol consumption is prohibited by law. In Asian countries such as China, Japan and the Republic of Korea, use of illicit drugs including heroin, amphetamines and marijuana constitutes an offence, with personal experience of illicit drugs constituting a criminal act. Drug substitution programmes are generally regarded as 'spoiling a person'. Many people in Asia believe that 'cold turkey' detoxification experiences are helpful in assisting drug dependent persons to fight against their addiction.

Major Constraints

There are several constraints to the implementation of harm-reduction programmes in developing countries, including the lack of comprehensive national policies, shortage of manpower and the lack of necessary data. Comprehensive national policies and programmes for alcohol and drugs are essential to reduce these problems. However, in many countries and areas in the Western Pacific Region such programmes simply do not exist. Where alcohol and drug programmes do exist in the region, they are generally confined to law enforcement programmes for drug users. Demand and harm reduction policies and programmes for alcohol and drug problems are usually accorded a very low priority in developing countries. Income from alcohol excise and other economic benefits derived by governments from the alcohol beverage industry always weigh more heavily than health concerns. Governments are often interested in actually increasing alcohol consumption as this means increased government revenue from taxation. Surprisingly, few governments are aware of the health and social costs of alcohol which exceed tax revenues in the long run. Strong international and domestic marketing pressures to increase the sale of alcoholic beverages are an additional obstacle to the implementation of comprehensive national policies and programmes in developing countries. These conditions should be improved by the concerted efforts of experts and responsible government officials, including those of alcohol-exporting countries.

In many developing countries, very scarce resources are available for reducing demand for alcohol and drugs or minimising problems consequent on consumption of mood altering substances. Medical experts are fully occupied by providing treatment for diseases and very few are interested in reducing harm resulting from alcohol or drugs. Counselling skills for dealing with alcohol and drug problems are generally not included in educational curricula. However, several reports suggest that alcohol, drugs and HIV infection are affecting highly trained manpower in developing countries, such as political leaders and health professionals. In spite of the magnitude of the problems resulting from alcohol and drug use in developing countries, very limited information is available on the magnitude, trends and nature of these problems.

HIV Infection and Drug Abuse

In recent years, the number of HIV-infected injecting drug users in developing countries has increased rapidly and is expected to increase further especially in Asia (Li and Yeogh, 1992). HIV-infected injecting drug users have become major sources of HIV transmission in some

Asian countries. HIV spreads from infected injecting drug users to commercial sex workers who are often their sexual partners. Commercial sex workers transmit HIV to the general population through unprotected sex. HIV prevalence among drug injectors varies from country to country and, even within one country, the prevalence varies considerably between cities. For example, in New York, the prevalence is more than 50% whereas in San Franisco it has remained at 12%. The same phenomenon is observed in the United Kingdom; in Edinburgh, over 50% of injecting drug users are infected with HIV (Robertson et al., 1986) whereas only 5% have been infected so far in Glasgow .

The very rapid spread of HIV infection among injecting drug users in some developing countries is alarming: in Thailand, over 50% of injecting drug users in Bangkok and more than 70% of injecting drug users in the northern part of the country are HIV positive (Weniger et al., 1991; Patrick and Li, 1992). Even in the People's Republic of China, 1690 HIV antibody tests in drug users showed 391 positive cases during 1989–1991 (21.4%) (country reports from China to WHO Manila). These cases are mostly from Yunnan province bordering the so-called 'Golden Triangle', which is the major world source of opium. In Malaysia, a survey of 1500 injecting drug users in 1991 found 169 infected with HIV (11.3%) (country reports from Malaysia to WHO Manila). These figures are likely to increase in the near future unless effective programmes on harm reduction are established.

In the Western Pacific Region, the cumulative number of reported AIDS cases and HIV infections as of 1 January, 1992 was 4066 and 22 100 respectively. Among reported AIDS cases, those from the developed countries of Australia, New Zealand and Japan accounted for 3757 cases (92.4%). There were 2479 reported deaths from AIDS. The number of AIDS cases comprising injecting drug users (80) was relatively small. However, this group and cases attributed to heterosexual transmission are the fastest growing categories of AIDS cases in the Region. The distribution of estimated and projected annual adult AIDS cases indicates that in the near future, Europe and North America will bring the HIV/AIDS epidemic under control. But AIDS will become a growing problem in developing regions such as Africa, Asia and Latin America (Chin, 1991). In this regard, harm-reduction programmes for drug users in developing countries will be a key determinant of the magnitude of the global epidemic of HIV infection in the twenty-first-century.

Conclusions

First, concepts and terminology relevant to harm reduction should be considered as part of a comprehensive national policy and programme on alcohol and drugs. However, it is dangerous only to stress harm reduction as supply reduction and demand reduction should be developed in harmony, particularly in developing countries with scarce resources.

Second, the magnitude of alcohol- and drug-related problems is very serious in developing countries undergoing rapid socio-economic changes. In addition, the prevalence of these problems is increasing rapidly and most developing countries are unable to cope with the increasing magnitude of alcohol and other drug problems.

Third, harm reduction is a necessary and relevant component of comprehensive efforts aimed at reducing a variety of adverse consequences of mood altering drugs, including injuries, violence, crimes and HIV infection.

Fourth, developing countries are increasingly targeted by multinational industries for the sale of legal drugs such as alcohol and tobacco, as the consumption of these commodities declines in developed countries.

Fifth, alcohol-related problems are very serious in the South Pacific including Papua New Guinea. Developed countries should provide technical and financial assistance for less well-resourced countries to assist in the implementation of sound national policies and programmes to reduce alcohol and drug-related harm. Responsible marketing practices should be established by multinational industries for the sale of legal drugs to developing countries.

Sixth, the restoration of cultural identities and traditional values are of paramount importance in efforts to reduce harm related to legal drugs in developing countries among minorities such as American Indians, Alaskan Eskimos and Australian Aborigines.

Seventh, harm reduction for injecting drug users is necessary even in developing countries in view of the possible spread of HIV infection among this population. However, the introduction of these programmes requires careful assessment of the country's socio-cultural background and the concurrence of the Government at the highest political level.

Eighth, unless the demand for drugs in affluent countries is halted, drug problems in developing countries will continue. Developing countries on drug trafficking routes experience spill-over effects and this may be a major cause of increasing drug consumption and drug problems among local people.

National policies on alcohol and drugs should be 'humanistic, cost-effective and socio-culturally relevant'. Community support and strong political will are indispensable for the success of national policies on alcohol and drugs. Each country should develop a national policy taking into account the above principles. Also, national policy should be consistent with international agreements. The legalisation of a scheduled substance in one country may have a major impact on neighbouring countries. Such issues should be discussed thoroughly in appropriate international forums.

References

Chin, J. (1991). Global estimates of HIV infection and AIDS cases: 1991. *AIDS*, 5 (Suppl. 2), 57–61.

Li, E.K.Y. and Yeogh, E.Y. (1992). Current epidemiological trends of HIV infection in Asia. In P. Volberding and M.A. Jacobson (Eds), *AIDS Clinical Review*. New York: Marcel Decker Inc.

Programme on Substance Abuse (1991). *Inter-regional Meeting on Alcohol-related Problems, Tokyo, 2–8 April, 1991*. Geneva: WHO

Robertson, J.R., Bucknall, A.B.V., and Welsby, P.D. et al. (1986). Epidemic of AIDS related virus (HTLV-III/LAV) infection among intravenous drug users. *British Medical Journal*, 292, 527–529.

Weniger, B.G., Limpakarnjanarat, K., Ungchusak, K., Thanprasertsuk, S., Choopanya, K., Vanichseni, S., Uneklabh, T., Thongcharoen, P. and Wasi, C. (1991). The epidemiology of HIV infection and AIDS in Thailand. *AIDS*, 5 (Suppl 2), 71–85.

Chapter 20
Implementing Policies to Reduce Harm Associated with Legal Drug Use in the Developing Countries of the Pacific: Who Can Help?

SALLY CASSWELL

As the markets for alcohol and tobacco in parts of the industrialised world have become somewhat saturated, public health practitioners have watched expansion of sectors of the industry into the developing world with concern. The Pacific region has been no exception and use of alcohol and tobacco in the small island states is now facilitated by the production and marketing practices of commercial industries. There has been some documentation of consumption and associated harm in the region and the World Health Organization (WHO) has received requests from governments in the region for assistance with the prevention of harm associated with alcohol use.

This chapter is based on participant observation at a number of WHO and other meetings concerned with alcohol problem prevention, the published literature and field work carried out by the author in the 1980s to research alcohol issues in several Pacific Islands.

Alcohol and Tobacco Markets in the Developing Countries of the Pacific

Neither alcohol nor tobacco, the two legal drugs which contribute most to drug-related harm in many industrialised countries, were present in the developing nations of the Pacific prior to their introduction by Asian and European visitors and colonisers. Their incorporation into Pacific Island societies has been inextricably linked with the process of colonisation and modernisation (Marshall, 1982). The implications drawn by indigenous people from watching tourists' behaviour and from mass media portrayal of life in industrialised countries must have been that alcohol and tobacco use are an integral part of a modern Western society.

The industrialised world, which introduced alcohol and tobacco to the Pacific, continues to play a major role in the supply of alcohol, though the supply takes a number of different forms. These include: importation from industrialised countries (Australia and, to a lesser extent, New Zealand play a major role); local production dependent on the importation of capital and expertise from industrialised countries (a major global player, Heineken, has involvement in the region, as have Australian and some smaller European breweries); and local production under license (both San Miguel and Heineken are brewed under license in the Pacific) (Casswell, 1985).

The technology imported from the industrialised world has meant that much of the brewing in the Pacific, as elsewhere in the developing world (Kortteinen, 1990), is very modern. In Tahiti, for example, the brewery is highly automated (*Islands Business Pacific*, July 1991). The breweries often have the capacity to produce well in excess of national consumption and look to exports elsewhere in the Pacific.

Alcohol consumption in the Pacific is predominantly beer, and commercially produced beer rather than home-brew almost certainly makes up the bulk of this. Accurate figures on informal sector production are not available, and there are traditions of local production that date from colonisation times (Casswell, 1989) but these are probably not as culturally ingrained or as widespread as elsewhere – in Africa, for example (Kortteinen, 1990). Commercially produced beer, with all its overtones of modernisation, often combined with a nationalistic brand image, seems to be the preferred beverage of the majority of drinkers (Casswell, 1986).

The statistics on the production, imports and exports of alcohol in the Pacific suggest that consumption in many of the island states rose during the decade 1970–1980 (Casswell, 1989; Smart, 1991). Vanuatu was a notable exception, probably influenced to some extent by the outflux of expatriates after Independence. Many of the countries for which data are available showed a fairly slow increase, and their estimated per capita consumption remained at or below two litres of absolute alcohol per head. This can be compared with New Zealand and Australia at about seven to nine litres per head. The French territories were much higher than the other developing countries, as were relatively affluent states like Belau.

A comparable exercise drawing together the statistics for tobacco production, imports and exports to estimate levels of per capita consumption does not appear to have been done for developing countries of the Pacific region.

Alcohol- and Tobacco-Related Harm

The comparison with Australasia in terms of estimated per capita consumption of alcohol cannot be interpreted as indicating that little or no harm is associated with alcohol use in the developing countries of the Pacific. Higher proportions of the population are abstainers in the island states than in Australasia (Casswell, 1986), and the quantities drunk by individual drinkers are probably similar to those in industrialised countries (Ringrose and Zimmet, 1979; Marshall, 1983).

Furthermore, the cultural, political and economic context of use is obviously very different from industrialised countries in ways which impact on the experience of and ways of handling alcohol-related problems. The quality of roads and motor vehicles is an obvious example. Another is the disruption of traditional patterns of participation in the community and replacement by a monetary economy from which significant numbers of young men are excluded. A combination of alcohol and unemployment were behind rioting by Kanaks in New Caledonia in early 1992 according to newspaper reports (*Dominion*, March 16, 1992) and a study of palm wine drinking in Bali suggested that unusually high levels were related to lack of work opportunities (Suryani, Adnyana and Jensen, 1990).

Alcohol can contribute to issues of public order and security, to lowered work productivity and economic performance, and to impairment of the public health (Makela and Viikari, 1977). All of these three areas of potential alcohol-related harm would seem to apply in the developing countries of the Pacific.

Only limited research data exist on alcohol-related harm in the Pacific, a notable exception being the ethnographic data collected in Papua New Guinea in the 1970s with Mac Marshall's encouragement (Marshall, 1982). Anecdotal evidence from key informants in a number of countries and from the popular media discussion of the issue support the limited research data available in suggesting an impact in all three areas. For example, in 1977 the Asian and Pacific Centre for Women and Development stated: '...the issue of drunken and violent husbands and the associated squandering of money stands out as the most heartfelt and desperate problem of women in the region' (Marshall and Marshall, 1990).

The involvement of alcohol in public disorder is certainly a continuing theme (Marshall, 1979; Casswell, 1986). Media coverage of crime in the tiny island country of Tuvalu in 1991, for example, emphasised the relative lack of crime in a society which still adhered closely to traditional ethics and ways of living. However, the crime which did occur was seen to be related to alcohol use and alcohol was described by the police as public enemy number one (*Islands Business Pacific*, April, 1991). In countries which have experienced greater socio-cultural change alcohol is also cited repeatedly as a major factor in crime and particularly in violent crime, including domestic violence. It is an indication of the widespread perception that alcohol plays a causal role in such violence that many police forces in the region routinely record categories such as 'major offences arising from the consumption of liquor' (Casswell, 1986). Ethnographers point out that a high level of non-alcohol-related violence exists, but have also provided insight into the way in which drunken comportment tends to increase the likelihood of violence (Mahoney, 1974; Lindstrom, 1982; Sexton, 1982; Walter, 1982; Warry, 1982).

Violent crime, while a public order issue, also impacts on the health services because of the injuries involved. A series of post-mortem examinations carried out in Papua New Guinea 1976–1980 on all trauma deaths showed that almost half were caused either by blunt instruments wielded in brawls and domestic fights, or by sharp penetrating weapons such as axes which were used in fights or attacks by unknown assailants. About one in five of these fatalities had blood alcohol levels at or above 80 mg/100 ml (an underestimate because of the time delay occurring before the sample was taken) (Sinha et al., 1981).

The other half of the post-mortem series was of deaths in motor vehicle crashes. In this sample blood alcohol was measured at or above 80 mg/100 ml in one third (Sinha et al., 1981). Similar research data are not available from elsewhere in the Pacific but the clustering of crashes and anecdotal evidence suggest alcohol involvement elsewhere. The levels recorded in Papua New Guinea are similar to those of industrialised countries (Roizen, 1982) where per capita consumption levels are much higher. This reflects both the pattern of heavy consumption during a drinking occasion suggested by survey data from Nauru (Ringrose and Zimmet, 1979) and Papua New Guinea (Marshall, 1983) and probably also the state of the roads and habitual patterns of driving.

In virtually all developing countries the relative importance of injury to the medical system has increased over the past 15 years due to both increased prevalence of injury hazards and improved control of infectious and parasitic diseases (Stansfield, Smith and McGreevy, 1990).

In marked contrast to alcohol, tobacco does not contribute to problems of public order and injury. It does, however, have very significant effects on the smoker (and those exposed to sidestream smoke) from the physical effects of chronic exposure. Passive smoking increases the risk of respiratory disease (United States Public Health Service, 1986; Kawachi, Pearce and Jackson, 1989).

These relationships have led to tobacco emerging as the most significant contributor to drug-related premature mortality in many industrialised countries and now in developing countries. A projection for tobacco-related deaths given at the 8th World Conference on Tobacco or Health, March 1992, was of seven million deaths in developing countries in the year 2025 (compared with two million in industrialised countries). Cardiovascular disease and cancer are now emerging as leading causes of death in many of the Pacific states (Taylor, Lewis and Levy, 1989).

In contrast with alcohol where women's experience of harm is probably predominantly related to men's consumption, tobacco use is a more direct source of harm. This is certainly the case in industrialised countries where increasingly men's tobacco consumption is declining leaving women consuming an increasing share (Graham, 1989) and may become the case in developing countries. The first International Conference on Women and Smoking held in 1992 stated that 'women's tobacco use is a serious global issue... The transnational tobacco companies have openly identified women as a key target group. This is reflected in advertising and promotional strategies, the development of brands designed to appeal to women...'.

In relation to the third category of drug associated harm, the effect on productivity and economic performance, there is little information available about the role of either alcohol or tobacco in the Pacific. All South Pacific countries import more tobacco than they produce (Stanton, 1990). This deficit balance of trade in tobacco will have an adverse effect on economic performance.

There has been little discussion of the impact of alcohol production on the macro-economic level in the region. Most of the alcohol globally consumed in developing countries is produced locally (Kortteinen, 1989) and this is true for many of the Pacific island states. An economic issue then arises over the use of resources required to produce beverage alcohol.

Commercially produced alcohol and tobacco, whether imported or produced locally, is expensive relative to disposable income. In 1990 up to 25% of Fijian villagers' income was being used for the purchase of cigarettes (L. Leslie, G. Groth-Marnat and M. Renneker, 1992, unpublished data) and the Bureau of Statistics figures showed 6% of family budgets spent on alcohol and tobacco across the country (Duignan and Casswell, 1990). A number of studies of household expenditure in the Papua New Guinea highlands in the 1970s and early 1980s were consistent in suggesting that about 30% of expenditure was spent on alcohol (Townsend, 1977; Grossman, 1982; Sexton, 1984). In Western Samoa in 1991 it was reported that it took a person on the average wage three hours to earn enough money to buy one beer (*Islands Business Pacific*, March, 1991). (This compares with an estimate of about 15 minutes for New Zealanders in 1991.)

Women in particular express concern about expenditure on alcohol, presumably because of their responsibilities for supplying food and shelter for children. However, concern over the economic effects is more widespread and when local governments have attempted to curtail access to alcohol, the reasons given have included the desire to redirect money elsewhere (Piau-Lynch, 1982; Casswell, 1986).

Productivity at the individual level can also be affected by alcohol consumption and while no research data are available key informants sometimes expressed concern over this aspect. Injury is highest among young males and this group makes up the bulk of the agricultural labouring sector. Informants also pointed out that those in the public service and commercial sector who are in the cash economy are those with greatest access to commercially produced alcohol.

Much of the tobacco- and alcohol-related harm described for the developing countries of the Pacific is similar to that found in the industrialised countries in the region, although the lack of resources in the poorer countries may mean a greater relative impact on the health and public order systems, for example.

Harm-reduction Strategies

To some extent the strategies which have been found to be effective in industrialised countries will also be valuable in reducing harm associated with alcohol and tobacco in developing countries. However, the effect of policies in any country depends on a complex web of interaction between the cultural, political, economic and social characteristics of a community. The small amount of information we have available for the Pacific illustrates that there is not likely to be a direct and simple transfer of technology of harm-reducing alcohol and tobacco policies from industrialised to developing countries. At the same time, however, there are some lessons to be learned from the experiences of industrialised countries which have struggled to contain the effects of much higher levels of per capita use than the developing countries have yet experienced.

One of the strategies which has been shown to be relatively cost-effective in industrialised countries is control of the price of alcohol and tobacco relative to the cost of other commodities by means of taxation policy (Kendell et al., 1983; Cook, 1987; Grossman, Coate and Arluck, 1987; Grossman, 1989; Laugesen and Meads, 1991a). In New Zealand, for example, the policy of inflation-adjusted taxation on both alcohol and tobacco, which was introduced in 1989, ensured that neither drug became easier to afford. Econometric analyses have shown that the decrease in aggregate levels of consumption of both alcohol and tobacco in New Zealand have been, in part, the result of the taxation policy (Laugeson and Meads, 1991b; Wette et al., 1993). There is also evidence for both drugs that in industrialised countries teenagers are particularly responsive to price increases (Grossman, Coate and Arluck, 1987; Grossman, 1989).

The evidence from studies of real price in developing countries shows that people there are also constrained by price and income. Econometric analyses of beer prices in Kenya have suggested that elasticities are larger than those often found in industrialised countries, suggesting a difference in the prestige value of beer; however, long term elasticities do show an impact of price increases (Partanen, 1991). Data exists in the Pacific region, for Fiji, which suggest a relationship between alcohol consumption and real price (Casswell, 1986).

Changes in the availability of alcohol have also been shown to have effects on consumption and related problems in industrialised countries. Sharp reductions in availability have been shown to decrease consumption (Osterberg and Saila, 1991). However, in recent years sharp reductions in availability have not been politically feasible and more common have been small increases in availability, many of which have been shown to increase alcohol-related problems (Osterberg and Saila, 1991). The only politically feasible major reduction in availability in recent years in free market industrialised countries was one directed at a specific, relatively powerless sector of the population: youth. Enactment of an older minimum drinking age has been shown in north America to reduce consumption and prevent alcohol-related traffic crashes among youth (O'Malley and Wagenaar, 1991).

Sharp decreases in availability have, however, occurred in developing countries in the Pacific during the past two decades (Marshall and Marshall, 1990). Particularly well documented, but by no means an isolated case, was the experience on the island of Moen in Truk (Millay, 1985; Marshall and Marshall, 1990).

This prohibition, introduced in 1978, was based on a coalition of interests of older men and women. In this way it bears some relationship to the passing of minimum drinking laws in industrialised countries. Both symbolise a social norm opposed to the drinking and drunkenness of young males. In Truk the drunken violence characteristic of young male drinking in the 1970s prior to prohibition was described by Marshall (1979) in *Weekend Warriors*. Alcohol provided a legitimate time out from normal moral standards and the need of the young Melanesian male to display bravery and risk taking was met by drunken fighting instead of earlier traditional warfare (Marshall, 1979). Women were opposed to the public violence and deaths in traffic accidents and murders, to the spending of money which could have gone for the support of families, to being themselves beaten by drunken husbands and to the abuse of their children (Marshall and Marshall, 1990).

In the five years following the passing of prohibition three attempts at repeal were defeated and ten years later, in 1988, there was still sufficient support for the prohibition to be maintained (Marshall and Marshall, 1990). Drinking was by no means absent from Moen, which has been described as the 'wettest dry island in the Pacific' (Millay,

1985). A thriving black market supplied alcohol to those able to pay the inflated prices. However, the law had resulted in major changes to the drinking. It had moved from public places to the bush or private homes and took place among friends and family groups. While drunken violence did occur, it did so outside the public arena and 'no longer commanded the attentive and appreciative audience it once had' (Marshall and Marshall, 1990). There was also a shift in the social climate surrounding drinking in Truk, such that public drunkenness had been redefined as something shameful (Marshall and Marshall, 1990). Women perceived improvements both from the reduction in the public violence and also in domestic violence.

It seems likely that prohibition on Moen, while not eliminating access to alcohol had a positive effect on alcohol-related problems by increasing the price and by influencing societal norms.

A somewhat similar, and equally fascinating, example of prohibition exists for tobacco in the Fijian village of Nabila (L. Leslie, G.Groth-Marnat and M. Renneker, 1992, unpublished data). In this case the village determined that the entire village would abstain from smoking and it was proposed that the money saved would be put towards the cost of building a community centre. Prior to the introduction of a formal taboo all the smokers gathered together. After collecting all the cigarettes in the village they chain smoked to the point of nausea; the few remaining cigarettes were destroyed. That night a long *kava* drinking ceremony was performed and a taboo was set in place. Four individuals relapsed and each of them had a negative consequence occur. The first one stood up after smoking a cigarette, tripped and lacerated his scalp. The second was attacked by a dog shortly after commencing smoking and the third developed an unspecified testicular swelling within two days after relapse. The fourth one collapsed unconscious immediately after smoking a cigarette while he was drinking his *kava*. Nine months later smoking was described as 'almost nonexistent' (L. Leslie, G. Groth-Marnat and M. Renneker, 1992, unpublished data).

The prohibition on tobacco took place in a cohesive community which was described as 'highly respectful of authority'; it was backed up by a strong belief in the power of the taboo produced through the *kava* ceremony (L. Leslie, G. Groth-Marnat and M. Renneker, 1992, unpublished data). In the case of Moen, the societal group was bigger, was in a state of rapid socio-cultural change and was less cohesive. All these factors probably contributed to the more partial outcome of the alcohol prohibition and the development of a black market which met the needs of the drinkers and the elite which made money from it (Marshall and Marshall, 1990).

However, the researchers who documented the policies in Nabila and on Moen draw some similar conclusions about the factors which led to both the acceptance and the success of the prohibition strategy.

In both cases it can be noted that, relative to people in industrialised countries, there was a much greater willingness to place moral judgements on the behaviour. Similarly, relative to industrialised countries, there was a greater acceptance of collective values and a willingness to support laws that constrain individual behaviour.

These two case studies illustrate that culturally appropriate solutions which have been found to ameliorate some of the harm associated with the use of introduced modern drugs into the Pacific can be very different from policies likely to be implemented in industrialised countries. They serve to remind researchers and consultants from the industrialised world that the nature of the solutions sought and found in developing countries will sometimes be very different from those found appropriate in their own countries. Of course, the policies operating in developing countries will change to meet changing circumstances and policies found appropriate in Moen and Nabila in the 1980s will not necessarily be appropriate in the same setting in the future.

Research and Public Health Advocacy in Developing Countries

To turn to the question posed in the title of this chapter, 'Who Can Help?', the differences illustrated above do not mean that input from the outside is entirely inappropriate or unhelpful. In the two case studies cited the impact of outside advocates was an important catalyst to policy development in the short term. The health professionals (the Surfers' Medical Association) in Fiji worked to establish health promotion activity in the village of Nabila, and the Women's Board of Missions for the Pacific Islands held a conference in 1976 at which temperance and prohibition were emphasised as important social causes for Micronesian women to pursue in their communities; women from Truk who attended played an important role in the establishment of prohibition on Moen some months later.

However, this outside influence was taken by the indigenous people and incorporated into the development of culturally embedded policy. The most appropriate input from researchers and consultants will often be that which recognises and assists the local ongoing policy process.

The research on alcohol in developing countries has largely been descriptive surveys of drinkers and some studies of emergency room patients (Odejide et al., 1990). These research approaches reflect a particular disciplinary approach, and while the data collected in such studies do have a potentially valuable role to play in policy and programme development, the links are not always direct or obvious. In the past two decades a major development in the field of social alcohol research has been a new emphasis on change. It is recognised that major changes occur, in whole populations as well as in individual lives, and research has now focused on the processes underlying these changes (Institute of Medicine, 1987). Case studies of policy development and evaluations of programmes designed to reduce harm are examples of this kind of research. However, in developing countries there is little evidence of this kind of research as yet.

One model which might be useful for researchers from industrialised countries and for WHO to adopt is one we have developed in New Zealand for working with community groups in the alcohol harm-reduction area (L. Stewart, S. Casswell and P. Duignan, 1992, unpublished data). This is known as a formative evaluation approach (McClintock, 1986). The formative evaluation approach is one in which research methods and research-based knowledge are used to assist people working in a community to define their objectives and strategies; and to help redefine and refine them in a dynamic on-going process as they develop appropriate ways to decide on and implement harm-reduction strategies in their community.

This research input provides a way of facilitating local key players to take an ongoing role in developing harm-reduction policies. It ensures that research effort is directed towards small scale, strategic research which is locally relevant. This approach contrasts with some previous research input into developing countries which has emphasised collection of descriptive data which are comparable across countries. This has usually measured consumption and experience of alcohol-related problems. This approach provides useful comparisons but may be at the expense of local relevance and timeliness, and may reduce the value of the training experience for local researchers and problem prevention actors.

There is also a need for research input from disciplines able to examine alcohol and drug issues from the perspective of economic and social development, since this is likely to feed into development of appropriate and feasible harm-reduction policy (Kortteinen, 1989; Swantz, 1990).

A need has also been recognised to promote research into global alcohol questions, particularly the import of alcohol beverages to developing countries (Maula, Linblad and Tigerstedt, 1990). The increasing globalisation of alcohol and tobacco promotion has also been recognised as a key issue and was in 1992 the subject of a recommendation from the WHO 28th Expert Committee on Drug Dependence. The Committee discussed ways of controlling international broadcast of health-relevant messages and included this topic among its recommendations. At the 8th World Conference on Tobacco or Health held in March 1992, the Papua New Guinea delegate expressed pleasure at the move to end Winfield sponsorship of the Australian rugby league competition as this is closely followed by a large percentage of the Papua New Guinean population.

The WHO Expert Committee on Drug Dependence, meeting in 1992, unlike its predecessors, included tobacco within its remit; this is perhaps an indication of increasing acceptance of the need for international organisations to focus attention and efforts on legal drugs which are commercially produced and marketed and which are responsible for considerable harm in both industrialised and developing countries.

Researchers from industrialised countries also have a role to play in assisting efforts to reduce drug-related harm which, as this chapter has suggested, is present in developing countries in the Pacific region, as elsewhere. For this outside assistance to provide maximum possible help, the research must be designed to facilitate change and to involve local players, both researchers and public health actors, in its design, implementation, analysis and dissemination. The policies appropriate to the cultural setting of developing countries may be somewhat different to those found appropriate in industrialised countries, and the research methodologies may also differ somewhat, but the potential value of research to assist the development and implementation of harm-reducing drug policies is probably universal.

References

Casswell, S. (1985). The alcohol industry in developing economies of Oceania. In J. Cavanagh, F. Clairmonte and R. Room (Eds), *The World Alcohol Industry with Special Reference to Australasia and Oceania*. University of Sydney: Transnational Corporations Research Project.

Casswell, S. (1986). *Alcohol in Oceania*. University of Auckland: Alcohol Research Unit.

Casswell, S. (1989). Alcohol-related casualties in Oceania. In N. Giesbrecht, R. Gonzalez, M. Grant, E. Osterberg, R. Room, I. Rootman and L. Towle (Eds), *Drinking and Casualties, Accidents, Poisonings and Violence in an International Perspective*. London: Tavistock/Routledge.

Cook, P.J. (1987). The impact of distilled-spirits taxes on consumption, auto fatalities and cirrhosis mortality. In H. Holder (Ed.), *Advances in Substance Abuse: Behavioural and Biological Research*. Suppl.1. Greenwich, Connecticut: JAI Press Inc.

Duignan, P. and Casswell, S. (1990). *A Report on the Workshop on the Prevention of Alcohol-related Injury in the Pacific Islands*. University of Auckland: Alcohol Research Unit.

Graham, H. (1989). Women and smoking in the United Kingdom: The implications for health promotion. *Health Promotion*, 3, 371–382.

Grossman, L. (1982). Beer drinking and subsistence production in a Highland village. In M. Marshall (Ed.), *Through a Glass Darkly: Beer and Modernization in Papua New Guinea*, Monograph 18. Boroko, Papua New Guinea: Institute of Applied Social and Economic Research.

Grossman, M. (1989). Health benefits of increases in alcohol and cigarette taxes. *British Journal of Addiction*, **84**, 1193–1204.

Grossman, M., Coate and D., Arluck, G. (1987). Price sensitivity of alcoholic beverages in the United States: Youth alcohol consumption. In H. Holder (Ed.), *Control Issues in Alcohol Abuse Prevention: Strategies for States and Communities*. Greenwich, Connecticut: JAI Press Inc.

Institute of Medicine. (1987). *Causes and consequences of alcohol problems: An agenda for research*. Report of a Study by a Committee of the Institute of Medicine, Division of Health Sciences Policy. Washington DC: National Academy Press.

Kawachi, I., Pearce, NE. and Jackson, RT. (1989). Deaths from lung cancer and ischaemic heart disease due to passive smoking in New Zealand. *The New Zealand Medical Journal*, **102**, 337–340.

Kendell, R.E., de Roumanie, M. and Ritson, E.B. (1983). Influence of an increase in excise duty on alcohol consumption and its adverse effects. *British Medical Journal*, **287**, 809–811

Kortteinen, T. (1989). *Agricultural Alcohol and Social Change in the Third World*. Helsinki, Finland: The Finnish Foundation for Alcohol Studies.

Kortteinen, T. (1990). Alcohol and urbanisation in Africa. In J. Maula, M. Lindblad, C. Tigerstedt (Eds), *Alcohol in Developing Countries: Proceedings from a Meeting in Oslo, Norway*. Helsinki, Finland: Nordic Council for Alcohol and Drug Research.

Laugesen, M. and Meads, C. (1991a). Advertising, price, income and publicity effects on weekly cigarette sales in New Zealand supermarkets. *British Journal of Addiction*, **86**, 83–89.

Laugesen, M.and Meads, C. (1991b). Tobacco advertising restrictions, price, income and tobacco consumption in OECD countries, 1960–1986. *British Journal of Addiction*, **86**, 1343–1354.

Lindstrom, M. (1982). Grog blong yumi: Alcohol and kava on Tanna, Vanuatu. In M. Marshall (Ed.), *Through a Glass Darkly: Beer and Modernization in Papua New Guinea*, Monograph 18. Boroko, Papua New Guinea: Institute of Applied Social and Economic Research.

Mahoney, F.B. (1974). *Social and Cultural Factors Relating to the Cause and Control of Alcohol Abuse Among Micronesian Youth*. Prepared for the Government of the Trust Territory under contract with James R. Leonard Assn. Inc., Trust Territory of the Pacific, Taipan.

Makela, K. and Viikari, M. (1977). Notes on alcohol and the state. *Acta Sociologica*, **20**, 155–179.

Marshall, M. (1979). *Weekend warriors: Alcohol in a Micronesian culture*. Palo Alto: Mayfield Publishing Co.

Marshall, M. (Ed.). (1982). *Through a Glass Darkly: Beer and Modernization in Papua New Guinea*. Monograph 18. Boroko, Papua New Guinea: Institute of Applied Social and Economic Research.

Marshall, M. (1983). Patterns of alcohol use in Port Moresby, Papua New Guinea: A quantity frequency survey. Paper presented to Symposium on Alcohol Use and Abuse: Meanings and Context, Vancouver.

Marshall, M. and Marshall, LB. (1990). *Silent Voices Speak: Women and Prohibition in Truk*. Belmont, California: Wadsworth Publishing Company.

Maula, J., Lindblad, M. and Tigerstedt., C. (Eds) (1990). *Alcohol in Developing Countries: Proceedings from a Meeting in Oslo, Norway*. Helsinki, Finland: Nordic Council for Alcohol and Drug Research.

McClintock, C. (1986). Toward a theory of formative program evaluation. *Evaluation Studies Review Annual*, 11, 205–223.

Millay, J.R. (1985). The wettest dry island in the Pacific: The prohibition experience in Truk. Paper prepared for the Alcohol Policies Symposium, International Congress on Anthropological and Ethnological Sciences, Zagreb, Yugoslavia.

Odejide, O.A, Ohaeri, J. U., Ikuesan, B.A. and Adeikan, M.L. (1990). A need for cross-cultural collaborative research activities: The promotion of alcohol research in Nigeria. In J. Maula, M. Lindblad and C. Tigerstedt, (Eds). *Alcohol in Developing Countries: Proceedings from a Meeting in Oslo, Norway*. Helsinki, Finland: Nordic Council for Alcohol and Drug Research.

O'Malley, P.M. and Wagenaar, A.C. (1991). Effects of minimum drinking age laws on alcohol use, related behaviours and traffic crash involvement among American youth: 1976–1987. *Journal of Studies on Alcohol*, 52, 478–491.

Osterberg, E. (1991). Current approaches to limit alcohol abuse and the negative consequences of use: A comparative overview of available options and an assessment of proven effectiveness. Expert meeting on the Negative Social Consequences of Alcohol Use, Oslo, 27–31 August, 1990.

Osterberg, E. and Saila, S.L. (Eds) (1991). *Natural Experiments with Decreased Availability of Alcoholic Beverages: Finnish Alcohol Strikes in 1972 and 1985*. Helsinki, Finland: The Finnish Foundation for Alcohol Studies.

Partanen, J. (1991). *Sociability and Intoxication: Alcohol and Drinking in Kenya, Africa and the Modern World*. Helsinki, Finland: The Finnish Foundation for Alcohol Studies.

Piau-Lynch, A. (1982). The Simbu liquor ban of 1980–1981. In M. Marshall, (Ed.), *Through a Glass Darkly: Beer and Modernization in Papua New Guinea*. Monograph 18. Boroko, Papua New Guinea: Institute of Applied Social and Economic Research.

Ringrose, H. and Zimmet, P. (1979). Nutrient intakes in an urbanised Micronesian population with a high diabetes prevalence. *American Journal of Clinical Nutrition*, 32, 1334–1341.

Roizen, J. (1982). Estimating alcohol involvement in serious events. *Alcohol Consumption and Related Problems*, 82, 179–219.

Sexton, LD. (1982). New beer in old bottles: An innovative community club and politics as usual in the Eastern Highlands. In M. Marshall (Ed.), *Through a Glass Darkly: Beer and Modernization in Papua New Guinea*. Monograph 18. Boroko, Papua New Guinea: Institute of Applied Social and Economic Research.

Sexton, LD. (1984). Social and economic impact of the colonial introduction of alcohol into Highland Papua New Guinea. Paper presented at the Conference on the Social History of Alcohol, Berkeley, CA, USA.

Sinha, E.H, Sengupta, S.K. and Ramesh, R.C. (1981). Five year review of deaths following trauma. *Papna New Guinea Medical Journal*, 24, 222–228.

Smart, R.G. (1991). World trends in alcohol consumption. *World Health Forum*, 12, 99–103.

Stansfield, S., Smith, G. and McGreevy, W. (1990). Injury and poisoning. In D. Jamison and W. Mosley (Eds), *Disease Control Priorities in Developing Countries*. The World Bank: Population, Health and Nutrition Division.

Stanton, H. (1990). Tobacco promotion in the Pacific Islands: An exploitation of human addiction. In B. Durston and K. Jamrozik (Eds), *The Global War: Proceedings of the Seventh World Conference on Tobacco and Health*. Perth, Australia: Health Department of Western Australia.

Suryani, LK., Adnyana, T. and Jensen, G. (1990). Palm wine drinking in a Balinese village: Environmental influences. *The International Journal of the Addictions*, **25**, 911–920.

Swantz, M. (1990). Alcohol research in developing societies from the point of view of development studies. In J. Maula, M. Lindblad and C. Tigerstedt (Eds), *Alcohol in Developing Countries: Proceedings from a Meeting in Oslo, Norway*. Helsinki, Finland: Nordic Council for Alcohol and Drug Research.

Taylor, R., Lewis, N. and Levy, S. (1989). Societies in transition: Mortality patterns in Pacific Island populations. *International Journal of Epidemiology*, **18**, 634–646.

Townsend, D. (1977). The 1976 coffee boom in Papua New Guinea. *Australian Geographer*, **13**, 419–422.

United States Public Health Service. (1986). *The Health Consequences of Involuntary Smoking: A Report of the Surgeon General*. Rockville, MD: Department of Human and Health Services.

Walter, M. (1982). Drink and be merry for tomorrow we preach: Alcohol and the male menopause in Fiji. In M. Marshall (Ed.), *Through a Glass Darkly: Beer and Modernization in Papua New Guinea*. Monograph 18. Boroko, Papua New Guinea: Institute of Applied Social and Economic Research.

Warry, W. (1982). Bia and bisnis: The use of beer in Chuave ceremonies. In M. Marshall Ed.), *Through a glass darkly: beer and modernization in Papua New Guinea*. Monograph 18. Boroko, Papua New Guinea: Institute of Applied Social and Economic Research.

Wette, H., Zhang, J.F., Berg, R.J. and Casswell, S. (1992). The effects of taxes on alcohol consumption, New Zealand 1983–1991. *Drug and Alcohol Review*, in press.

Chapter 21
An Evolving Public Health Crisis: HIV Infection Among Injecting Drug Users in Developing Countries

ALEX WODAK, ROBERT FISHER and NICK CROFTS

Injecting drug use is now known to exist in over 80 countries. Human immunodeficiency virus (HIV) infection among injecting drug users (IDUs) is recognised to be a problem in over 50 of these countries (Stimson, 1992). HIV infection in IDUs is being reported from an increasing number of countries and also continues to spread, albeit more slowly in recent years, within countries where it was first reported several years ago. The rapid spread of HIV infection amoung populations of IDUs in less developed countries (LDCs) in recent years has been one of the most ominous and unjustly neglected developments in the history of illicit drug use. Drug injecting with frequent needle sharing, the common use of prostitutes, an important 'male oriented' tourist industry, ignorance of the risk of HIV infection associated with injecting drug use (IDU), mobile populations and the merging of these characteristics within populations of IDUs are all factors known to influence the rapidity of spread of HIV infection.

The first LDC found to have a major epidemic of HIV among IDUs was Thailand. HIV infection spread extremely rapidly among injecting drug users in Thailand during the mid 1980s shortly after the first 'official' case was reported in 1984 (Smith, 1990). However, for various reasons, the Thai Government did not begin to respond to the problem until 1986–1987. The association of an epidemic of HIV with IDUs was already well known at that time but had only been reported from developed countries in Europe and North America (Carballo and Rezza, 1990).

The combination of IDU and LDCs involves other regions and periods of history. It appears that heroin began to move across south west China in the early 1980s (Fisher, 1991; Fisher, Ch'ien and Kittelsen, 1991). When HIV testing began in China in 1986, many infected individuals, generally IDUs, were soon detected. In October 1989, 12.5% of 1167 IDUs tested in China were reported to be infected with HIV

(Li and Yeogh, 1992). During the early 1980s, evidence began to appear of HIV infection in IDUs in the northern reaches of Malaysia bordering on southern Thailand (Edstrom, unpublished data). In 1990, HIV prevalence in IDUs increased rapidly in Myanmar (Burma) with positive tests confirmed in 63% of 701 individuals tested (Li and Yeogh, 1992). In 1990 54% of 1564 IDUs in the states of Manipur and Mizoram in north eastern India were also found to have been infected (Li and Yeogh, 1992).

By the early 1990s, the HIV epidemic had also spread to involve IDUs in LDCs in central and South America, including Honduras, the Dominican Republic, Brazil, Argentina, Venezuela, Chile and Paraguay. Documentation of IDU in Egypt extends back to the 1920s (Biggam, 1929). Some recent reports have appeared of IDU in Nigeria, Senegal, South Africa and Tunisia, with earlier reports indicating heroin use in Mauritius (Stimson, 1992). Although the risk of HIV associated with IDU in other developing countries is still uncertain, it is likely that a substantial proportion of the IDU population in other developing countries will sooner or later become infected (Senay, 1991; World Health Organization, 1991).

The concept of harm reduction has proved to be an important component of public health efforts to control the spread of HIV among IDUs in a number of developed countries. In this chapter, we review the possible relevance for developing countries of harm-reduction activities intended to reduce the spread of HIV in IDUs.

The Gathering Storm

The estimated annual global production of opium increased 9% in 1991 to reach 3785 metric tons. Seventy per cent of global production was in the 'Golden Triangle' in south-east Asia, 28% in the 'Golden Crescent' in south-west Asia and the remaining 1–2% in South America (Bureau of International Narcotics Matters, 1992). It is now known that substantial populations of IDUs exist in the Golden Triangle, particularly in Thailand and Myanmar. Although there is limited information available about the use of opium or its derivatives within Laos, it is unlikely that a sizeable population of IDUs exists in that country (Bureau of International Narcotics Matters, 1992).

In the period following the Second World War, opium produced in the Golden Triangle was usually destined for export. It was refined in laboratories in Bangkok, Hong Kong or Marseille to morphine and then further processed to heroin. Within the Golden Triangle countries, opium was generally consumed unrefined and heroin was unavailable locally until the 1960s. Within the last two decades, increased enforcement pressures on the laboratories outside the Golden Triangle has led to their closure. At the same time, improvements in laboratory techniques and the availability of cheap production chemicals have enabled heroin refinement laboratories to be moved closer to the opium fields. This relocation allowed a major reduction in refinement costs and decreased the chance of detection since heroin takes up less volume and is easier to hide than its parent opium. As a result, abundant and cheap heroin became available for the first time in the small towns and villages of the south-east Asian countries. Initially only the less pure grade IV heroin, which is usually smoked, was available. Recently, availability of the more expensive and potent grade III heroin has exceeded that of grade IV heroin.

Grade III heroin can be smoked or injected and is mainly consumed by young men using medical syringes or makeshift instruments to inject the drug. Social controls, which originally had restricted the consumption of opium to elderly men and occasionally elderly women within opium dens, and then to younger men, began unravelling rapidly. During the transition to injecting, young men who almost invariably first smoked tobacco began smoking heroin; they might then begin their injecting career by being 'fixed' by a friend or attending a 'professional injector' who had appropriate equipment and expertise. The advantages for the user of fixing at a specific 'common' house are significant; he (or less commonly, she) does not have to carry injection equipment around which can be a serious criminal offence in some developing countries; he can also avoid having to carry the drug itself. The disadvantages, however, are considerable. These facilities are equivalent to the 'shooting galleries' found in inner city areas of some developed countries, which have so efficiently disseminated HIV, HTLV-II and hepatitis viruses.

Until recent times, the heroin from production countries in south-east Asia principally made its way to the outside world by transit through Bangkok. This became more difficult in the mid to late 1980s when the (then) Burmese military began cracking down on dissident ethnic groups. These groups were known to generate income, later used to fund the purchase of guns, by transporting opium and heroin. Further, the cost of the corruption of public officials, usually associated with the large scale transport of illicit commodities, increased significantly. The economics of the heroin trade resemble that of any other coveted commodity. Such a valuable product soon found alternative ways of reaching the lucrative markets of the western world. Heroin began to find its way overland from important opium and heroin production areas not controlled by the government in south-east Myanmar, across the border into Yunnan Province of China, and thence to Hong Kong (Lindner, 1990; Fisher, 1991; Fisher, Ch'ien and Kittelsen, 1991). Hong Kong has a significant population of IDUs as well as serving as a major trans-shipment port to the Philippines and eventually Australia and North America. Another major route opened

into the north-eastern states of India. Some heroin, of course, continued to be sent to Bangkok and some made its way into Malaysia and
Singapore to supply local consumers. Severe penalties and vigorous
law enforcement seem to have confined IDU to relatively few individuals in Singapore; however, generalizing from the experience of this
unique and tightly controlled island state to other countries is probably
of doubtful value.

Heroin traffickers are constantly searching for new, safer and thus
more cost-effective ways to ship their goods. To evade detection, heroin
destined for developed and thus more profitable countries has also
been sent by courier to transit through ports not generally associated
with the international drug trade. Lagos (Nigeria) is probably the best
known of such ports. In the Pacific, Noumea (New Caledonia), Nadi
(Fiji), the Solomon Islands, Manila (the Philippines) and Colombo (Sri
Lanka) are some of the many ports which have been used for this purpose. Just as illicit drug profits are 'laundered' to reduce the possibility
of detection, drugs are often shipped to neutral ports to mask their origin and evade detection. However, countries through which large
quantities of intravenous illicit drugs transit are themselves at risk if
indigenous populations begin to use the drugs, as they almost invariably do. Local transit markets are then created which also helps smooth
out the uncertainties associated with more distant destinations. Some
contries, such as Malaysia, have introduced severe penalties to deter
the local population from experimenting with drugs known to be transiting through their ports, although the effectiveness of these measures
is unknown (Antidadah Task Force, 1991; Scorzelli, 1992). It is exceedingly difficult to establish whether stringent enforcement of prohibition
laws decreases the likelihood of experimentation, as is usually presumed, or whether it inadvertently increases the risk because of the
sizeable economic incentives introduced. However, recent developments in Asia would suggest that, while law enforcement is able to disrupt stable trade routes of drugs for injecting, this merely exposes
larger populations to the hazard of HIV infection associated with needle sharing as new trade routes open when older routes become too
dangerous.

Heroin produced in south-west Asia mainly supplies the European
market. The number of persons using heroin in Pakistan grew dramatically in the 1980s, and has been estimated to have reached 1.2–1.7 million heroin addicts (Bureau of International Narcotic Matters, 1992)
with an apparently increasing proportion mainly injecting the drug.
There is now a large population of IDUs in India and Nepal. The injection of cocaine in some South American countries is also a new development. Although opium had not been cultivated in South America
before, in 1991 opium from Colombia began to reach the United States
of America for the first time (Bureau of International Narcotic Matters,

1992; Anonymous, 1992). This trade is estimated to be ten times more lucrative for traffickers than cocaine. It is difficult to predict which developing countries are now most at risk for HIV through the sharing of injection equipment as the cultivation, production, transit and mode of administration of illicit, potentially injectable drugs is very unstable. What is more certain is that a proportion of the at-risk populations in countries where drugs are available will continue to seek psychoactive drugs as an alternative to an often depressing reality. As populations in LDCs gain more financial resources to purchase drugs, consumption of psychoactive substances may increase.

Alternatively, declining national income and rising indebtedness of developing countries may increase the need to generate income and increase the likelihood of illicit drug cultivation, production, trafficking or consumption. Medical problems including HIV, hepatitis and a variety of other disorders and social problems, such as family break-up and violence, are likely to soon follow any increase in drug injection (Bewley, Ben-Aire and James, 1968; Plat, 1986; Perucci et al., 1991; Selwyn, 1991). Apart from a lack of money to purchase illicit drugs, the Philippines has all of the necessary social ingredients for a major heroin problem, including easy access to transiting heroin. Most Filipinos however cannot affort heroin so it simply passes through local ports destined for developed countries with more lucrative markets.

Potential Consequences

That IDUs are important vectors for the HIV was acknowledged early in the epidemic, first in North America and later in Europe (Gossop, 1987; Des Jarlais, Friedman and Stoneburner, 1988; Lange et al., 1988; Miller, Turner and Moses, 1990). In both Europe and North America, spread of HIV to populations of IDUs was followed within a few years by the rapid spread of the epidemic to non-drug using heterosexuals (Homes, Karon and Kreis, 1990; Miller, Turner and Moses, 1990). Substantial numbers of HIV-infected children born to drug using parents soon began to present or be detected in screening programmes. In New York City in 1988, IDUs were the source of HIV infection for more than 90% of the heterosexual transmission cases of AIDS and more than 80% of the maternal transmission cases (Des Jarlais, Friedman and Casriel, 1990). AIDS may then indeed be accurately portrayed as a 'family' disease (Sherer, 1990).

The spread of HIV infection to prostitutes became evident in Thailand within one year of the epidemic spreading through the IDU population; the following year, spread of HIV infection to the non-drug using heterosexual population was apparent (Weniger et al., 1991). In Thailand and Myanmar, rapid spread through the population was facilitated by sexual transmission and widespread prostitution (Edstrom, 1989; Smith, 1990). In any developing country where high risk sexual and drug use behaviours converge in populations who are poorly informed about the risks of HIV, as occurred in Thailand and Myanmar, the probability of extremely rapid spread of HIV must be a major concern.

Special Features of HIV among IDUs in Developing Countries

The epidemic of HIV infection in IDUs that is proceeding in a number of LDCs has potentially far-reaching ramifications. Developing countries have fewer resources than developed countries to meet greater needs. Health is invariably not a high priority for public expenditure. Due to the general impoverishment of LDCs, reflected in poor nutrition and basic health care, inadequate transportation and over-crowded housing, any threat to public health is therefore of even greater significance than in developed countries. For example, in many developing countries a number of diseases such as tuberculosis, leprosy and malaria have only recently come under control or are still only beginning to come under control. A poorly controlled epidemic of HIV threatens many recent, hard-won public health gains, including control of tuberculosis.

The long term control of HIV infection for the general community in many countries depends on the effectiveness of efforts to control the spread of HIV among IDUs; this in turn depends on the success of efforts to restrict the proportion exposed to the risk of HIV infection from sharing of injection equipment. As prevalence of HIV rises amoung IDUs, unprotected sexual intercourse contributes increasingly to spread of infection among and from IDUs.

In many developing countries, those most affected by HIV early in the epidemic have been the well-educated, well-travelled occupiers of senior positions of authority who represent just the populations developing countries can least affort to lose. In addition, the police and military have been severely affected by HIV in many less developed African countries. Infection and illness affecting the police or military could possibly have serious implications for the stability of these countries. In LDCs in Asia, the spread of HIV to involve both female and male prostitutes could also damage the tourism industry. Many of these countries rely on the tourism industry for precious foreign exchange. Since a substantial proportion of the customers of the prostitutes come from other countries, their international movements after becoming infected will also contribute to rapid contagion.

Most developed countries have known about their populations of IDUs for many decades. During this time, significant clinical and policy expertise has been acquired in health and other public sectors, even though a comprehensive understanding of drug use has not yet developed. When it was evident in industrialised countries that HIV placed IDU populations at particular risk, this expertise could then be harnessed in efforts to control the epidemic. In contrast, few developing countries were either aware of the full extent of their IDU populations before the epidemic or had implemented appropriate drug prevention and treatment programmes. Their public health response to HIV therefore originated from a significantly less advanced position.

In all developed countries where HIV infection has spread to populations of IDUs, the preferred drug for injection has been heroin. This is also true for south-east Asian developing countries gripped or threatened by the epidemic. In Brazil and Argentina, the preferred drug of injection is cocaine, presumably reflecting proximity to the Andean source of the drug. Methadone maintenance treatment has been recognised to slow the spread of HIV infection, probably by reducing the frequency of injections. However, methadone maintenance treatment may be unaffordable for many developing countries and will be of little value in countries where cocaine is the most commonly injected drug.

Most developed countries with substantial populations of IDUs were able to divert some of their resources previously allocated for the treatment of drug users to specific efforts to control the HIV epidemic, while also strengthening their drug prevention and treatment programmes. Attempts to estimate the size and characteristics of the IDU population in developed contries have often been valuable in planning prevention strategies, clinical interventions and anticipated health service requirements.

The rapid and often major changes in policy emphasis required to control the epidemic have frequently encountered strong opposition arising from philosophical and moral values. Gaining support in time for implementation of sensitive, but critical, prevention strategies has proved difficult to achieve even in some developed countries such as the United States of America. Introducing sensitive but critical prevention strategies is generally even more difficult to achieve in developing countries as traditional and religious values are often woven more tightly into government policy. Moveover, the media are less extensive and more fettered, and thus information available to the public is usually more limited.

The effectiveness of education in the prevention of illicit drug use, particularly IDU, remains contentious. To the extent that lack of correct knowledge is the missing component in the process of deciding whether or not to take or inject drugs, education may be sufficient. However, euphorogenic drug use is one of the most potent psychological reinforcers known and knowledge about a drug is rarely adequate as a prevention strategy (Sorensen et al., 1991). Indeed, a number of studies have shown that knowledge about the dangers of IDU or awareness of HIV serostatus has little impact on the initiation of drug use (Des Jarlais, Friedman and Casreil, 1990) or a substantial reduction of high risk injecting or sexual behaviours (O'Conner and Stafford-Johnson, 1987; Baxter and Schlecht, 1990; Klee et al., 1990a; Memon, 1990; Cleary et al., 1991; McCaig, Hardy and Winn, 1991; Calsyn et al., 1992; Van den Hoek, van Haastrecht and Coutinho, 1992). Educational campaigns are often insentitive to the social and cultural factors that contribute to the initiation of illicit drug use in the first place and whose recognition is absolutely indispensable to successful primary prevention in the particular society.

However, an increasing number of studies suggest that, as more is learned about HIV and IDUs, as target populations are more precisely identified and strategies developed that reflect both a better understanding of high-risk behaviour and media capabilities, education is becoming more effective (Catania, Kegeles and Coates, 1990; Dryfoos, 1990; Alcohol, Drug Abuse and Mental Health Administration, 1991; Leukefeld and Bukoski, 1991). As emphasised elsewhere by Des Jarlais and Friedman (see Chapter 22), early dissemination by both official and unofficial sources of information about the hazards of HIV/AIDS and especially about the risks of sharing injection equipment has probably altered the course of the epidemic. The epidemic preceded dissemination of this information in San Francisco, New York City, and some cities in Scotland, Italy and Spain, but IDU populations in most developed countries had the benefit of early warning. In contrast, HIV had already infected many IDUs in Thailand, Myanmar, Malaysia and China (Yunnan) before they were aware of the dangers of sharing injection equipment.

Mass campaigns of the past have been supplanted recently in many developed countries by more costly but also more targeted and possibly more effective educational interventions. Also, successful campaigns have been carefully explicit without offending important sectors of the population. As with the general population, education of the IDUs is far more difficult to achieve in developing countries. Mass media reach a far smaller section of the population in LDCs, although radio has been used effectively where sets are affordable and can be made available. Posters and pamphlets are produced in abundance in developed countries despite a general lack of evidence of effectiveness. For LDCs, production and distribution of posters and pamphlets is much more problematic. Also, printed matter is probably less effective in developing countries as IDUs are far more likely to be illiterate. Acquiring the essentials for daily living understandably receives a higher priority in LDCs than concerns about preventing a socially abhorrent disease that only affects a none too popular population. Authorities in developing countries are also far more likely to be cautious about offending conservative forces; treading the fine line between disseminating information essential to allow people to protect themselves from HIV infection without appearing to condone an illegal and usually highly disapproved practice is even more difficult in traditional communities.

Distribution of sterile injection equipment to IDUs has been one of the most commonly adopted approaches to HIV prevention in developed countries attempting to respond vigorously to this major threat to public health. In many developing countries, there are insufficient supplies of injection equipment for routine medical uses. Before needles and syringes can be re-used, they must be sterilised. This requires a reliable source of electricity to operate sterilising apparatus. Reliable electricity supplies are rarely a feature of life in developing countries. Developing countries thus face agonising choices. For example, should a government in a developing country decide to divert sterile needles and syringes previously reserved for treating patients with, for example, tuberculosis to try to prevent the potential threat of an epidemic? This is even harder to justify when the epidemic is only known to occur in some far off countries. Also, if needles and syringes were to suddenly become freely available in a developing country where heroin or cocaine is cheap and abundant, how could authorities persuade themselves that administration by injection would not eventually become more common and replace self-administration by smoking and snorting?

The provision of a drug of addicition to addicted persons as a legal therapeutic exercise still causes considerable discomfort in many developed countries. In most developing countries, substitution therapy is often regarded with even greater suspicion. Stringent enforcement of the law reflects cultural mores that drug addiction is more a crime than an illness; culturally syntonic traditional (and religious) forms of treatment of IDUs are more readily supported by the community and political circles. Although the cost of pharmaceutical methadone, approximating US$150 per person per year, might be considered insignificant in a developed country, this is a not inconsiderable cost for a developing country where the mean annual income may be only a few times larger.

Methadone maintenance has been well accepted in Hong Kong for more than ten years. Following the explosive spread of HIV in Thailand, authorities in that country extended the use of methadone from brief detoxification to maintenance with little apparent opposition. Therefore, the possibility remains that other developing countries might adopt either methadone maintenance or local variants based on cheaper oral forms of opium which are readily available in some of the LDCs surrounding opium production regions.

What Should Be Done?

Psychoactive drug use is an extraordinarily complex phenomenon. It involves some of the most primitive and profound of human appetites and frailties. Unless correct decisions are made soon and implemented skilfully and vigorously, the future of large populations living in developing and developed countries could be adversely affected for generations. The first step involves recognition that 'changing high risk behaviours is the only means of preventing transmission of the HIV' (Catania, Kegeles and Coates, 1990). There are no panaceas. Solutions found to be effective in one country do not necessarily apply in another country with very different conditions. Most experience in controlling the epidemic of HIV was initially gained in developed countries which were the first to be affected. Extrapolating from the special conditions which apply in many developed countries is unwise. Compared to LDCs, more developed countries are some distance from the major opium and cocaine production areas, family structures and cultural mores in some of their sub-populations are often significantly weakened, and financial resources are more available.

Social changes required to respond adequately and sufficiently quickly to the threat of HIV in a society can only proceed at a pace determined by the readiness of that community to accept change. Until recently, with some minor exceptions, illicit drug use in LDCs has usually involved types of drugs consumed without injection. The risk of rapid spread of injecting and the serious consequences associated with parenteral drug use were relatively limited. However, unlike any previous historical period, the public health repercussions of the current HIV epidemic involving IDUs do not allow the luxury of time.

There is compelling evidence to suggest that persons engaged in one high risk behaviour are more likely to be engaged in other risky behaviours; people who self-administer illicit psychoactive drugs are likely to share syringes and needles as well as engage in unprotected sexual activities (Coates, 1990; Klee et al., 1990b; Nemoto et al., 1990; McCaig, Hardy and Winn, 1991; Van der Hoek, van Haasbrecht and Coutinho, 1992). Both psychoactive drug use and sex, as powerfully reinforcing behaviours, may 'cross-over' in behavioural reinforcement so that treatment becomes much more difficult (Plant et al., 1989; Sorenson et al., 1991).

It is vital, especially for LDCs, that prevention research is undertaken urgently and leads to more effective methods of reducing and delaying the initiation of drug injecting (Leukefeld and Burkowki, 1991). Improved methods of inexpensively acquiring epidemiological and socio-demographic information are needed so that the nature and extent of drug use in each country and its exposure to the risk of HIV can be forecast (Gossop and Grant, 1990; Allen, Onorato and Green,

1992; Hartwall, 1992; Working Group on Demand Reduction Regarding Drug Abuse in Europe, 1991). It is also important that countries with an established population of IDUs and countries threatened by this development determine the factors within their own sub-populations that exacerbate drug use and HIV transmission, and the factors that may assist in effective prevention (Cheung, 1990; Klee et al., 1990b; Alcohol, Drug Abuse and Mental Health Administration, 1991). Identifying high-risk groups and directing major interventions to these persons is a cost-effective approach to conserving often scarce resources.

Prevention and treatment strategies should accurately reflect the magnitude of potential problems but also be in sympathy with the social, cultural, religious and philosophical characteristics of the community they are intended to protect. Educational modalities that have been demonstrated to be effective transcend the mere distribution of information and adopt multi-modal approaches. These interventions should be meaningful not only throughout society, but also throughout a person's life-time. They may be more effective if based on and within powerful social institutions (such as the family, church or even peer group) (Coates, 1990; Miller, Turner and Moses, 1990; Alcohol, Drug Abuse and Mental Health Administration, 1991; Grund, Kaplan and Adriaans, 1991; Sorensen et al., 1991).

Readily available and effective treatment must be a critical component of a national illicit (and licit) drug problems prevention strategy (Hubbard et al., 1988; Cates and Bowen, 1989; Brettle, 1991; Miller, Turner and Moses, 1990; Working Group on Demand Reduction Regarding Drug Abuse in Europe, 1991; Allen, Onorato and Green, 1992). To reduce problems resulting from drug use and minimise the spread of HIV, effective drug treatment programmes which are attractive to the target population should be readily available to all who seek help. Policies which dictate that the identity of all persons undergoing treatment for drug-related problems must be entered in a national register, reduce the attractiveness of treatment to illicit drug users and thus hinder efforts to minimise the spread of HIV.

In essence, all prevention and treatment efforts attempt to be 'harm reducing'. Some proceed on the assumption that decreasing drug use will result in fewer problems whereas others assume that a reduction in drug consumption for some individuals or societies is unachievable, at least in the short term. It is argued therefore that efforts should be directed specifically to minimising harm without requiring a prior reduction in consumption. The current use of the term 'harm reduction', however, acknowledges the fact that the harm that individuals do to themselves (and others) lies on a continuum. Some disorders are far more serious than others; HIV infection clearly represents the most serious potential complication of IDU both for individuals and the community they live in. Health workers may find themselves drawn into participating with aspects of drug use which engender considerable discomfort, such as providing sterile needles and syringes to drug dealers, to reduce the damage that IDU can cause to individuals and societies. They do so fully recognising that injection of unknown quantities of preparations of unknown concentration and purity is always inadvisable. But without an alternative intervention, such behaviour could result in even more unhealthy behaviours (Strang, 1988).

Considerations of this kind form the basis of drug substitution programmes such as methadone maintenance, and needle and syringe cleansing and exchange programmes to prevent the spread of the HIV. Although such programmes appear to contribute to a reduction in high risk behaviours (Ingold and Ingold, 1989; Klee et al., 1991), single approaches are generally considered to be inadequate. Drug users have often been injecting drugs for a number of years before seeking any form of assistance (Oppenheimer, Sheehan and Taylor, 1988; Stimson et al., 1988; McKeganey and Watson, 1989). If the treatment provided is attractive, demand usually outstrips supply. Rehabilitation efforts must therefore be combined with a variety of other approaches.

Attempts to restrict illicit drug supplies have generally been costly, associated with substantial unintended negative consequences and rarely providing any significant and sustained reduction in illicit drug problems. However, when the demand for drugs is low, detection is difficult to evade and substitutes are not readily available, restricting drug supplies can be effective in reducing drug problems. This suggests that supply reduction will only become a successful harm-reduction strategy when effective demand-reduction methods have been identified.

In essence, harm reduction, shorn of its 'drug' trimmings, is nothing more than pragmatism. Most societies practice pragmatism, albeit in very different forms. A senior leader of the largest country in Asia is fond of quoting a saying that it does not matter whether a cat is black or white as long as it still catches mice. The challenge facing national and international health policy-makers now is how to adapt national traditions of pragmatism to the protection of public health. Terms such as 'harm reduction' presumably sound quite alien to more traditional audiences, yet local variants of the same spirit of pragmatism probably exist within many cultures and could be readily exploited to control this most dangerous of epidemics.

References

Alcohol, Drug Abuse and Mental Health Administration (DHHS) (1991). *Preventing Adolescent Drug Use: From Theory to Practice*. Washington DC: OSAP Prevention Monograph 8.

Allen, D.M., Onorato, I.M. and Green, T.A. (1992). HIV infection in intravenous drug users entering drug Treatment, United States, 1988 to 1989. *American*

Journal of Public Health, **82**, 541–6.

Anonymous (1992). Next heroin. *The Economist*, May 2, 47.

Antidadah Task Force (National Security Council, Prime Minister's Department) (1991). *Narcotics Report, 1991*. Malaysia: Task Force.

Baxter, D.N. and Schlecht, B. (1990). Patterns of behaviour amongst injecting drug users: Implications for HIV. *Public Health*, **104**, 321–325.

Bewley, T.H., Ben-Aire, O. and James, I.P. (1968). Morbidity and mortality from heroin dependence. I. Survey of heroin addicts known to Home Office. *British Medical Journal*, **1**, 725–726.

Biggam, A.G. (1929). Malignant malaria asociated with the administration of heroin intravenously. *Transactions of The Royal Society of Tropical Medicine and Hygiene*, **23**, 147–153.

Brettle, R.P. (1991). HIV and harm reduction for injection drug users. *AIDS*, **5**, 125–36.

Bureau of International Narcotics Matters (US Department of State) (1992). *International Narcotics Control Strategy Report*. Washington DC.

Calsyn, D.A., Saxon, A.J., Freeman, G. and Whittaker, S. (1992). Ineffectiveness of AIDS education and HIV antibody testing in reducing high risk behaviours among injection drug users. *American Journal of Public Health*, **82**, 573–5.

Carballo, M. and Rezza, G. (1990). AIDS, drug misuse and the global crisis. In J. Strang and G. Stimson (Eds), *AIDS and Drug Misuse: The Challenge for Policy and Practice in the 1990s*. London: Routledge.

Catania, J.A., Kegeles, S.M. and Coates, T.J. (1990). Towards an understanding of risk behaviour: An AIDS Risk Reduction Model (ARRM). *Health Education Quarterly* (Spring), **17**, 53–72.

Cates, W. and Bowen, G.S. (1989). Education for AIDS prevention: Not our only voluntary weapon. *American Journal of Public Health*, **79**, 871–874.

Cheung, Y.W. (1990–91). Overview: Sharpening the focus on ethnicity. *International Journal of the Addictions*, **25**, 573–579.

Cleary, P.D., Van De Vanter, N., Rogers, T.F., Singer, E., Shipton-Levy, R., Steilen, M., Stuart, J. and Pindyck, J. (1991). Behaviour changes after notification of HIV infection. *American Journal of Public Health*, **81**, 1586–1590.

Coates, T.J. (1990). Strategies for modifying sexual behavior for primary and secondary prevention of HIV disease. *Journal of Consulting and Clinical Psychology*, **58**, 57–69.

Des Jarlais, D.C., Friedman, S.R. and Stoneburner, R.L. (1988). HIV infection and intravenous drug use: Critical issues in transmission dynamics, infection, outcomes and prevention. *Review of Infectious Diseases*, **10**, 151–158.

Des Jarlais, D.C., Friedman, S.R. and Carriel, C. (1990). Target groups for preventing AIDS among intravenous drug users: 2. The hard data studies. *Journal of Consulting and Clinical Psychology*, **58**, 50–56.

Dryfoos, J. (1990). *Adolescents at Risk: Prevalence and Prevention*. New York: Oxford University Press.

Fisher, R.B. (1991). *Prevention and Control of Drug Dependence (People's Republic of China). Mission Report (revised)*. Manila: World Health Organization.

Fisher, R.B., Ch'ien, J.M.N. and Kittelsen, J. (1991). *Prevalence and Control of Drug Dependence (People's Republic of China). Mission Report*. Manila: World Health Organization.

Gossop, M. (1987). *Living with Drugs*, pp. 156–159. Aldershot: Wildwood House.

Gossop, M. and Grant, M. (Eds) (1990). *Preventing and Controlling Drug Abuse*. Geneva: World Health Organization.

Grund, J.C., Kaplan, C.D. and Adriaans, N.F.P. (1991). Needle sharing in the Netherlands: An ethnographic analysis. *Americal Journal of Public Health*, **18**, 1602–1607.

Hartwall, R. (1992). Epidemiological approaches to drug misuse in Britain. *Journal of Addictive Diseases*, **11**, 37–45.

Homes, U.K., Karon, J.M. and Kreiss, J. (1990). The increasing frequency of heterosexually acquired AIDS in the United States, 1983–88. *American Journal of Public Health*, **80**, 58–63.

Hubbard, R.L., Marsden, M.E., Cavanaugh, E., Rachal, J.V. and Ginsburg, H.M. (1988). Role of drug-abuse treatment in limiting the spread of AIDS. *Review of Infectious Diseases*, **10**, 377–84.

Ingold, F.R. and Ingold, S. (1989). The effects of the liberalization of syringe sales on the behaviour of intravenous drug users in France. *Bulletin on Narcotics*, **XLI**, 67–81.

Klee, H. Faugier, J., Hayes, C., Boulton, T. and Morris, J. (1990a). Sexual partners of injecting drug users: The risk of HIV infection. *British Journal of Addiction*, **85**, 413–418.

Klee, H., Faugier, J., Hayes, C., Boulton, T. and Morris, J. (1990b). Factors associated with risk behaviours among injecting drug users. *AIDS Care*, **2**, 133–145.

Klee, H., Faugier, J., Hayes, C. and Morris, J. (1991). The sharing of injecting equipment among drug users attending prescribing clinics and those using needle-exchanges. *British Journal of Addiction*, **86**, 217–223.

Lange, R.W., Snyder, F.R., Lozovsky, O., Kaistha, V., Kaczanluk, M.A. and Jaffe, J.J. (1988). Geographic distribution of human immunodeficiency virus markers in parenteral drug abusers. *American Journal of Public Health*, **78**, 443–446.

Leukefeld, C.G. and Bukoski, W.J. (1991). Drug abuse prevention evaluation methodology: A bright future. *Journal of Drug Education*, *21*, 191–201.

Leukefeld, C.G. and Burkowki, W.J. (Eds) (1991). *Drug abuse prevention intervention research: Methodological issues*. NIDA Research Monograph 107. Washington DC: Alcohol, Drug Abuse and Mental Health Administration (DHHS).

Li, E.K.Y. and Yeogh, E.Y. (1992). Current epidemiological trends of HIV infection in Asia. In P. Volberding and M.A. Jacobson (Eds) *AIDS Clinical Review*. New York: Marcel Decker, Inc.

Lindner, B. (1990). Roads from Mandalay. *Far Eastern Economic Review*, June 18, 27.

McCaig, L.F., Hardy, A.M. and Winn, D.M. (1991). Knowledge about AIDS and HIV in the US adult population: Influence of the local incidence of AIDS. *American Journal of Public Health*, **81**, 1591–1595.

McKeganey, B.M. and Watson, H. (1989). HIV-related behaviours among a non-clinical sample of injecting drug users. *British Journal of Addiction*, **84**, 1481–1490.

Memon, A. (1990). Young people's knowledge, beliefs and attitudes about HIV/AIDS: A review of research. *Health Education Research, Theory and Practice*, **5**, 327–335.

Miller H.G., Turner, C.F. and Moses, L.E. (Eds) (1990). *AIDS: The Second Decade*. Washington DC: National Academy Press.

Nemoto, R. Brown, L.S. Jr, Fostor, K. and Chu, A. (1990). Behavioural risk factors of human immunodeficiency virus infection among intravenous drug users and implications for preventive interventions. *AIDS Education and Prevention*, **2**, 116–26.

O'Conner, J.J. and Stafford-Johnson, S. (1987). AIDS and intravenous drug abuse (Letter). *British Journal of Addiction*, **82**, 813.

Oppenheimer, E., Sheehan, M. and Taylor, C. (1988). Letting the client speak: Drug misusers and the process of help seeking. *British Journal of Addiction*, **83**, 635–648.

Peucci, C.A., Davoli, M., Rapitie, E., Abeni, D.D. and Forastiere, F. (1991). Mortality of intravenous drug users in Rome: A cohort study. *American Journal of Public Health*, **81**, 1307–1310.

Plant, M.L., Plant, M.A., Peck, D.F., Setter, B.A. and Setter J. (1989). The sex industry, alcohol and illicit drugs: Implications for the spread of HIV infection. *British Journal of Addiction*, **84**, 53–59.

Plat, J.J. (1986). *Heroin Addiction: Theory, Research and Treatment*, 2nd edn. Malabar, Florida: Robert E. Kreiger:

Scorzelli, R. (1992). Has Malaysia's anti-drug effort been effective? *Journal of Substance Abuse Treatment*, **9**, 171–176.

Selwyn, P. (1991). Injection drug use, mortality and the AIDS epidemic. *American Journal of Public Health*, **81**, 1247–1249.

Senayl E.C. (1991). Drug abuse and public health: A global perspective. Drug Safety, **6**, 1–15.

Sherer, R. (1990). AIDS policy in the 1990s (editorial). *Journal of the American Medical Association*, **263**, 1982–1984.

Smith, D.G. (1990). Thailand: AIDS crisis looms. *The Lancet*, **355**, 781–782.

Sorensen, J.L., Wermuth, L.A., Gibson, D.R., Choi, K-H., Juydish, J.R. and Batki, S.L. (1991). *Preventing AIDS in Drug Users and Their Sexual Partners*. New York: Guilford Press.

Stimson, G.V. (1992). *The global diffusion of injecting drug use: Implications for HIV infection*. Eighth International Conference on AIDS/III STD, World Congress, 22 July, Amsterdam.

Stimson, G.V., Alldritt, L., Dolan, K. and Donoghoe, M. (1988). Syringes exchange schemes for drug users in England and Scotland. *British Medical Journal*, **296**, 1717–1719.

Strang, J. (1988). Changing injecting practices: Blunting the needle habit. *British Journal of Addiction*, **83**, 237–239.

Van den Hoek, J.A.R., van Haastrecht, H.J.A. and Coutinho, R.A. (1992). Little change in sexual behaviours in injecting drug users in Amsterdam. *Journal of the Acquired Immune Deficiency Syndrome*, **5**, 518–22.

Wenigern, B.G., Limpakarnjanarat, K., Ungchusak, K., Thanprasertsuk, S., Choopanya, K., Banichseni, S., Uneklabh, T., Thongcharoen, P. and Wasi, C. (1991). The epidemiology of HIV infection and AIDS in Thailand. *AIDS*, **5**, S71–S85.

Working Group on Demand Reduction Regarding Drug Abuse in Europe (1991). *Current Programs and Opportunities for Further Development*, Geneva: World Health Organization.

World Health Organization (1991). *Current and Future Dimensions of the HIV/AIDS Syndrome: A Capsule Summary*. Geneva: World Health Organization.

Part VI
Harm Reduction and
HIV/AIDS

Chapter 22
AIDS, Injecting Drug Use and Harm Reduction

DON C. DES JARLAIS and SAMUEL R. FRIEDMAN

As a previous volume on harm reduction (O'Hare et al., 1992) has amply demonstrated, the harm-reduction perspective can encompass many aspects of psychoactive drug use, from designated driver programs, to restricting advertising of cigarettes, to hepatitis B vaccination programs for injecting drug users. As Berridge (Chapter 5, this volume) has shown, there were many examples of harm reduction in the United Kingdom prior to the AIDS epidemic. Methadone maintenance treatment for heroin addiction should also be added as an important example of harm reduction prior to AIDS. Nevertheless, the prevention of HIV infection and AIDS among injecting drug users (IDUs) may be the most important problem to be addressed to date by the harm-reduction approach.

Concern about the possible spread of HIV among IDUs has led many conservative as well as many liberal political leaders to experiment with the harm-reduction approach. In many countries, harm-reduction initiatives to prevent HIV infection have been relatively well-funded. The funding standard has often been influenced by the actual level of need.

The ease with which HIV infection rates can be measured among samples of injecting drug users (albeit unrepresentative samples) will provide a relatively clear evaluation test for harm reduction. However, if harm-reduction programs are not able to successfully reduce the spread of HIV among IDUs, then the approach as a whole is likely to lose its current political credibility. Indeed, it is unlikely that any other successes in reducing overall drug-related harm could overcome the loss of credibility that would thereby occur.

What is 'Harm Reduction'?

There is no single, generally accepted definition of harm reduction at present. The field of harm-reduction activities is growing rapidly, and it may be too soon to formulate a definition that draws clear lines of demarcation between the harm-reduction perspective and other perspectives on the problems associated with psychoactive drug use. Despite the current lack of a clear definition of harm reduction, there are some common elements that have been included in almost all attempts at defining the term (Stimson, 1990a; Des Jarlais and Sotheran, 1990; Brettle, 1991; Strang, Chapter 1, this volume). It will be useful to briefly examine the implications of these common components of harm-reduction programs for the prevention of HIV infection among IDUs.

First, harm reduction emphasizes short-term pragmatic goals over long-term idealistic goals. *There is certainly a pragmatic urgency to the prevention of HIV among IDUs*. At the community level, HIV can spread very rapidly among populations of IDUs, so that efforts to stop transmission need to be implemented as quickly as possible. At the individual level, HIV infection is almost always fatal, so that if infection is not prevented, then achieving other goals, such as abstinence or vocational rehabilitation, could become meaningless.

Second, harm reduction involves establishing a scale of means to achieving specific goals. From the broadest perspective, prevention of HIV infection among injecting drug users could be accomplished through having drug injectors completely stop using illicit drugs. A second method would be through stopping illicit drug injection. If this is not possible, then a third method would be through ensuring that injecting occurs without any multi-person use ('sharing') of injection equipment. If this too is not possible, then a fourth method would be ensuring that whenever two or more persons did use the same injection equipment, it would be disinfected before each person used it. This hierachical methods approach to attaining the same specific goal is part of the pragmatism of harm reduction, but it has an additional important implication for prevention programing. *The number of alternative methods inherent in harm reduction suggests that a variety of different AIDS prevention programs need to be implemented simultaneously*. That is, different programs are considered to be complementary rather than in conflict. This inclusion of a variety of programs is in contrast to implementing only the most politically acceptable type of prevention program, or seeking to find the single 'best' prevention program.

Third, the harm-reduction perspective views illicit drug users as full members of the community, worthy of respect, and capable of both rational and altruistic behavior. Although the harm-reduction perspective recognizes the restrictions on free choice that occur with drug dependence, drug users are still considered capable of rationality and of altering their behavior. *Rather than being passive recipients of services, they are considered to have an important role in both planning and implementing AIDS prevention programs*. Indeed, they have often been credited with being responsible for changing the social norms within the drug injection group towards AIDS risk reduction, and drug users' organizations make important contributions to strategy development in several countries.

Harm Reduction as a Hegelian Synthesis

While the harm reduction perspective has been elaborated to the point where there is now a wide variety of harm-reduction programs for the prevention of HIV infection among drug users and for the prevention of many other types of drug-related harm, further conceptual development of the perspective will also be needed. One of the present shortcomings of the perspective, as noted even by its advocates (see Strang, Chapter 1, this volume), is the difficulty in formulating positive statements of the conceptual/philosophical/ethical bases of the perspective. Too often statements about harm reduction are phrased in terms of what harm reduction is not rather that what it is. The difficulties that harm reduction advocates have in articulating the values and ideals embodied within the perspective have greatly limited the political appeal of the perspective (see Hawks, Chapter 8, this volume.).

Towards this goal of conceptual/philosophical development, we would propose thinking of harm reduction as a Hegelian synthesis of the 'utilization of psychoactive drugs to celebrate human potential' perspective (the thesis) and the 'zero-tolerance prohibition' perspective (antithesis). (See Musto (1991) for a discussion of the alternation of these two perspectives in the United States of America.) The 'celebratory' perspective utilizes the potential of psychoactive drugs within religious and secular ceremonies to create a sense of positive community. At a less exalted level, psychoactive drugs are also used for increasing economic productivity and for recreation. In contrast, the 'prohibition' approach sees psychoactive drug use as immoral in itself as well as leading to multiple other harms. Because of the inherent danger that psychoactive drug use may increase beyond the control of the individual, no level of psychoactive drug use is considered to be acceptable within the prohibition perspective.

A true Hegelian synthesis must be more than a simple combination of some parts of the thesis and some parts of the antithesis. It must create a whole that is greater than the simple sum of its parts. Both the celebratory and prohibition approaches imply a uniformity of psychoactive drug use in society – everyone using drugs constructively in the celebratory perspective versus no one using psychoactive drugs at all in the prohibition perspective. The great advantage of the harm-reduction approach is that it recognizes the actual diversity in psychoactive drug use. Many people in many different societies will use psychoactive drugs, and a substantial minority of users – but certainly not all users – will use drugs in ways that are harmful to the individual users, to their immediate social networks, and to the society as a whole. Harm reduction starts from acknowledging this diversity of use and then proceeds to examine ways in which the drug-use-related harm might be pragmatically reduced. Because it recognizes the diversity in psychoactive drug use, harm reduction may be particularly appropriate for the economically complex, multicultural societies that may well become the norm in the next century.

That the harm-reduction perspective may be developed to incorporate a positive value on diversity within societies could become critical for AIDS prevention efforts among persons who inject psychoactive drugs. One of the major limitations of AIDS prevention efforts has been the tendency to stigmatize persons with AIDS in many different societies. This stigmatization has often been particularly acute with respect to injecting drug users with AIDS, and has limited AIDS prevention efforts in many different countries. As HIV continues to spread among injecting drug users throughout the world, it will be necessary for prevention programs to overcome the double stigmatization associated with AIDS and the injection of psychoactive drugs.

Current Scope of the HIV/Drug Injection Problem

In the decade since AIDS was first observed in injecting drug users, it has become clear that this is truly a multi-national problem. HIV infection among IDUs has occurred in North America (USA and Canada), Europe (virtually all countries of western Europe as well as Yugoslavia and Poland in eastern Europe), South America (Brazil and Argentina), and Asia (Thailand, China, Myanmar and India), along with Australia and New Zealand. Although there is not yet documentation of significant HIV infection among IDUs in Africa, the problem appears to occur at all levels of industrialization and among all political systems.

While HIV infection has occurred among drug injectors in a large number of countries, the level of infection among IDUs (i.e. of HIV seroprevalence) varies at least as much within countries as it does across countries. Many countries with HIV infection among their IDUs have some cities with moderate to high seroprevalence rates (30%–50+%) and other cities with very low seroprevalence (rates less than 5%). The greatest contrast may be that in Scotland between Edinburgh, with a seroprevalence rate of approximately 50% (Robertson et al., 1986), and Glasgow, less than 80 kilometers away, with a seroprevalence of less than 5% (Goldberg et al., 1988).

There are at least two factors that have been associated with rapid transmission of HIV among drug injectors leading to high seroprevalence. First, rapid transmission has usually occurred prior to awareness of an AIDS threat among the local drug injectors. In some instances, for example, New York City, the rapid spread occurred prior to the discovery of AIDS (Des Jarlais et al., 1989). In other cities, however, the rapid spread occurred after the presence of AIDS among drug injectors had been well-established, but before any prevention programs had been implemented in the city. The second factor that has been associated with rapid transmission is the presence of a mechanism for 'efficient mixing' within the population of drug injectors. Efficient mixing refers to contact patterns such that transmission of HIV occurs within large, loosely defined groups of otherwise unacquainted individuals, rather than within small friendship groups. 'Shooting galleries', where many different drug injectors may rent and use the same injection equipment, provide an obvious mechanism for efficient mixing. 'Dealer's works' (injection equipment that sellers of illicit drugs lend to many different customers) provide another good mechanism for efficient mixing. Efficient mixing may also occur in situations where large numbers of injectors meet on a casual basis, pool resources to obtain drugs (since better prices can usually be obtained when larger quantities of drugs are purchased), and then all use the same injection equipment.

Given that illicit drug injection (and HIV infection among drug injectors) has occurred in very different national, cultural and political settings, and that there are substantial variations in HIV seroprevalence among drug injectors in different areas, one might expect that there would also be very great differences with respect to HIV transmission behaviors. In order to test this hypothesis, the World Health Organization has been conducting a study of AIDS risk behavior among injecting drug users in 13 widely dispersed cities. The cities include sites in North and South America, Europe, and Australia. (It is important to note that some AIDS prevention programs are already in operation in all of these cities, and the data on AIDS risk behavior undoubtedly reflect widespread knowledge of AIDS among the subjects as well as other effects of the prevention programs.)

Despite the great diversity in the economic, political and cultural settings, the preliminary data show strong similarities with respect to potential HIV transmission (WHO, 1993). All the cities noted some continued drug injection risk behavior. The percentage of subjects who reported that they had used someone else's injection equipment in the previous six months ranged from approximately 20% to approximately 45%. Cleaning of injection equipment was common in all cities, but water was the most common method of cleaning in all but three of the cities. Since cleaning with water also permits re-use of the needle and syringe – and is not reliable for decontaminating the equipment – it is not clear whether merely cleaning with water increases or decreases the likelihood of HIV transmission.

There were also indications of potential heterosexual transmission of HIV from drug injectors to non-injecting sexual partners. In all the cities there were more male than female drug injectors, with the male:female ratio ranging from approximately 2:1 to 19:1. The average age at which the person began injecting drugs was between 18 and 21 for all of the cities. The subjects were thus injecting at the time when they were quite likely to be sexually active and having children. At least half of the sexually active subjects reported that they had never used condoms in the previous six months with regular partners. Condom use was slightly higher with casual partners, but at least 35% of subjects in all the cities reported that they had never used condoms with casual partners in the previous six months.

The general pattern emerging from these similarities can best be summarized as evidence of risk reduction – not risk elimination – with considerable potential for further HIV transmission, if not at a very rapid rate. These commonalities across cultures are important for strategies of prevention. They suggest that many of the same types of prevention programs could be effective in diverse settings and that it will not be necessary to develop unique prevention strategies for the wide variety of places where HIV infection is a threat to injecting drug users. Indeed, much of the variation in existing prevention programs throughout the world is not based on differences in the behavior of IDUs at risk for HIV infection, but on what types of prevention are popular with the political leaders of the area.

HIV Prevention Programing

A wide variety of programs have been implemented to prevent HIV infection in injecting drug users. These include: information-only programs (Jackson and Baxter, 1988; Ostrow, 1989; Pott, 1990); drug abuse treatment programs (Ball et al., 1988; Yancovitz et al., 1988; Sorensen et al., 1989); outreach/bleach distribution programs (Watters, 1988; Thompson et al., 1990; Wiebel, Chene and Johnson, 1990); syringe-exchange programs (Stimson and Lart, 1990; O'Keefe, Kaplan and Khoshnood, 1991; van Haastrecht et al., 1991); over-the-counter sales programs (Espinoza et al., 1988; Ingold and Ingold, 1989); and HIV counseling and testing (Casadonte et al., 1990; Roggenburg et al., 1990; Rugg and MacGowan, 1990).

Evaluation studies have indicated that all these programs will lead to some degree of behavior change/AIDS risk reduction. At present it is not possible to compare the relative effectiveness of the different types of programs for several reasons. First, most of the programs that have been evaluated have utilized more than a single type of prevention activity. Second, the specific units of measurement for assessing the behavior change vary widely across the different studies. Third, very few studies have used control or comparison groups; indeed, most have used only pre-post designs. Fourth, the characteristics of the subjects participating in the studies generally have not been described in sufficient detail that one could statistically control for subject differences in comparing across studies. Finally, very few studies have used HIV transmission as an outcome variable, so that even if it were possible to construct common metrics for behavior change (e.g. percent of injections in shooting galleries, percent of injections with one's own equipment, percent of injections with disinfected equipment, etc.) there would still be the problem of extrapolating from the behavior change to actual HIV transmission.

Despite these many methodological limitations, however, a number of working generalizations have emerged from the evaluation studies (Des Jarlais and Friedman, 1992):

1. Providing information about AIDS and HIV transmission is critical but not sufficient.
2. Providing means for behavior change is also critical.
3. Multiple means for behavior change are needed for different subsets of injecting drug users and for the same drug injectors at different points in time.
4. Coordination of different programs, either through referral or through multiple 'programs' offered at the same site, is important in providing the needed variety of means for behavior change.
5. AIDS prevention programs must also address other needs of injecting drug users, including needs for drug abuse treatment and for social and medical services.
6. Risk reduction is usually a social process, with drug injectors influencing each other to change behavior.

None of the above generalizations have been rigorously tested scientifically, although all of them are certainly consistent with the epidemiological and evaluation studies. Many of them were developed from the practical experience of operating prevention programs rather than from prevention theories. As noted in the earlier discussion of harm reduction, several of these working generalizations are fundamental to current conceptualizations of harm reduction: for example, offering alternative means to the same specific goals, and encouraging drug injectors to influence each other to change behavior.

Prevention 'Successes'

While the aforementioned methodological difficulties in most prevention evaluation studies make it difficult to assess the effects of prevention programs on actual transmission of HIV among injecting drug users, there are at least two geographical areas where prevention programming appears to be successful. In the Skane province of southern Sweden, prevention programming was begun even before HIV became

established among local IDUs (Ljungberg et al., 1991). These prevention programs included a syringe exchange, drug abuse treatment programs, and extensive HIV counseling and testing. (The extensiveness of
the counseling and testing in turn provides much of the evidence as to
the effectiveness of the prevention effort. HIV-positive test results are
reported to public-health authorities, and the authorities estimate that
over 90% of the local injecting drug users have been tested for HIV.)
Indeed, even though HIV-positive drug users are known to have moved
into the area, there has been remarkably little local transmission of HIV.
The current seroprevalence in the province is estimated to be approximately 2%, but only 20% of those HIV-positive drug injectors were
infected while residing in the province. The rest were infected outside
of the province, including already HIV-positive IDUs who have recently
moved into the area. Thus, seroprevalence for local transmissions is
actually under 0.5%. Although it is not possible to determine the relative effectiveness of the individual components of the prevention
efforts in Skane, it is clear that, to date, there has been successful prevention of an HIV epidemic among injecting drug users in the area.

On a nationwide basis, Australia probably has had the most effective
prevention programing in regard to HIV among injecting drug users
(Bowtell, 1992; Crofts, 1992; Wodak, 1992). Again, an important part of
this prevention effort was that it was initiated before HIV infection was
well-established among drug injectors in the country. The components
of the prevention programming were: (1) methadone maintenance
treatment for heroin addiction was greatly expanded; (2) laws restricting the sale of injection equipment were repealed; (3) large numbers
of syringe exchanges were established; and (4) users' groups were
funded in order that injecting drug users could actively participate in
the planning and implementation of AIDS prevention activities. Indeed,
risk behaviors among IDUs in Australia have been at low to moderate
levels, and HIV seroprevalence has remained under 5%, since the start
of these prevention activities in 1986–1987.

One of the most important questions arising from the research on
such evidently successful prevention programs is, 'What proportion of
the active IDUs need to directly participate in the prevention activities
in order to prevent epidemic spread of HIV among the entire group?'.
Based on the Swedish, Australian and Tacoma, Washington (Hagan et
al., 1991) studies – all of which were conducted in low seroprevalence
areas – it would appear that, while it is necessary for all (or almost all)
IDUs at least to know (1) that HIV is a local threat and (2) how it is
transmitted, perhaps only a quarter to a third of the IDUs need to be
regular participants in prevention programs such as syringe exchanges.
(It should be noted that many participants in syringe exchanges also
serve as 'satellite' agents by providing sterile injection equipment to
drug injectors who do not attend the exchange. These indirect partici-

pants are *not* included in this fraction.) Many drug injectors who are not directly and regularly participating in prevention programs will, of course, also be practicing HIV risk reduction. *Much more research is clearly needed on this question.* It is time, however, to realize that in order to keep a low HIV seroprevalence at a stable level, it is not necessary to have all IDUs in the area participating regularly in prevention programs. Low HIV seroprevalence rates may remain stable even without complete participation of all drug injectors in regular prevention activities.

Challenges for the Future

While there clearly have been some areas that have avoided epidemics of HIV among drug injectors, there are also difficult challenges both for future research and for the harm-reduction/HIV prevention programs themselves. While there has been much research showing that IDUs will change their behavior to reduce the risk of AIDS, there has been little research on maintaining behavior change over time. One New York City study found that approximately one third of those who had changed their behavior reported that they had failed to maintain the change (Des Jarlais, Abdul-Quader and Tross, 1991). Whether failure to maintain change should be conceptualized as episodic 'lapses' or as full 'relapse', and how to increase maintenance of change, are urgent topics for investigation.

At a political level, there is a parallel question of maintenance of public commitment. To the extent that HIV prevention programs appear to have succeeded, there could arise a perception that they are no longer needed. The terminology of 'AIDS education', with its implication that once people learn about AIDS they have all that is needed to change their behavior, may be actively misleading in this regard. Discontinuation of the programs may subsequently lead to the rapid spread of HIV that the programs had prevented.

Although the present programs appear capable of preventing HIV epidemics before they spread in low seroprevalence areas, there are special problems for high seroprevalence areas. In such areas, residual levels of risk behavior will be much more likely to lead to substantial new HIV infections because of the much greater probability that, whenever multi-person use of injection equipment does occur, one or more of the persons involved will be carrying HIV. Therefore, a second generation of prevention programs may be needed for high seroprevalence areas.

For reasons that have not yet been fully determined, current programs have had much less effect on changing the sexual behavior of IDUs as compared to their drug-injection behavior (Des Jarlais and Friedman, 1992; Stimson, 1990b). For low seroprevalence areas, prevention of sexual transmission may best be accomplished by preventing infections in the first place, through reduction in the multi-person use of injection equipment. For high seroprevalence areas, however, the problem of sexual transmission needs to be addressed directly.

An additional prevention task that needs to be addressed is the problem of new persons starting to inject illicit drugs. While persons who started to inject after the AIDS epidemic emerged are more likely to practice safer injection than persons who began injecting before AIDS emerged (Neaigus et al., 1991; Vlahov et al., 1991), new injectors still exhibit disturbing levels of risk behavior. New injectors are also less likely than experienced injectors to utilize syringe exchanges and other AIDS prevention programs (Stimson, 1989). The harm-reduction perspective probably offers several advantages over a 'zero tolerance' perspective for preventing HIV infection among new injectors because, without requiring complete cessation of drug use, it can encourage the more modest, attainable goals of either 'safer injection' or non-injected use of illicit drugs as alternatives to high-risk injection of illicit drugs. At present, however, we do not have an adequate empirical knowledge base to apply harm-reduction strategies to the problem of new drug injectors (Strang et al., 1992; Des Jarlais et al., 1992).

The final challenge to the use of a harm-reduction perspective for preventing HIV infection among drug injectors may be the most difficult. Harm reduction has been developed, and harm-reduction programs have been implemented, primarily in industrialized countries. The problems of illicit drug injection and HIV infection among injecting drug users are, however, particularly acute in developing/newly industrializing countries. It is difficult to foresee how harm reduction might be implemented or expanded in many of these countries. Harm reduction appears antithetical to the political and religious cultures of many developing countries (as it is in some industrialized countries too). There is also a question of resources. Does it make sense to propose a syringe exchange for injecting drug users in countries that cannot afford enough sterile injection equipment for regular medical use? Earlier in this chapter, the importance of HIV prevention to the entire harm-reduction movement was discussed. If harm reduction cannot be applied successfully to the problems of illicit drug injection and HIV transmission among injecting drug users in developing countries, many persons will see this as due to not merely the tactical limitations of harm reduction, but as a fundamental failure of the entire approach.

References

Ball, J.C., Lange, W.R., Myers, C.P. and Friedman, S.R. (1988). Reducing the risk of AIDS through methadone maintenance treatment. *Journal of Health and Social Behavior*, **29**, 214–226.

Bowtell, B. (1992). Development of policy relating to the prevention of HIV among injecting drug users. Presented at the Third International Conference on the Reduction of Drug Related Harm, Melbourne, Australia.

Brettle, R.P. (1991). HIV and harm reduction in injection drug users. *AIDS*, **5**, 125–136.

Casadonte, P.P., Des Jarlais, D.C., Friedman, S.R. and Rotrosen, J.P. (1990). Psychological and behavioral impact among intravenous drug users of learning HIV test results. *International Journal of the Addictions*, **25**, 409–426.

Crofts, N. (1992). *Epidemiology of HIV among injecting drug users in Australia.* Presented at the Third International Conference on the Reduction of Drug Related Harm, Melbourne, Australia.

Des Jarlais, D.C., Friedman, S.R., Novick, D., Sotheran, J.L., Thomas, P., Yancovitz, S., Mildvan, D., Weber, J., Kreek, M., Maslansky, R., Bartelme, S., Spira, T. and Marmor, M. (1989). HIV-1 infection among intravenous drug users in Manhattan. *Journal of the American Medical Association*, **261**, 1008–1012.

Des Jarlais, D.C. and Sotheran, J.L. (1990). The public health paradigm for AIDS and drug use: Shifting the time frame. *British Journal of Addiction*, **85**, 348–349.

Des Jarlais, D.C., Abdul-Quader, A. and Tross, S. (1991). The next problem: Maintenance of AIDS risk reduction among intravenous drug users. *International Journal of the Addictions*, 26, 1279–1292.

Des Jarlais, D.C., Casriel, C., Friedman, S.R. and Rosenblum, A. (1992). AIDS and the transition to illicit drug injection: Results of a randomized trial prevention program. *British Journal of Addiction*, 87, 493–498.

Des Jarlais, D.C. and Friedman, S.R. (1992). AIDS prevention programs for injecting drug users. In: G.P. Wormser (Ed.), *AIDS and Other Manifestations of HIV Infection*, 2nd edn, pp. 645–658. New York: Raven Press

Espinoza, P., Bouchard, I., Ballian, P. and Devoto, J. (1988). *Has the open sale of syringes modified the syringe exchanging habits of drug addicts?* Presented at the Fourth International Conference on AIDS, Stockholm, Sweden.

Goldberg, D., Watson, H., Stuart, F., Miller, M., Gruer, L. and Follett, E. (1988). *Pharmacy supply of needles and syringes: The effect on spread of HIV in intravenous drug misusers.* Presented at the Fourth International Conference on AIDS, Stockholm, Sweden.

Hagan, H., Des Jarlais, D.C., Purchase, D., Reid, T.R. and Friedman, S.R. (1991). *Lower HIV seroprevalence, declining HBV incidence and safer injection in relation to the Tacoma syringe exchange.* Presented at the Seventh International Conference on AIDS, Florence, Italy,

Ingold, F.R. and Ingold, S. (1989) . The effects of the liberalization of syringe sales on the behaviour of intravenous drug users in France. *Bulletin on Narcotics*, 41, 67–81.

Jackson, J. and Baxter, R. (1988). *Inner-city mobile units: AIDS education and prevention.* Presented at the Fourth International Conference on AIDS, Stockholm, Sweden.

Ljungberg, B., Christensson, B., Tunving, K., Andersson, B., Landvall, B., Lundberg, M. and Zäll-Friberg, A.-C. (1991). HIV prevention among injecting drug users: Three years of experience from a syringe exchange program in Sweden. *Journal of Acquired Immune Deficiency Syndrome*, 4, 890–895.

Musto, D.F. (1991). Opium, cocaine and marijuana in American history. *Scientific American*, **265**, 40–47.

Neaigus, A., Friedman, S.R., Stepherson, B., Jose, B., Sufian, M. and Des Jarlais,

D.C.. (1991). *Declines in syringe sharing during the first drug injection*. Presented at the Seventh International Conference on AIDS, Florence, Italy.

O'Hare, P., Newcombe, R., Matthews, A., Buning, E.C. and Drucker, E. (Eds) (1992). *The Reduction of Drug-related Harm*. London: Routledge.

O'Keefe, E., Kaplan, E. and Khoshnood, K. (1991). *Preliminary Report: City of New Haven Needle Exchange Program*. New Haven, CT: New Haven Health Department.

Ostrow, D.G. (1989). AIDS prevention through effective education. *Daedalus*, **118**, 229–254.

Pott, E. (1990). *AIDS prevention and health education in the Federal Republic of Germany*. Presented at the Sixth International Conference on AIDS, San Francisco, CA.

Robertson, J.R., Bucknall, A.B.V., Welsby, P.D., Roberts, J.J.K., Inglis, J.M., Peutherer, J.F. and Brettle, R.P. (1986). Epidemic of AIDS related virus (HTLV-III/LAV) infection among intravenous drug users. *British Medical Journal*, **292**, 527–529.

Roggenburg, L., Sibthorpe, B., Tesselaar, H., Gould, J. and Fleming, D. (1990). *IDUs' perception of the effect of HIV counseling and testing on behavior*. Second Annual NADR National Meeting, Bethseda, MD.

Rugg, D.L. and MacGowan, R.J. (1990). *Assessing the effectiveness of HIV counseling and testing: A practical guide*. Background paper for WHO Global Programme on AIDS (GPA). WHO: Geneva.

Sorensen, J.L., Gibson, D.R., Heitzmann, C., Dumontet, R., Constantini, M. and Melese-d'Hospital, I. (1989). *Pyschoeducational group approach to AIDS prevention with drug abusers in residential treatment: Impact 6 months after intervention*. Presented at the Fifth International Conference on AIDS, Montréal, Canada.

Stimson, G.V. (1989). Syringe-exchange programmes for injecting drug users. *AIDS*, **3**, 253–260.

Stimson, G.V. (1990a). *The prevention of HIV infection in injecting drug users: Recent advances and remaining obstacles*. Presented at the Sixth International Conference on AIDS, San Francisco, CA.

Stimson, G.V. (1990b). AIDS and HIV: The challenge for British drug services. *British Journal of Addiction*, **85**, 329–339.

Stimson, G.V. and Lart, R. (1990). *National survey of syringe-exchanges in England*. Presented at the Sixth International Conference on AIDS, San Francisco, CA.

Strang, J., Des Jarlais, D.C., Griffiths, P. and Gossop, M. (1992). The study of transitions in the route of drug use: The route from one route to another. *British Journal of Addiction*, **87**, 473–483.

Thompson, P.I., Jones, T.S., Cahill, K. and Medina, V. (1990). *Promoting HIV prevention outreach activities via community-based organizations*. Presented at the Sixth International Conference on AIDS, San Francisco, CA.

van Haastrecht, H.J.A., van den Hoek, J.A.R., Bardoux. C., Leentvarr-Kuypers, A. and Coutinho, R.A. (1991). The course of the HIV epidemic among intravenous drug users in Amsterdam, the Netherlands. *American Journal of Public Health*, **81**, 59–62.

Vlahov, D., Anthony, J.C., Celentano, D., Solomon, L. and Chowdhury, N. (1991). Trends of HIV-1 risk reduction among initiates into intravenous drug use, 1982–1987. *American Journal of Drug and Alcohol Abuse*, **17**, 39–48.

Watters, J.K., Case, P., Huang, K., Cheng, Y.-T., Lorvick, J. and Carlson, J. (1988). *HIV seroepidemiology and behavior change in intravenous drug users: Progress report on the effectiveness of street-based prevention*. Presented at the Fourth International Conference on AIDS, Stockholm, Sweden.

Wiebel, W., Chene, D. and Johnson, W. (1990). *Adoption of bleach use in a cohort of street intravenous drug users in Chicago*. Presented at the Sixth International Conference on AIDS, San Francisco, CA.

Wodak, A. (1992). *Implementation of policy into programs*. Presented at the Third International Conference on the Reduction of Drug Related Harm, Melbourne, Australia.

Yancovitz, S., Des Jarlais, D.C., Peyser, N., Senie, R., Drew, E. and Mildvan, D. (1988). *Innovative AIDS risk reduction project: Interim methadone clinic*. Presented at the Fourth International Conference on AIDS, Stockholm, Sweden.

Chapter 23
Assessing the Risk of HIV-1 Transmission in Correctional Centres

MATT GAUGHWIN and DAVID VLAHOV

Infection with HIV-1, the cause of AIDS, is a major public health problem in prisons throughout the world. AIDS has become the leading cause of death in some correctional systems (Salive, Smith and Brewer, 1990; Hammett, Moini and Daugherty, 1991).

Seroprevalence of HIV-1 infection in correctional systems varies geographically within and between countries. In the United States of America seroprevalence at entrance to prison ranges from 0% among women in states such as Wyoming to 19% among women entering prisons in New York (Truman et al., 1988; Hammett, Moini, and Daugherty 1991). Similar variations are seen in Europe (Harding, 1987), while limited evidence from Australia suggests point prevalences are less than 2% and vary from 0% in the Northern Territory to 1.2% in South Australia (Heilpern and Eggar, 1991).

Where temporal trends in the prevalence of HIV-1 infection have been examined, a few studies have shown stable prevalence both at entry to prison and within prisons (Vlahov et al., 1989; Vlahov et al., 1990; Gaughwin et al., 1991).

Outside prisons, rapid increases in the prevalence of HIV-1 infection among injecting drug users (IDUs) have been observed in the USA, Europe, Scotland and Asia but apparently not in Australia (Des Jarlais and Friedman, 1989; Bell, Fernandes and Batey, 1990; Donovan et al., 1990; Wolk et al., 1990). There is evidence of stabilisation of prevalence at well below 100% in New York and elsewhere. However, stable prevalence does not necessarily mean that transmission does not occur (Des Jarlais et al., 1989).

Risk Factors and Requirements for HIV-1 Infection and Transmission in the Correctional Setting

The main risk factor for having HIV-1 infection and AIDS in the correctional setting is intravenous drug use prior to incarceration; a number of studies from the USA and Europe have replicated this observation. Intravenous drug users entering prisons in Maryland were eight times more likely to be infected with HIV-1 than non-injectors in 1987 (Vlahov et al., 1989). Within the New York State prison system, which conducts risk factor investigations on diagnosed cases of AIDS, approximately 95% of inmates with AIDS report a history of intravenous drug use compared with 3% who claim to be exclusively homosexual (Bureau of Communicable Disease Control, 1989). In South Australia 85% of infected individuals are known to be IDUs (Gaughwin et al., 1991).

Substantial proportions of prisoners in correctional systems in many parts of the world have a history of engaging in risk behaviours which predispose them to becoming infected with communicable diseases. The predominant predisposing behaviour among prisoners in general is intravenous drug use. Several studies have reported that up to 53% of prisoners have a history of injecting drugs while up to 28% have engaged in homosexual activity at some time in their lives (Gaughwin, Douglas and Wodak, 1991).

There is also evidence that when in prison those who have a history of intravenous drug use may continue to inject themselves and share needles at some time during their imprisonments. A few individuals commence injecting in prisons. A recent review of studies of risk behaviours in prisons indicated that on average about 33% of all prisoners injected themselves and about 12% engaged in homosexual activity while in prison (Gaughwin, Douglas and Wodak, 1991).

Studies of intravenous drug users indicate that when in prison about 42% on average inject themselves, that about 80% of those who inject in prison share equipment at some time, and less than 30% clean shared equipment adequately with bleach or boiling water (Gaughwin, Douglas and Wodak, 1991).

A few studies of intravenous drug users suggest however that the frequency of injection in prison is substantially lower than outside prison, about once per week on average (Gaughwin, Douglas and Wodak, 1991).

Evidence for HIV-1 Transmission in Prisons

So, given that the risk of HIV-1 transmission appears to be substantial in prisons, what is the evidence for actual HIV-1 transmission occurring during incarceration? Epidemiologic evidence from a small number of incidence studies in the USA shows infrequent transmission of HIV-1 in prison systems (Kelly, Redfield and Ward, 1986; Brewer et al., 1988; Horsburgh et al., 1990; K. Castro, personal communication, 1992).

Outside prisons, cross-sectional studies of IDUs have found that injecting practices strongly associated with HIV-1 infection are increased frequency of injection, sharing equipment with strangers, sharing equipment with many other injectors and the use of shooting galleries (Friedland and Klein, 1987; Schoenbaum et al., 1989). Frequent injection could increase the risk of HIV-1 infection by increasing the chance of any exposure to the virus and by exposing an individual to multiple innocula of HIV-1 infected blood.

While the prevalence of infection in some prisons appears to be substantial, the prevalence and frequency of injection among IDUs is lower than outside prison (Gaughwin, Douglas and Wodak, 1991) and may partly explain the finding of infrequent HIV-1 transmission in prisons.

It is probably unrealistic to conceptualise HIV-1 transmission in correctional institutions as occurring in some uniform way. While the prevalence of HIV-1 infection at entry to prison systems may give an indication of the extent of infection within prisons, it may be different from the point prevalence in the system as a whole and from that in particular institutions. In Australia, prisons tend to aggregate those who have committed serious crimes and consequently receive long sentences, whereas those entering prisons are predominantly individuals who have received short sentences for minor crimes (Walker, 1989). One study of hepatitis B transmission in a US correctional system noted that inmates who remained in prison were more likely to have engaged in risk behaviours while incarcerated than those who had been discharged (Decker et al., 1985).

Another consideration is the distribution of HIV-1 infected prisoners within a correctional system. There is no a priori reason to expect that infected prisoners will be evenly distributed throughout any system. Factors such as policies of segregation of infected prisoners and policies relating to security arrangements may at times aggregate HIV-1 infected prisoners in some institutions. Although the prevalence of infection in the prison system as a whole may be low, it may be particularly high in some institutions. Thus, in South Australia in 1989, some prisons had never housed a known HIV-1 infected prisoner whereas others, at times, had up to 5% prevalence of infection. In contrast, the overall correctional system prevalence in South Australia was about 1.2% in 1989 (Gaughwin et al., 1991).

Prevalence and Incidence of HIV-1 Infection in Prisons

There is some evidence that higher prevalence of infection in prisons is associated with greater rates of HIV-1 transmission (Table 23.1). This observation suggests that prisons in high HIV-1 prevalence areas such as New York may be contributing substantial numbers of HIV-1 infected individuals to their communities. By extrapolating the US data we estimate that an Australian prison system such as the South Australian system may be contributing up to two new infections per 1000 prisoners per year. The estimates have wide confidence limits and we are aware of the limitations of such extrapolations, but in the absence of adequate surveillance of HIV-1 transmission in Australian prison systems, they are a useful guide.

Table 23.1 Point estimates for prevalence and incidence of HIV seropositivity among prison inmates, United States of America

Prison system	Prevalence (%)	Incidence per 10^3 prison years	95% confidence interval incidence
Military*	1.0	0.0	0.0–2.0
Nevada†	2.4	1.7	0.1–7.4
USA§	3.3	3.3	1.2–7.0
Maryland¶	7.0	4.2	0.1–16.3

* Kelly, Redfield and Ward (1986).
† Horsburg et al. (1990).
§ K. Castro, personal communication (1992).
¶ Brewer et al. (1988).

It is also likely that HIV-1 transmission within prisons will occur in an episodic manner when the conjunction of risk behaviours and prevalence of infection is such that localised transmission is facilitated. Such conditions may occur rarely and transiently. Evidence that this may be the pattern of transmission comes from studies of hepatitis B transmission in correctional systems. Two studies in the USA have shown infrequent hepatitis B transmission in prisons (Decker et al., 1985; Hull et al., 1985). These outcomes are cause for some optimism in regard to HIV-1 since hepatitis B is thought to be more infectious than HIV (Friedland and Klein, 1987). It is not however cause for complacency. Studies in US correctional systems report short-lived outbreaks of extensive hepatitis B transmission (Decker et al., 1984).

A Scenario for an Outbreak of HIV-1 Infection in a Prison

What are the circumstances which may precipitate outbreaks of HIV-1 in prisons among intravenous drug users? One may be local high prevalence of infection and risk behaviours. For example, a unit or cell block of 10 individuals may contain mostly injectors with one or two infected. If there were only one or two needles available for use, preconditions for an outbreak are present. If there is no bleach in the cell block with which to adequately disinfect equipment, the situation is worse. These prisoners may usually wash their equipment with water before injecting but on one night, just after an infected prisoner has injected, the others hear a prison officer approaching; the choice is not to inject or to inject quickly. Rather than miss an opportunity, the next prisoner cursorily cleans the equipment and receives a relatively large innoculum of blood containing HIV-1 and so becomes infected. He remains relatively well apart from an influenza-like illness at which time he has a pronounced HIV-1 viremia. He continues to inject and share equipment for injection but, because of the viremia, even small volumes of blood remaining in the syringe contain many virions. These conditions may facilitate extensive transmission of HIV-1 (Barry et al., 1990).

Such a scenario is not fanciful. During our discussions with prisoners some have described similar circumstances, with comments such as 'I saw blood in the syringe but it was inject or miss out'.

Further, high viremia during primary HIV-1 infection is now well-documented (Clark et al., 1991). Symptoms may be mild, and viral titres may be substantial before symptoms develop. Given little change in health and the observation that most primary infections go unnoticed (Clark et al., 1991), it would be unlikely that injection behaviour would be altered. There may be no obvious sign of infection and no way that a prisoner who uses a syringe after someone he regards as not infected can be sure that that prisoner is not indeed infected.

The scarcity of needles in prisons compounds the situation. There are few data on how many needles are available to injectors in prisons. In South Australia, analysis of data on the numbers of syringes found in a year and former prisoners' estimates of the numbers of needles suggest a ratio of about one needle for every four to five injectors (Gaughwin et al., 1991). Further, needles and syringes circulate from unit to unit and cell to cell in prisons. In many cases it is not possible to have any idea who used a needle previously.

Although the scenario suggested here is realistic, it is important to note that there are no reports of outbreaks of HIV-1 transmission in prisons. However, the apparent infrequency of a pronounced clinical syndrome during primary infection, the infrequency of serological testing for HIV-1, the relatively long incubation period, and the extensive movement of prisoners between prisons and to communities all mitigate against detecting HIV-1 outbreaks.

Prisons as Facilitators of HIV-1 Transmission

Prison systems throughout the world are, with few exceptions, facilitating potential HIV-1 and other disease outbreaks by failing to assist prisoners to either stop injecting drugs or to provide adequate means to make injection practices safe (Harding, Manghi and Sanchez, 1990).

Only one or two correctional systems in Australia provide bleach. To date, no prison anywhere in the world has permitted distribution or exchange of needles and syringes (Harding, Manghi and Sanchez, 1990; Gaughwin, Douglas, and Wodak, 1991).

As noted previously, the circumstances of injecting may be crucial to whether injection occurs safely. Surveillance of prisoners by officers may precipitate hasty and very unsafe injection practices. Unfortunately there are few data which describe and quantify the prevalence and frequency of such circumstances which may well be keys to understanding communicable disease transmission in prisons and other low prevalence environments. In many prison systems, contraband which invariably includes needles and syringes is searched for in cells and elsewhere. When needles are in such short supply the confiscation of one may dramatically increase the sharing of the remaining needles until such time as other needles get into a prison.

Condoms are not available in Australian prisons but are available in a few prisons in the USA, Canada and elsewhere, without adverse consequences (Harding, Manghi and Sanchez, 1990; Hammett, Moini and Daugherty, 1991). There are few data on the nature and frequency of sexual behaviour in prisons although some authors have described sociological associates of such behaviour and focus on dominance relationships between prisoners; these studies have been reviewed by Heilpern and Eggar (1989). The occurrence of rape in prisons has been documented and as such may be a special circumstance in which localised frequent transmission of communicable diseases could occur. Should an HIV-1 infected male prisoner be a homosexual rapist or promiscuous, the possibility of extensive local transmission is present. Condoms are unlikely to be used during rape (Gaughwin et al., 1990) and hence the best hope for prevention may be understanding the determinants of prison rape and adjusting housing practices so that potential perpetrators and susceptibles do not come in contact with each other. Understanding prison sexuality more comprehensively will help make prisons safer places for prisoners. That gonorrhoea transmission has been documented within male prisons (van Hoeven, Rooney and Joseph, 1990) confirms that anal intercourse occurs and is transmitting infectious agents.

The Wider Role of Prisons in Helping to Prevent HIV-1 Epidemics

For most prisoners, prisons are half-way houses where they live for relatively short periods before returning to their communities. Because injecting drug use is a criminal activity, many prisoners have a history of drug injection and many drug injectors have a history of imprisonment.

Various surveys have reported pre-incarceration injecting drug use of up to 50% among prison inmates (Gaughwin, Douglas and Wodak, 1991). Large numbers of individuals pass through prison systems in a year, up to five times the numbers in prison at any one time (van Hoeven, Rooney and Joseph, 1990). This large turnover of prisoners means that prisons have the potential to communicate with and assist many people.

That the instability of the prison-to-community-to-prison lifestyle is a recipe for catastrophe is perhaps no better illustrated than by the high mortality from drug overdose of recently released prisoners (Harding-Pink and Frye, 1988). Prisons, because they house many individuals and because they are pivotal points in prisoners' lives, have a responsibility to minimise the chances that individuals and communities suffer as a result of their interactions with prison systems.

Meeting this responsibilty requires a pragmatic approach to a number of vexed questions, including particularly what to do about drugs in prisons. Specifically, multifaceted approaches to rehabilitation, including adequate education, adequate medical care including treatment for drug problems, and adequate planning for and assistance on release from prison, are required

Inmates and IDUs in general appear to have adequate knowledge about HIV-1 although some confusion persists among prisoners about unlikely routes of transmission (Celentano et al., 1990; Gaughwin et al., 1990; Celentano et al., 1991). But knowledge alone is no guarantee that risk behaviours will not occur (Wolk et al., 1990). Injecting drug use is a complex phenomenon which has personal and situational determinants. South Australian prisoners are of the opinion that injection will continue in prisons despite the presence of HIV-1 infection (Gaughwin et al., 1990). In the light of such evidence, a pragmatic realisation that a harm-reduction approach rather than an abstinence-only approach is needed. Harm-reduction has prevented HIV-1 transmission outside prisons (Brettle, 1991). Appropriately designed and instituted, such a philosophy and approach has the same potential inside prisons. It follows that efforts at prevention should take account of the markedly different conditions of prisons compared to outside prisons. There is some evidence that therapeutic communities within prison settings can reduce drug-related recidivism (Gerstein and Lewin, 1990).

In Australia, an international conference of correctional workers, health workers, academics and a representative of prisoners agreed to and advocated a pragmatic approach to the prevention of HIV-1 transmission, including a trial of needle provision (Douglas, 1991).

In addition to basic requirements for prevention of infection, institutional activities which bear on the risk of transmission should be reviewed. There is a need to further describe and characterise high-risk events in prisons so that preventive practices are appropriate. It is useful to conceptualise HIV-1 transmission in prisons in terms of out-breaks of small clusters of infection due to the conjunction of rare events. Development of additional prevention strategies may benefit from keeping such a concept in mind.

Prisons have one advantage over the community in that they can regulate the movement and placement of inmates. Modelling of whether more infections occur when HIV-infected prisoners are aggre-gated or dispersed in a system needs to be done. Such knowledge might be useful to prison administrations and still avoid the problems of segregating infected from non-infected prisoners. Intuitively, if sus-tained high prevalence in any prison can be avoided, then it may be possible to avoid escalated transmission.

In areas where the prevalence of HIV-1 infection among prisoners is low, it is clear that a focus of prevention efforts on those who are infect-ed may be an efficient way of minimising the risk of transmission. Such an approach relies of course on a serological surveillance mechanism but does not imply that it should be mandatory. Compassionate assis-tance and the highest quality of medical care to those who are infected may be rewarded by improvements to their health and reduction of the risk of transmission.

In summary, we have argued that HIV-1 transmission has occurred infrequently in some prisons but that it may occur more frequently in prisons where the prevalence of infection is high. We argue that HIV-1 transmission in prisons probably occurs in an episodic manner as small clusters of infection. Prison conditions, and policies related to provi-sion of condoms and bleach, could substantially alter the risk of trans-mission. But the special circumstances in prisons which predispose to very unsafe behaviours need also to be considered when designing pre-vention strategies.

Prisons have a responsibility and the opportunity to contribute sub-stantially to preventing HIV-1 transmission. Managers and administra-tors of prisons, and the politicians who direct them, should accept the responsibility and grasp the opportunity to help decrease the risk of HIV-1 transmission both inside and outside prisons. Such action may require them to divest themselves of their own metaphorical shackles but if they do so, it is likely to benefit us all.

References

Barry, M., Gleavy, D., Herd, K., Schwingl, P. and Werner, B. (1990). Prevalence of markers for hepatitis B and hepatitis D in a Municipal House of Corrections. *American Journal of Public Health*, 80, 471–473.

Bell, J., Fernandes, D. and Batey, R. (1990). Heroin users seeking methadone treat-ment. *Medical Journal of Australia*, 152, 361–364.

Brettle, R. (1991). HIV and harm reduction for injection drug users. *AIDS*, 5, 125–136.

Brewer, T., Vlahov, D., Taylor, E., Hall, H., Munoz, A. and Polk, B. (1988). Transmission of HIV-1 within a statewide prison system. *AIDS*, **2**, 363–367.

Bureau of Communicable Disease Control. (1989). *AIDS Surveillance Monthly Update*. New York State Department of Health, Albany: New York.

Celentano, D,. Brewer, T., Sonnega, J. and Vlahov, D. (1990). Maryland inmates knowledge of HIV-1 transmission and prevention: a comparison with the US general population. *Journal of Prison and Jail Health*, **9**, 45–54.

Celentano, D., Vlahov, D., Menon, A. and Polk, B. (1991). HIV knowledge and attitudes among intravenous drug users – comparisons to the US population and by drug use behaviours. *Journal of Drug Issues*, **21**, 647–661.

Clark, S., Saag, M., Decker, W., Campbell-Hill, S., Roberson, J., Veldkamp, P., Kappes, J., Hahn, B. and Shaw, G. (1991). High titres of cytopathic virus in plasma of patients with symptomatic primary HIV-1 infection. *New England Journal of Medicine*, **324**, 954–960.

Decker, M., Vaughn, W., Brodie, J., Hutcheson, R. Jr and Schaffner, W. (1984). Seroepidemiology of Hepatitis B in Tennessee prisoners. *Journal of Infectious Disease*, **150**, 450–459.

Decker, M.D., Vaughn, W.K., Brodie, J.S., Hutcheson, R.H. Jr and Schaffner, W. (1985). Incidence of hepatitis B in Tennessee prisoners. *Journal of Infectious Disease*, **152**, 215–217.

Des Jarlais, D. and Friedman, S. (1989). AIDS and IV drug use. *Science*, **245**, 578.

Des Jarlais, D., Friedman, S., Novick, D., Sotheran, J., Thomas, P., Yancovitz, S., Mildvan, D., Weber, J., Kreek, M., Maslansky, R., Bartelme, S., Spira, T. and Marmor, M. (1989). HIV-1 infection among intravenous drug users in Manhattan, New York City, from 1977 through 1987. *Journal of the American Medical Association*, **261**, 1002–1008.

Donovan, S., Finlayson, R., Mutimer, K., Price, R., Robertson, M., Nelson, M., Slade, M., Reece, I. and Nogare, J. (1990). HIV infection in sexually transmissable disease practice in Sydney: The effects of legislation, public education and changing clinical spectrum. *International Journal of STD and AIDS*, **1**, 21–27.

Douglas, R. (1991). AIDS in Australian prisons. What are the challenges? In J. Norberry, M. Gaughwin and S. Gerull (Eds), *HIV/AIDS and Prisons. Conference Proceedings No. 4*, Canberra: Australian Institute of Criminology.

Friedland, G. and Klein, R. (1987). Transmission of the human immunodeficiency virus. *New England Journal of Medicine*, **317**, 1125–1135.

Gaughwin, M., Douglas, R., Liew, C., Davies, L., Mylvaganam, A., Treffke, H., Edwards, J. and Ali, R. (1991). Human immunodeficiency virus (HIV) prevalence and risk behaviours for its transmission in South Australian prisons. *AIDS*, **5**, 845–851.

Gaughwin, M., Douglas, R. and Wodak, A. (1991). Behind bars-risk behaviours for HIV transmission in prisons, a review. In J. Norberry, M. Gaughwin and S. Gerull (Eds), *HIV/AIDS and Prisons. Conference Proceedings No. 4*, Canberra: Australian Institute of Criminology.

Gaughwin, M., Douglas, R., Davies, L., Mylvaganam, A., Liew, C. and Ali, R. (1990). Preventing human immunodeficiency virus (HIV) infection among prisoners: Prisoners' and prison officers' knowledge of HIV and their attitudes to options for prevention. *Community Health Studies*, **14**, 61–64.

Gerstein, D. and Lewin, L. (1990). Treating drug problems. *New England Journal of Medicine*, **323**, 844–848.

Hammett, T.M., Moini, S. and Daugherty, A. (1991). HIV/AIDS in US prisons and gaols: Epidemiology, policy, and programs. In J. Norberry, M. Gaughwin and S.

Gerull (Eds), *HIV/AIDS and Prisons. Conference Proceedings No. 4,* Canberra: Australian Institute of Criminology.

Harding, T.W. (1987). AIDS in prisons. *The Lancet*, 2, 1260–1264.

Harding, T., Manghi, R. and Sanchez, G. (1990). *HIV/AIDS and Prisons.* Report for the WHO Global Programme on AIDS. University Institute of Legal Medicine: Geneva.

Harding-Pink, D. and Frye, O. (1988). Risk of death after release from prison: A duty to warn. *British Medical Journal*, 297, 596.

Heilpern, H. and Eggar, S. (1989). *AIDS in Australian Prisons – Issues and Policy Options.* Canberra: Department of Community Services and Health.

Heilpern, H. and Eggar, S. (1991). HIV/AIDS and Australian prisons. In J. Norberry, M. Gaughwin and S. Gerull (Eds), *HIV/AIDS and Prisons, Conference Proceedings No. 4,* Canberra: Australian Institute of Criminology .

Horsburgh, C. Jr, Jarvis, J., McArthur, T., Ignacio, T. and Stock, P. (1990). Seroconversion to human immunodeficiency virus in Prison inmates. *American Journal of Public Health*, 80, 209–210.

Hull, H., Lyons, L., Mann, J., Hadler, S., Steece, R. and Skeels, M. (1985). Incidence of hepatitis B in the penitentiary of New Mexico. *American Journal of Public Health*, 75, 1213–1214.

Kelly, P., Redfield, R. and Ward, D. (1986). Prevalence and incidence of HTLV-111 infection in a prison. *Journal of the American Medical Association*, 256, 2198–2199.

Salive, M., Smith, G. and Brewer, T. (1990). Death in prison: Changing mortality patterns among male prisoners in Maryland, 1979–87. *American Journal of Public Health*, 80, 1479–1480.

Schoenbaum, E., Hartel, D., Selwyn, P., Klein, R., Davenny, K., Rogers, M., Feiner, C. and Friedland, G. (1989). Risk factors for human immunodeficiency virus infection in intravenous drug users. *New England Journal of Medicine*, 321, 874–879.

Truman, B., Morse, D., Mikl, J., Lehman, S., Forte, A., Broaddus, R. and Stevens, R. (1988). HIV seroprevalence and risk factors among prison inmates entering New York State Prisons. *Fourth International Conference on AIDS*, Stockholm, Sweden, p. 311.

van Hoeven, K., Rooney, W. and Joseph, S. (1990). Evidence for gonoccocal transmission within a correctional system. *American Journal of Public Health*, 80, 1505–1506.

Vlahov, D., Brewer, F., Munoz, A., Hall, D., Taylor, E. and Polk, F. (1989). Temporal trends of human immunodeficiency virus type 1 (HIV-1) infection among inmates entering a statewide prison system, 1985–1987. *Journal of Acquired Immune Deficiency Syndrome*, 2, 283–290.

Vlahov, D., Lee, H., Taylor, E., Canavaggio, M., Canner, C., Burczak, J. and Saah, A. (1990). Antibody to human T-lymphotropic virus type I/II (HTLV-I/II) among male inmates entering Maryland prisons. *Journal of Acquired Immune Deficiency Syndrome*, 3, 531–535.

Walker, J. (1989). *Prison Sentences in Australia: Trends and Issues in Crime and Criminal Justice.* Canberra: Australian Institute of Criminology.

Wolk, J., Wodak, A., Morlet, A., Guinan, J. and Gold, J. (1990) HIV-related risk-taking behaviour, knowledge and serostatus of intravenous drug users in Sydney. *Medical Journal of Australia*, 152, 453–458.

Chapter 24
Peer-based User Groups:
The Australian Experience

DAVID HERKT

The changes that have occurred to the Australian communities of drug users as a direct result of national HIV/AIDS policies have been nothing short of revolutionary. This is true not only with regard to the lives of individuals within those communities but also with regard to the relationship between those communities of drug users and the general population.

In Australia in 1982, it would have been inconceivable that, within a decade, drug users would be utilising government-funded needle and syringe exchanges, often staffed by fellow drug users employed in full knowledge that they were current drug users. It would have also been unthinkable for either drug users or service providers that within a few years drug users would be able to enter these facilities and receive, at no cost, large numbers of syringes, alcohol swabs, ampoules of sterile water, sharps containers and a government-funded 160 page book (Australian IV League, 1990), which included information on how to inject drugs without transmitting HIV and how to avoid other problems associated with either specific injecting techniques or particular drug types.

It would also have been inconceivable that the Australian State and Commonwealth governments would be funding user-groups in all jurisdictions bar one by 1989 – peer-based user groups which would often be based around a needle exchange programme and would employ users in education projects (both for the user community and for service providers to that community) in advocacy positions and in administration roles.

Further, it would have been a violation of all medical thought current in 1982 to even consider that users on methadone programmes and in drug treatment centres would be able to obtain syringes from the same agency that was dispensing methadone or providing abstinence-directed therapy.

The growth of organisations of drug users in several developed countries during the last decade has occurred in response to the epidemic of HIV and the need to minimise this potentially most serious of complications of drug use. These organisations have had the unanticipated effect of changing both societies' views about drug users and drug users' views about themselves. This chapter traces the development in Australia of organisations of drug users – referred to in this chapter by the colloquial term 'users' – to identify principles that may well apply in other countries. User organisations were conceived to facilitate the harm reduction of HIV prevention. By extending the community's conceptual framework, by organising users' own experience to serve utilitarian ends and by developing education strategies both with regard to the user communities and those who service them, these organisations of users may well take on a life beyond AIDS.

Changes in Intravenous Drug Use in Australia

Changes in drug injecting practices in Australia as a result of national policies have been well documented. Before 1987, most Australian drug users would inject with the same syringe if necessary and cleaning practices were not satisfactory for either HIV or hepatitis B or C. Alcohol swabs were rarely used.

By the early 1990s, new syringes were used by the majority of users in almost all episodes of drug use. It is anecdotally reported that, for many drug users, the smell of alcohol swabs has become associated with the administration of illicit drugs. The most important change in drug using practices in Australia, as elsewhere, has been a reduction in the sharing of injection equipment. Before 1987, sharing was common practice when two or more drug users were present. Syringes were generally cleaned with hot water although some users boiled their syringes between injections. Cleaning techniques rarely effectively eradicated the hepatitis viruses or HIV. By the early 1990s, sharing occurred infrequently and, when equipment was shared, cleaning was now usually effective, involving either bleach or alcohol.

The various Australian user communities have also been accepted as recognised communities with representative mechanisms and formal structures. The relationship between these communities, government committees and health organisations has now become well-established on an official level. Users are represented on a wide range of policy-making and service-providing agencies. By 1992, it was possible in all but one state of Australia to contact a current user employed, not only because of their personal background, but also for other important skills in such areas as education, administration and counselling.

Government policy-making bodies and organisations providing direct services to injecting drug users (IDUs) have had to substantially alter their relationships both with individual IDUs and that community.

In many cases, this has necessitated a re-evaluation of service philoso-
phies in facilities as diverse as detoxification, methadone maintenance,
rehabilitation and crisis counselling.

These organisational changes were required because of the realisation that, in order to prevent transmission of HIV, it was necessary for
experienced users to alter their injecting practices and, for those experimenting with drug injecting, knowledge of how to avoid HIV infection
associated with drug use was required from the outset. As the majority
of drug users are *not* in contact with treatment agencies, this required
new strategies of contact to conduct the new research agenda. Peer-
based education models were generally considered to have been highly
successful in the gay community in Australia. Consequently Australian
authorities were influenced by their example to adopt similar
approaches for drug users. This peer-based strategy was to dominate
HIV education amongst users in Australia from 1988 to 1992.

As a result of these changes in policy, HIV prevention, drug treatment and research, the perception of users has changed from that of
dysfunctional individuals requiring substantial therapeutic support to
individuals capable of acquiring education and gaining employment
while still using drugs. This dramatic reversal in the perception of users
was also apparent in the funding of groups of users. These groups not
only reflected the need for peer-based groups in the HIV area but also
the need for representative groups that could be consulted by state
government in the area of policy production and implementation.
Thus, in addition to HIV, user groups have been consulted on a broadening range of issues from legal issues to health policy.

Mechanisms of Change

Policy

HIV infection and the subsequent development of AIDS must be considered from a broader perspective than simply that of a complex virus
and a collection of symptoms. HIV transmission occurs as a result of
specific intimate behavioural practices which are, for the most part,
unacceptable to the majority of society. Not only are the sexual and
drug use practices involved in the transmission of HIV socially problematic, but they are also often illegal. Consequently, AIDS is perceived
by some as a just reward for moral and legal transgressions, while others see HIV as a human-engineered virus with some eugenic properties
that will conveniently remove 'deviant' members from society. The conservative perceptions of HIV as a just punishment of sin, a natural consequence of an unnatural act or as a social purifier have been balanced
by other perceptions which view HIV as an agent of social reform in an
essentially conservative society. Although many expected that HIV/AIDS

would lead to a resurgence of conservative values in Australian society, with even stronger emphasis on chastity, heterosexuality and non-drug use, somewhat surprisingly HIV has been a catalyst for far-reaching social change, including greater tolerance for minority sexual and drug-use practices.

Many of the developments described in this chapter could not have happened without the influential White Paper on the Australian Government's policy on HIV/AIDS (Department of Community Services and Health, 1989).

This strategy was developed following extensive nation-wide consultations involving panels on specific subjects. The role that peer-based user groups would play in the completed strategy was clearly demonstrated by the inclusion in the panel convened to deal with the area of intravenous drug use of a representative of one of the earliest peer-based user groups. The resulting strategy, as ratified by all State and Territory Governments, now forms the basis of Australian policy in this area.

While this document recognises that the most effective strategy for preventing HIV infection among drug-users is one that reduces the number of users, which is the Government's long-term goal in addressing drug-use in the community, it is also seen as imperative that strategies are developed which minimise harm among existing IV drug users. Measures advocated included needle distribution and disposal centres operated to ensure their effective utilisation by IDUs. Changes were recommended to laws which reduced the effectiveness of needle and syringe exchange programmes (NSEPs). These changes have included the removal of possession of syringes from the list of criminal offences and non-custodial sentencing for drug users. The transformation of drug treatment programmes from abstinence-based models to harm-reduction objectives was also recommended. These legal changes were proposed to safeguard public health. Previously punitive practices were common in abstinence-based drug treatment programmes, resulting in rewards or punishments for patients; various models of drug dependence provided the rationale for these practices and their ethical aspects were at the time rarely considered. However, with the transformation of the perception of drug users in the National HIV/AIDS Strategy and the practical recommendations of the policy, a new era of harm reduction has been implemented which has involved the examination of a broader range of treatment modalities.

The education initiatives advocated by the National HIV/AIDS Strategy implied recognition of a multitude of diverse communities, each with their own values, behaviours and community standards. The Strategy recognised both the gay and IDU communities as possessing values worthy of attention. It was recommended that specific material be made available for these diverse communities, even where it may have offended or contravened presumed general community standards which form the basis of national censorship laws.

The consequences of these government policies on IDUs and IDU communities were swiftly felt. By 1989, all but one of the eight jurisdictions in Australia had needle and syringe exchanges. By 1990, for example, the state of New South Wales had 32 primary needle and syringe exchange programme (NSEP) outlets and a further 80 secondary outlets for needles and syringes which also provided other health services. The 32 primary outlets in New South Wales exchanged and distributed 88 000 syringes in the month of August 1990 alone. Victoria offered 102 programmes including mobile, late night and weekend services (Inter-goverment Committee on AIDS, 1992).

Community attitudes to these programmes were surveyed in New South Wales (NSW Department of Health, 1990). Substantial community support was demonstrated with 90% of respondents agreeing that NSW should continue to have NSEP, 94% believing that NSEP will play an important part in the control of the epidemic, 78% agreeing that teaching drug users to use safely is important to stop the spread of AIDS and 72% agreeing that teaching drug users how to use safely is important in stopping health risks like overdoses. Thus actions taken by authorities in Australia to prevent the spread of HIV appear to have also changed community attitudes to government policies on drug use and IDUs. Preventing the spread of HIV among IDUs was perceived by a majority of respondents as sufficient justification for more tolerant attitudes to illicit drug use.

The change in philosophy of drug treatment programmes from an abstinence-orientation to a harm-reduction objective has permitted a range of alternative approaches, including client-demanded abstinence programmes and low-intervention, low-threshold methadone programmes. Even some strict abstinence-oriented programmes now incorporate harm-reduction features, albeit with an element of uncomfortable contradiction. Some methadone programmes which withdraw take-away methadone doses in response to urinalysis evidence of continuing illicit opiate use, for example, also conduct a NSEP which is available to the patients of the unit. Although the process of change in some agencies has often been slow and at times contradictory, all drug and alcohol treatment programmes have had to consider changing their protocols to some extent to reflect the need for more harm minimisation.

Previously, views of drug users in 'treatment' were disregarded routinely 'for their own good'. Even the floor layout of methadone clinics was designed to control users who were perceived to be dangerous to both staff and themselves. While traces of this attitude remain, the changes that have occurred as a result of the adoption of harm reduction have been dramatic.

The endorsement in the National HIV/AIDS Strategy of organisations of intravenous drug users and the presumption that IDUs were educable were major departures from the stereotypical image of users fostered during the previous policy of total prohibition. The education strategy of the national policy emphasised that 'members of the target group and community based organisations will be involved in developing and implementing programmes' (National HIV/AIDS Strategy, Department of Health and Community Services, 1989). Funding for state IDU organisations and a national body (The Australian IV League) was inevitable given the strong endorsement in the National HIV/AIDS Strategy.

Research

The advent of HIV/AIDS required a new research agenda focusing on the behaviour of current injecting drug users. This required researchers to collaborate with the IDU community to develop a conceptual framework for research and to gain access to the required data. Considerable consultation with IDUs resulted in researchers being funded for the first time to examine the structures, behaviours and individual lifestyles of that community.

As in most countries, research in Australia had previously been predominantly conducted with drug users recruited from treatment or detoxification centres. Consequently conclusions were often badly skewed. The Australian National AIDS and Injecting Drug Use Study (ANAIDUS) commenced in 1988 as a pilot project to examine risk behaviours of IDUs relevant to HIV infection (Australian National AIDS and Injecting Drug Use Study, 1991; Wodak et al., 1992). Respondents recruited included IDUs currently receiving treatment and others attending NSEP many of whom had never entered treatment and had no intention of entering treatment in the future. This study recruited 2482 IDUs from five cities in 1989 and 700 IDUs from two cities in 1990 to establish the first substantial national data base of user demographics, user injecting behaviour and an assessment of user knowledge of HIV/AIDS risks. In addition to the ANAIDUS study, a Victoria Injecting Drug-User Cohort Study (VICS), a longitudinal cohort study of IDUs, was subsequently established in Melbourne. In contradistinction to the ANAIDUS study, the VICS study involved considerable consultation with users in the development of research protocols and programme questionnaires. IDUs believe that this study will be highly relevant to the needs of the IDU community. The project employs IDUs to administer surveys and recruit a network of urban and rural subjects. The adoption of a consultative process has reduced the influence of traditional preconceptions and stereotypical perceptions of users, and has resulted in the development of a questionnaire which is meaningful to those taking part. IDUs have often struggled in previous research to make sense of many questions that have employed corrupted versions of phrases used by IDUs to make bizarre inquiries bearing little relationship to their world.

In addition to these studies, there have been many smaller and more specifically focused research projects covering a diverse range and including ethnographic studies building on the previous more quantitative behavioural research. A project based at Macquarie University specifically examined the concepts of functional and dysfunctional drug use, concepts which have become increasingly important to harm-reductive practices (Sharp et al., 1991). Previous Australian research on drug use assumed that all drug use was dysfunctional. The greater the consumption, it was assumed, the more dysfunction was likely. By recruiting functional users, especially those not in treatment, the Macquarie study invited a conceptual re-evaluation of drug use, concluding that the change from a functional to a dysfunctional state mainly occurs because of changes in the drug users' patterns of beliefs and social behaviours. Drug use was represented as a complex of social and personal attitudes rather than a mere dependence on drugs resulting in an inevitable array of consequences ranging from predictable social interactions to physiological responses. A logical extension of this study is the conclusion that most of the harm caused by illicit drug use results from the social and legal framework rather than drug use itself.

As a result of these studies, perceptions of drug use from the individual context to generalised education campaigns are changing. Educational programmes, such as the Sydney 'Tribes' campaign, have begun to utilise this conception of 'functional' or successful drug users to contact many who bear no resemblance to the stereotypical user of previous research (Keys Young, 1991). This project contacted young, economically successful individuals unlikely to enter treatment, or to identify or be identified as users. Safer-using education was promoted employing the same methods of recruitment.

This campaign was based on a view that the IDU community comprises a number of major subgroups, called 'Tribes', each with their own approved and rejected behaviours, cultural heroes and social images. Members of the individual tribes were employed to design and implement HIV/AIDS information campaigns for their own tribe. This strategy enabled safer use and safer sex messages to be disseminated to individuals who would not previously have received such information from generalised IDU peer-based education. This campaign was evaluated and considered to be successful in terms of its original aims. Recently, responsibility for future 'Tribes' campaigns has been transferred to the New South Wales Users AIDS Association (NUAA), the peak user group in that state.

Research in the area of drug users in Australia continues to advance, as is evident by comparison with US studies and HIV/AIDS projects. The major and overwhelming difference is the conceptualisation of drug use and drug users. US research is conducted within boundaries erected by the 'zero-tolerance for drug use' policy of the Federal Government. Funding is denied to proposals which examine questions beyond these boundaries. From the Australian perspective, most US research into drug use, HIV/AIDS transmission and using behaviours are lessons in the dangers of close association between government and scientific researchers.

Peer-user Groups

The user community

Does an IDU community exist? This question has been debated by many academics and service providers. However, the prohibition of drugs must be considered to lead inevitably to the creation of a community of individuals who use drugs, much in the same way that the gay community was created by legislative discrimination. Users are defined by legislation which specifies that the use of illicit drugs is subject to a penalty. Although bonded as a result of these laws, forced to form economic networks to facilitate a continuing supply of their drugs, and despite a history and culture extending over half a century, the user community has only recently received official recognition.

The development of funded, peer-based user groups has created formal structures in this community for the first time, with elected management committees and user delegates to national user groups and non-user organisations. User representatives also provide experiential information to services and education strategies that involve the community. It is no longer unusual to see user delegates serving with police and medical representatives on many state advisory committees in the eastern and southern Australian states.

The need for IDUs to change their behaviour to avoid transmission of HIV is the basis of the social implications of Australia's national policy as discussed above. Whether the belated recognition of users results from a concern that the user community might provide the major gateway for HIV to enter the 'general' population is unclear. It is clear, however, that the need for IDUs to alter certain injecting behaviours has also compelled a change in behaviour of non-users to the user community. As the National HIV/AIDS Policy emphasised:

Education about HIV and IV drug-use also needs to be provided for all those in direct contact with IV drug-users including treatment, law enforcement and custodial officers and workers in the drug and alcohol field, to overcome attitudinal barriers to the implementation and prevention strategies and to enable them to work effectively with campaigns dealing with HIV infection and IV drug-use.

(Department of Community Services and Health, 1989)

The need to involve all members of this community, facilitating change in their behaviours and establishing services to perform tasks in conjunction with IDUs, has meant that those who are not IDUs but are involved in working with them have also had to make 'attitudinal' changes.

Government policy and peer-based involvement

The Australian experience of peer-based user groups has been an important component of a response to HIV/AIDS which has begun to be recognised internationally as effective. The formation, funding and assignment of official roles to these groups by the National HIV/AIDS Strategy has also involved substantial changes to the representation and standing of drug users both in a bureaucratic and social sense. Peer-based user groups have been one of the most effective elements in the education of the various Australian IDU communities.

Recognising the potential for rapid spread of HIV through the IDU community, the National Strategy states that 'public health objectives will be most effectively realised if the cooperation of people with HIV infection and those at risk is maintained' (National HIV/AIDS Strategy, Department of Health and Community Services,1989).

The National HIV/AIDS Strategy recognises that abstinence is an option and designates it as the *primary* long-term aim. But abstinence is presented as one of a number of options available. It recommends that promotion of abstinence must be complemented by a promotion of other objectives, including the reduction of harms which may occur before abstinence is achieved. This recognition of the reality of drug use and the failure of previous policies and practices to achieve abstinence has had far-reaching effects. A need for re-education is accepted for those in direct contact with drug users, including treatment, law enforcement and drug and alcohol workers, to overcome 'attitudinal' barriers to the implementation of new prevention strategies.

Evaluation of the peer-based response

The effectiveness of these policies is demonstrated by the fact that the prevalence of HIV among Australian IDUs remains low. Only 1.7% of the AIDS cases diagnosed in the period 1982–1990 are attributed to injecting drug use, with a further 1.6 % attributed to the combined injecting drug use – homosexual/bisexual categories. Thus at most, IDUs constitute 3.3% of the total national AIDS case load in Australia by

1990 (Inter-government Committee on AIDS, 1992). It is estimated that approximately 2% of IDUs in Australia are infected with HIV at present (Inter-government Committee on AIDS, 1992).

That this success is, in some measure, due to peer-based groups can be demonstrated by comparison of needle and syringe exchange programmes. The peer-based only NSEPs in South Australia are more successful in distributing needles and syringes and contacting new attendees than other programmes. Information can also be gained from a comparison within the same programme. A needle and syringe exchange programme in Victoria changed from a peer controlled to a non-peer controlled programme after allegations of financial impropriety. In the last year before the change, the number of clients attending per month increased steadily from 185 (January 1990), 210 (March), 300 (May) and 357 (July) to reach 503 in August (figures from VIVAIDS exchange). An appropriation of government money by a funded user group had long been feared and the response was swift. Responsibility for this alleged misappropriation is still unclear. Unfortunately, the user organisation was dismembered despite the fact that it had been operating extremely successfully in the areas of education and advocacy. After the NSEP had been transferred to a nearby community health centre, growth of services stopped. Client numbers initially remained stable with an average of 262 per month in 1991 and 261 per month in early 1992. However, with the establishment of a non-peer-based service and removal of all user workers, the numbers of clients attending on a monthly basis have dropped 30% between July and October 1992.

The traditional client-service focus of user groups in urban areas and their provision of crisis services is changing. One of the user organisations (NUAA) sought to replace this initial focus on crisis intervention work with more emphasis on effective advocacy and education at a state bureaucratic level, hoping to have a greater impact on a larger number of users' lives by this strategy. By educating service providers ('train the trainers') NUAA has also aimed to change the relationship of service providers to drug users. This change, which is being closely observed by other groups, indicates not only a step in the consolidation of the gains of the last decade, but also indicates a more effective route of service provision by these groups.

Conclusion

It is clear that Australia's peer-based groups played an integral role in the containment of HIV infection among IDUs. The small number of recent cases of HIV transmission involving IDUs is due at least in part to continuing programmes of prevention and education.

The basis of Australia's response to HIV/AIDS in the IDU community was established by the National HIV/AIDS Strategy. A change in behaviour required from IDUs also requires a change in attitudes and behaviour of those who relate to them through policy development, service provision and research. Changes in social relations between these specialised groups and IDUs has diffused into Australian society. This is apparent in most HIV/AIDS publicity campaigns and has also been communicated on an individual level through personal contact and altered organisational profiles.

Far from the reinforcing a conservative set of moral and social values, as was expected at the outset of the epidemic, Australia's response to HIV/AIDS in both policy and practice has strengthened progressive and, in some cases, revolutionary social changes. It is important to note that these changes have not disrupted or otherwise damaged the national social fabric. More changes are needed in medical, legal and social practices which are still rooted in the discredited and anachronistic policy of prohibition. The effectiveness of Australia's harm-reduction policy can be demonstrated by examining the epidemic of HIV infection. It is difficult to doubt its success. It remains therefore for the state and commonwealth policy makers of Australia to further extend this successful strategy in conjunction with community opinion in order to reduce the social and physical harm caused directly by prohibition.

References

Australian IV League (1990). *Handy Hints*. Stanmore: Social Change Media.

Australian National AIDS and Injecting Drug Use Study (1991). *Neither a Borrower nor a Lender be: The First Report of the Australian National AIDS and Injecting Drug Use Study, 1989 Data Collection*. Sydney: ANAIDUS.

Department of Community Services and Health (1989). *National HIV/AIDS Strategy: A Policy Information Paper*. Canberra: Australian Government Printing Service.

Inter-government Committee on AIDS (1992). *A Report on HIV/AIDS Activities in Australia 1990–1991*. Canberra: Australian Government Publishing Service.

Keys Young, M.S.J. (1991). *The Tribes Education Campaigns 1990–1991*. Sydney: AIDS Bureau, Department of Community Services and Health, NSW Department of Health..

NSW Department of Health (1990). *Community Attitudes to Needle and Syringe Exchange Programs*. (A90/6). Sydney: Directorate of the Drug Offensive.

Sharp, R., Davis, M., Dowsett, G.W., Kippax, S., Hewitt, K., Morgan, S. and Robertson, W. (1991). *Ways of Using: Functional Injecting Drug Users Project*. Sydney: Centre for Applied Social Research, Macquarie University.

Wodak, A., Dwyer, R., Ross, M.W., Drury, M.J., Gold, J. and Miller, M.E. (1992). *Life at the epicentre: Sexual and drug using behaviour in Sydney, 1989*. Second Report of the Australian National AIDS and Injecting Drug-Use Study. Sydney: ANAIDUS.

Index